Physical Assessment for
Nurses and Healthcare Professionals

Physical Assessment for

Nurses and Healthcare Professionals

Third Edition

EDITED BY

CAROL LYNN COX PhD, MSc, MA (Theology) MA (Education), PG Dip Education, BSc (Hons), RN, ENB 254, FHEA

Professor Emeritus, School of Health Sciences, City, University of London, London, UK
Clinic Manager and Director of Nursing, Health and Hope Clinics, Pensacola, FL, USA

Adapted from *Lecture Notes on Clinical Skills* (third edition) by:

THE LATE ROBERT TURNER MD, FRCP

Professor of Medicine and Honorary Consultant Physician
Nuffield Department of Clinical Medicine
Radcliffe Infirmary, Oxford, UK

ROGER BLACKWOOD MA, FRCP

Consultant Physician, Wexham Park Hospital, Slough,
and Honorary Consultant Physician at Hammersmith Hospital, London, UK

WILEY Blackwell

Registered Office(s)
John Wiley & Sons, Inc., 111 River Street, Hoboken, NJ 07030, USA
John Wiley & Sons Ltd, The Atrium, Southern Gate, Chichester, West Sussex, PO19 8SQ, UK

Editorial Office
9600 Garsington Road, Oxford, OX4 2DQ, UK

For details of our global editorial offices, customer services, and more information about Wiley products visit us at www.wiley.com.

Wiley also publishes its books in a variety of electronic formats and by print-on-demand. Some content that appears in standard print versions of this book may not be available in other formats.

Library of Congress Cataloging-in-Publication Data

Names: Cox, Carol Lynn, editor. | Based on (work): Blackwood, Roger. Lecture
    notes on clinical skills. 2003.
Title: Physical assessment for nurses and healthcare professionals / edited by Carol Lynn Cox.
Other titles: Physical assessment for nurses.
Description: Third edition. | Hoboken, NJ : Wiley-Blackwell, 2019. | Preceded
    by Physical assessment for nurses / edited by Carol Lynn Cox. 2nd ed.
    2010. | Based on Lecture notes on clinical skills / Roger Blackwood, Chris
    Hatton. 4th ed. 2003. | Includes bibliographical references and index. |
Identifiers: LCCN 2018044840 (print) | LCCN 2018045696 (ebook) | ISBN 9781119108986 (Adobe PDF) |
    ISBN 9781119108993 (ePub) | ISBN 9781119108979 (pbk.)
Subjects: | MESH: Nursing Assessment
Classification: LCC RT48 (ebook) | LCC RT48 (print) | NLM WY 100.4 | DDC 616.07/5–dc23
LC record available at https://lccn.loc.gov/2018044840

Cover Design: Wiley
Cover Images: © Martin Barraud/Getty Images, © Hero Images/Getty Images, © XiXinXing/Getty Images, © Blend Images - Jose Luis Pelaez Inc/Getty Images

Set in 10/12pt Myriad by SPi Global, Pondicherry, India
Printed and bound in Singapore by Markono Print Media Pte Ltd

10 9 8 7 6 5 4 3 2 1

Contents

Chapter 4 Examination of the Cardiovascular System **67**
Carol Lynn Cox and Carrie E. Boyd

Chapter 7   **Examination of the Male Genitalia**   **149**
Michael Babcock, Carol Lynn Cox, and Anthony McGrath

Contents

List of Contributors

Daniel Apau, MSc (Advanced Practice), PG Dip, BSc (Hons), RN, FHEA
Registered Nurse, Medical Intensive Care, Houston Northwest Medical Center, Houston, TX, USA

Michael Babcock, MD
College of Medicine, Florida State University, Pensacola, FL, USA

Graham M. Boswell, D Ed, MA Ed, BA (Hons), BSc (Hons) RGN, FHEA
Senior Lecturer, Department of Adult Nursing and Paramedic Science, Faculty of Education and Health, University of Greenwich, London, UK

Carrie E. Boyd, MSN, BSN, RN
Staff Nurse, Health and Hope Clinics, Pensacola, FL, USA

Patrick Callaghan, PhD, MSc, BSc (Hons), RN, FHEA
Professor of Mental Health Nursing and Chartered Health Psychologist
University of Nottingham and Nottinghamshire Health Care NHS Trust, Nottingham, UK

Carol Lynn Cox, PhD, MSc (Nursing), MA (Theology) MA Ed, PG Dip Ed, BSc (Hons), FD, RN, FHEA
Professor Emeritus, School of Health Sciences, City, University of London, London, UK
Clinic Manager, Health and Hope Clinics, Pensacola, FL, USA

Jennifer Edie, M Ed, MBA, TDCR, DMU
Senior Lecturer, Department of Allied Health Professions and Midwifery, School of Health and Social Work, University of Hertfordshire, Hatfield, Hertfordshire, UK

Helen Gibbons, MSc, PG Cert (Medical Education), ENB (Ophthalmic Practice), BA (Hons), RN
Clinical Nursing Lead (Education and Research), Moorfields Eye Hospital NHS Foundation Trust, London, UK
Course Director, PG Cert Ophthalmic Practice, University College London, London, UK

Jessica Ham, MSN, BSN, ASN, FNP, RN
Clinical Preceptor, College of Medicine, Faculty of Florida State University, Tallahassee, FL, USA
Clinical Director, Elevate Personalized Medicine, Pensacola, FL, USA

Siobhan Hicks, MSc (Advanced Practice), PG Cert (Academic Practice), PG Cert (Leadership), BSc (Hons), RN
Advanced Nurse Practitioner, Andrews Health Centre, London, UK
Lecturer in Advanced Practice, School of Health Sciences, City, University of London, London, UK

Victoria Lack, MSN, PG Dip (Academic Practice), BN (Hons), FNP, Non-Medical Prescriber, DN(Cert), RN
Lecturer in Primary Care, Department of Health Sciences, University of York, York, UK
Advanced Nurse Practitioner, Beech House Surgery, Knaresborough, North Yorkshire, UK

Brandy Lunsford, MSN, BSN, APRN
Clinical Director, Health and Hope Clinics, Pensacola, FL, USA

Anthony McGrath, MSc, PGCE, BA (Hons) RMN, RGN, FHEA
Principal Lecturer, Head of Adult Nursing and Midwifery
London South Bank University, London, UK

Nicola L. Whiteing, MSc, PG Dip HE, BSc (Hons), RN, RNT, ANP
Lecturer in Nursing, Southern Cross University, Lismore, New South Wales, Australia

Foreword

Underpinning the appropriate delivery of healthcare is the Physical Assessment. This structured physical examination allows the healthcare professional to obtain a comprehensive assessment of the patient and is critically important in that it leads to clinical decisions which are crucial for the patients' care.

This volume, *Physical Assessment for Nurses and Healthcare Professionals*, provides a clear and easy-to-use guide to achieving an excellent physical assessment. It is specifically intended for those embarking on a career in healthcare and contains the techniques used by specialist/advanced practitioners.

In this book the need for a comprehensive and holistic approach to the Physical Assessment is excellently presented by Professor Cox. Professor Cox shows how important it is to develop a rapport with the patient in order to carefully assess their perceptions and how this relationship must be established from the very first meeting when information is exchanged between the healthcare professional and the patient. Fundamental to gaining this perspective is to listen. The importance of guiding the healthcare practitioner to engage in active listening cannot be underestimated and this is reflected in the fact that not being heard is an issue which is often raised as a point of criticism of healthcare professionals by patients and their families.

Careful observation and reports of subjective symptoms are the window through which healthcare professionals gain knowledge of their patients. Following on from the opening chapters this volume is structured to enable the healthcare professional to learn how to systematically gather information before moving on to an initial diagnosis and further investigations. The tools of inspection, palpation, percussion, and auscultation are key to this assessment and excellently laid out in the chapters covering the examination of the different organs of the body, different age groups, and some specialist topics. Professor Cox has also helpfully included in the appendix a number of the widely used standardised instruments to assess such areas as disability, activities of daily living, reading, and mental state.

It is key for healthcare professionals to be able to communicate the outcomes of their Physical Assessment to their professional colleagues. In the final chapter Professor Cox demonstrates her experience and understanding of the world of healthcare when she talks about the importance of this communication between professionals and how the Physical Assessment can bring together disparate professional views which will underpin the diagnostic process.

Professor Cox is a consummate professional who has been an educator for most of her career with a focus on clinical practice and the patient experience. She couples her educational activity with an extensive research record on nursing practice. In *Physical Assessment for Nurses and Healthcare Professionals*, Professor Cox has created an invaluable guide that will not only support practitioners as they enter into a clinical career in healthcare but which can be used as an ongoing reference book to support their careers as they move into advanced practice.

Professor Stanton Newman

Preface

Over the past two to three decades, many changes have been seen in the roles of healthcare professionals. Significant changes have been seen in the allied health professions, nursing, and midwifery. It is common practice now to see the healthcare professional functioning as an independent practitioner with specialist/advanced practice qualifications. For example, to list but a few, it is not uncommon to find audiologists, nurses, midwives occupational therapists, opticians, physiotherapists, and radiotherapists with master's and doctoral degrees diagnosing and treating patients. These practitioners are expected to know how to provide expert holistic health-oriented care for culturally diverse populations. Specialist/advanced practice health professionals view the patient as an individual with physical as well as emotional, psychological, intellectual, social, cultural, and spiritual needs. A comprehensive assessment of the patient is the foundation upon which healthcare decisions are made. The best way to develop assessment skills is to learn them systematically. The systematic approach involves taking a full health history, conducting a physical examination, and reviewing diagnostic tests/laboratory data. Use of advanced assessment skills are essential in clinical decision making that leads to the formulation of a differential diagnosis and final diagnosis.

This text for healthcare professionals is based on Turner and Blackwood's *Lecture Notes on Clinical Skills* that was written for medical students. It is intended to be used as a reference book that can be reviewed near the patient in the clinical setting. In general, the pages are arranged with simple instructions on the left, with important aspects requiring action marked with a bullet (•). Subsidiary lists are marked with a dash (–). On the right are brief details of clinical situations and diseases that are relevant to abnormal findings. In this edition, colour photographs of assessment techniques have been added as well as case studies to assist healthcare practitioners in their assessment of the patient.

Turner and Blackwood's *Lecture Notes on Clinical Skills* has been used in the Oxford Clinical Medical School for over 40 years and is viewed as an essential guide for medical students globally. It should be noted that although some doctors may use slightly different techniques in taking a history and physical examination, it is recommended that healthcare practitioners embarking on a career as specialist/advanced practitioners use the techniques recommended in this text because they provide a sound approach for developing and employing clinical decision making.

Carol Lynn Cox, PhD, RN

Acknowledgements

Special thanks are extended to Robert Turner and Roger Blackwood for granting permission for their text, *Lecture Notes on Clinical Skills*, to be revised as a text originally for nurses. I am grateful to my students for encouraging me to revise the original text so that they could have an accessible resource for reference purposes in the clinical setting. The Turner and Blackwood text still serves as a reference for the third edition which has been expanded for all healthcare practitioners. Sincere gratitude is expressed to Sandra Kerka for thoroughly reviewing this book and correcting a multitude of errors therein and to Vincent Rajan, Production Editor, for efficiently bringing the book to completion. Finally, I am grateful to the Health and Hope Clinics of Pensacola Florida; City University, London, England; and the University of Latvia, Department of Optometry and Vision Science, Latvia, for supporting this project through their generous provision of physical assessment technique photographs. Any faults or omissions in this book are entirely my own.

Figures appearing on pp. 36, 37, 41, 49 (Figure 3.1), 52 (Figure 3.2), 53 (Figure 3.3), 54, 55 (Figure 3.4), 56 (Figure 3.5), 69 (Figure 3.11), 75 (Figures 4.1 and 4.2), 76 (Figure 4.3), 77 (Figures 4.4 and 4.5), 78 (Figure 4.6), 81 (Figure 4.7), 82 (Figure 4.9) and 83 (Figure 4.10) are reproduced with permission of City University from *Advanced Practice: Physical Assessment* (1997), Carol Lynn Cox, Professor, City University London, St Bartholomew School of Nursing and Midwifery, ISBN 1900804255, Reprinted 2002.

The visual acuity reading charts (Appendices A and B) are reproduced courtesy of Keeler Ltd.

Introduction

The First Approach

Carol Lynn Cox

General Principles

It is important to understand that for the purposes of examination, assessment, and diagnosis, doctors are framing their approach to the patient from the perspective of the medical model. However, you must recognise that as an allied healthcare practitioner, you are employing the medical model within your frame of practice. Therefore, to be wholistic, the approach incorporates all aspects of your particular discipline (e.g. audiology, nursing, midwifery, physiotherapy, occupational therapy, radiography, respiratory therapy, speech therapy).

General Objectives

When you approach a patient there are four initial objectives you should consider:

- Obtain a professional rapport with the patient and gain their confidence.
- Obtain all relevant information that allows assessment of the illness and provisional diagnoses.
- Obtain general information regarding the patient and their background, social situation, and problems. In particular, it is necessary to find out how the illness has affected the patient, their family, friends, colleagues, and life.
  - A wholistic assessment of the patient is of utmost importance.
- Understand the patient's own ideas about their problems, major concerns, and expectations of the hospital admission, outpatient, or general practice consultation.

Remember medicine is just as much about worry as disease. Whatever the illness, whether chest infection or cancer, anxiety about what may happen is often uppermost in the patient's mind (Clark 1999; Japp and Robertson 2013; NHS Wales 2010).

Listen Attentively (Engage in Active Listening.)

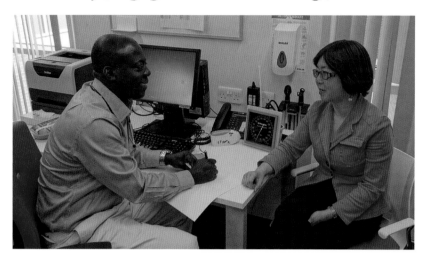

Engage in active listening

The following notes provide a guide as to how the healthcare practitioner obtains the necessary information.

Specific Objectives

In taking a history or conducting a physical examination there are several complementary aims:

- Obtain all possible information about a patient and the illness (a database) from both a subjective and objective perspective.
- Consider all possible differential diagnoses related to the patient and the illness.
- Formulate the diagnoses from the patient's subjective, objective physical examination and investigative tests (e.g. laboratory, radiologic, and other).
- Solve the problem as to the diagnoses (Bickley and Szilagyi 2013; Japp and Robertson 2013; Jarvis 2015).

Analytical Approach

For each symptom or sign you need to think of a differential diagnosis and of other relevant information (from the history, physical examination, and/or investigative tests) that will be needed to support or refute possible diagnoses. A good history, physical examination, and investigation include these two facets and can be viewed as either positive (support) or negative (refute) findings. To achieve a formal diagnosis, following differential diagnosis, critical thinking/clinical decision making is used to examine positive and negative findings. Healthcare practitioners frequently find that using the first two components of the Subjective, Objective, Assessment, and Plan (SOAP) (Clark 1999) format can help them formulate their diagnosis. You should never approach the patient with just a set series of rote questions. Frequently in preassessment clinics, ambulatory services (outpatient) clinics, or general practice settings, standard assessment forms within an electronic patient record (EPR) are used as a guide to history taking. However, there are some instances in which paper records are employed. These tools provide the necessary basis for a later, more inquisitive approach that should develop as knowledge about the patient's problem is acquired. Key to the process of achieving a diagnosis and formulating a plan of care is listening carefully to the patient, taking time, not assuming a diagnosis when the patient initially expresses their chief complaint, and understanding your own values, attitudes, and beliefs as they relate to diverse patient populations (Japp and Robertson 2013).

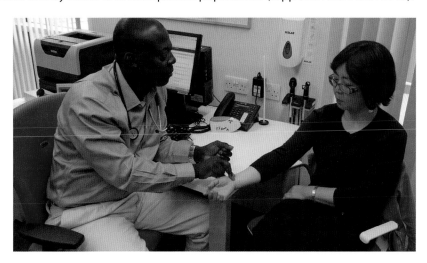

Focus on the patient

The 'subjective' and objective components of the SOAP format provide a basis for diagnosis. Within the subjective component, the patient's perspective of the problem/illness is stated in their own words. This is often listed as the patient's chief complaint. In addition, the patient's 'subjective' view of their health history (e.g. childhood diseases and immunisations) as well as family history, present medications, how and when the patient takes the medications, and chronological ordering of sequelae leading to the presenting problem are documented. The objective component consists of your physical examination and investigative tests. Assessment involves the formulation of a diagnosis from the history, physical examination, and investigative tests. Plan involves the development of the plan of care for the patient as well as where, when, how, and by whom the plan will be implemented (Bickley and Szilagyi 2013).

Self-Reliance – Getting Started

You must take your own history, make your own examination, and write your own clinical records. After a month or two you should be sufficiently proficient that your notes can become part of the final medical record. You should add a summary including your assessment of the problem list, provisional diagnoses, and preliminary investigations. Initially when developing your assessment/examination skills these will be incomplete and occasionally incorrect. Nevertheless, the exercise will help to inculcate an enquiring approach and to highlight areas in which further questioning, investigation, or study/reading is needed.

What Is Important When You Start?

At the basis of all practice is clinical competence. No amount of knowledge will make up for poor technique.

Over the first few weeks it is essential to learn the basics of history taking and physical examination. This involves:

- how to relate to patients
- how to take a good history efficiently, knowing which question to ask next and avoiding leading questions

- how to examine patients in a logical manner, in a set routine that will mean you will not miss an unexpected sign

You will be surprised how often healthcare practitioners can fail an exam, not because of lack of knowledge but because they have not mastered elementary clinical skills. These notes are written to try and help you to identify what is important and to help relate findings to common clinical situations.

There is nothing inherently difficult about history taking and physical examination. You will quickly become clinically competent if you:

- apply yourself
- initially learn the skills that are appropriate for each situation

Common Sense

Common sense is the cornerstone of good practice.

- Always be aware of the patient's needs.
- Always evaluate what important information is needed:
  - to obtain the diagnosis
  - to provide appropriate treatment
  - to ensure continuity of care at home.

Many mistakes are made by being sidetracked by aspects that are not important. Remain focused on the patient.

Learning

Your clinical skills and knowledge can soon develop with good organisation.

- **Take advantage of seeing as many patients** in acute care (hospital and ambulatory clinics) and in primary care (the community) as possible. It is particularly helpful to be present when patients are being admitted as emergencies or are being seen in an ambulatory clinic or general practice setting for the first time.
- **Obtain a wide experience of clinical diseases**, how they affect patients, and how they are managed.
  - The more patients you can clerk yourself, the sooner you will become proficient and the more you will learn about patients and their diseases.

Building Up Knowledge

At first history taking and physical assessment seem like a huge subject and each fact you learn seems to be an isolated piece of information. How will you ever be able to learn what is required? You will find after a few months that the information related to each system interrelates with other systems. The pieces of the jigsaw puzzle begin to fit together and then your confidence will increase. Although you will need to learn many facts, it is equally important to acquire the attitude of questioning, reasoning, and knowing when and where to go to seek additional information.

- Choose a medium-sized textbook in which you can read about each disease you see or each problem you encounter.
  - Attaching knowledge to individual patients is a great help in acquiring and remembering facts. To practice history taking and physical assessment/examination without a textbook is like a sailor without a chart, whereas to study books rather than patients is like a sailor who does not go to sea.

Understand the scientific background of disease, including the advances that are being made and how these could be applied to improve care. (The world wide web is a good resource as well as scientific journals for gaining knowledge that will assist you in building your knowledge.)

- Regularly read the editorials or any articles that interest you in scientific journals.
  - Even if at first you are not able to put information into context, they will keep you in touch with new developments that add interest. Nevertheless, it is not sensible to delve too deeply into any one subject when you are just beginning.

Relationships

Good relationships with patients and clinical colleagues are essential. You should maintain a natural, sincere, receptive, and supportive relationship with your patients and clinical colleagues. Your ultimate goal in working with patients and clinical colleagues is to achieve good care (Department of Health, Social Services and Public Safety in Northern Ireland 2016; Jarvis 2015).

Your Role as an Advanced Healthcare Practitioner

Your role as an advanced healthcare practitioner extends the boundaries of the scope of professional practice. The skills and practices associated with advanced practice involve using advanced clinical assessment techniques, interpreting diagnostic tests including diagnostic imaging, implementing and monitoring therapeutic regimes, prescribing pharmacological interventions, initiating and receiving appropriate referrals, and discharging patients (NMC 2005; HCPC 2013a, b; HCPC 2016).

Practice associated with the advanced practice role in healthcare involves:

- Assessment and management of patient illness/health status
- The healthcare practitioner–patient relationship
- Prescribing medicines, ordering diagnostic investigations and treatments
- An education function – including undertaking continuing education
- The professional role of the healthcare practitioner
- Managing and negotiating healthcare delivery systems
- Monitoring and ensuring quality of advanced healthcare practice
- Respecting culture and diversity (HCPC 2013a, b, 2016; NHS Wales 2010; RCN 2002, 2008, 2012; RCN Scotland 2015).

It is essential that you develop sound skills within the framework delineated here if you expect to be competent at the specialist/advanced practice level.

References

Bickley, L. and Szilagyi, P. (2013). *Bates' Guide to Physical Examination and History Taking*, 11e. New York: Wolters Kluwer/Lippincott Williams & Wilkins.

Clark, C. (1999). Taking a history. In: *Nurse Practitioners, Clinical Skills and Professional Issues* (ed. M. Walsh, A. Crumbie and S. Reveley). Oxford: Butterworth Heinemann.

Department of Health, Social Services and Public Safety in Northern Ireland (2016). *Advanced Nursing Practice Framework: Supporting Advanced Nursing Practice in Health and Social Care Trusts*. Belfast: NIPEC.

HCPC (2013a). *Standards of Proficiency*. London: Health & Care Professions Council.

HCPC (2013b). *Standards of Prescribing*. London: Health & Care Professions Council.

HCPC (2016). *Standards of Conduct, Performance and Ethics*. London: Health & Care Professions Council.

Japp, A. and Robertson, C. (2013). *Macleod's Clinical Diagnosis*. Edinburgh: Churchill Livingstone, Elsevier.

Jarvis, C. (2015). *Physical Examination and Health Assessment*, 7e. Edinburgh: Elsevier.

NHS Wales (2010). *Framework for Advanced Nursing, Midwifery and Allied Health Professional Practice in Wales*. Llanharan: National Leadership and Innovation Agency for Healthcare.

NMC (2005). Annex 1 domains of practice and competencies. In: *NMC Consultation on a Proposed Framework for Post-Registration Nursing*. London: Nursing and Midwifery Council.

RCN (2002). *Advanced Nurse Practitioners – An RCN Guide to the Nurse Practitioner Role, Competencies and Programme Accreditation*. London: Royal College of Nursing.

RCN (2008). *Advanced Nurse Practitioners – An RCN Guide to the Advanced Nurse Practitioner Role, Competencies and Programme Accreditation*. London: Royal College of Nursing.

RCN (2012). *Advanced Nurse Practitioners – An RCN Guide to the Advanced Nurse Practitioner Role, Competencies and Programme Accreditation*. London: Royal College of Nursing.

RCN Scotland (2015). *Nurse Innovators: Clinical Decision-Making in Action*. Edinburgh: Royal College of Nursing.

Chapter 1

Interviewing and History Taking

Carol Lynn Cox

General Procedures

Introduction

The patient's history is the major subjective source of data about their health status. Physiological, psychological, and psychosocial information (including family relationships and cultural influences) can be obtained which will inform you about the patient's perception of current health status and lifestyle. It will give you insight into actual and potential problems as well as providing a guide for the physical examination. History taking involves obtaining the patient's chief complaint, a full review of systems from the patient's perspective, exploration of patient problems associated with the chief complaint, and other (frequently associated) problems that require addressing from the patient's perspective (Ball et al. 2014a, b; Barkauskas et al. 2002; Bickley and Szilagyi 2007, 2013; Cox 2010; Dains et al. 2012, 2015; Epstein et al. 2008; Japp and Robertson 2013; Jarvis 2008, 2015; Seidel et al. 2006, 2010; Swartz 2006; Talley and O'Connor 2006, 2014).

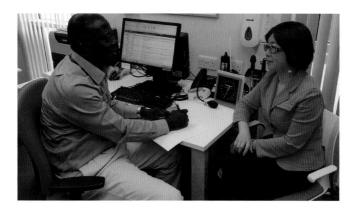

Ensure your patient is seated comfortably for the interview

Physical Assessment for Nurses and Healthcare Professionals, Third Edition. Edited by Carol Lynn Cox.
© 2019 John Wiley & Sons Ltd. Published 2019 by John Wiley & Sons Ltd.

Approaching the Patient

- Put the patient at ease by being confident and quietly friendly (Hatton and Blackwood 2003; Jackson and Vessey 2010; Rudolf and Levene 2011; Sawyer 2012).
- Greet the patient: 'Good morning, Mr/Mrs Smith'. (Address the patient formally and use the full name until the patient has given you permission for less formal address.)
- Shake the patient's hand or place your hand on theirs if the patient is ill. (This action begins your physical assessment. It will give you a baseline indication of the patient's physical condition. For example, cold, clammy, diaphoretic, or pyrexial.)
- State your name and title/role.
- Make sure the patient is comfortable.
- Explain that you wish to ask the patient questions to find out what happened.
  - Start the history taking by stating something like 'I will start the history by asking you some questions about your health'. (Always begin with general questions and then move to more specific questions (Cox 2010) Inform the patient how long you are likely to take and what to expect. For example, after discussing what has happened to the patient, explain that you would like to examine them.

Usual Sequence of Events

Figure 1.1 depicts the sequence of events in an examination.

Importance of the History

- It identifies:
  - what has happened
  - the personality of the patient
  - how the illness has affected the patient and family
  - any specific anxieties
  - the physical and social environment.
- It establishes the practitioner–patient relationship.
- It provides the foundation for your differential diagnoses.
- It often gives the diagnosis.
- Find the principal symptoms or symptom. Ask one of the following questions:
  - 'How may I help you?'
  - 'What has the problem been?'
  - 'Tell me why have you come to the surgery/clinic/hospital today?' or 'Tell me why you came to see me today?'

    Effective history taking involves allowing the patient to talk in an unstructured way whilst you maintain control of the interview. Use language that the patient can

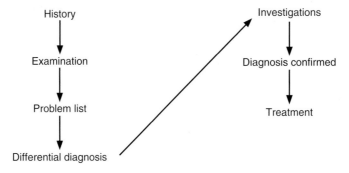

Figure 1.1   Usual sequence of events.

understand and avoid the use of medical jargon (Collins-Bride and Saxe 2013; Cox 2010; Sawyer 2012; Tally and O'Connor 2014). Avoid asking questions that can be answered by a simple 'yes' or 'no'. Ask questions that require a graded response. For example, 'Describe how your headache feels.' Avoid using multiple-choice questions that may confuse the patient (Cox 2010; Jackson and Vessey 2010). Ask one question at a time. Avoid asking questions like: 'What's wrong?' or 'What brought you here?' Use clarification to confirm your understanding of the patient's problem. Avoid forming premature conclusions about the patient's problem and above all remain nonjudgemental in your demeanour. Avoid making judgemental statements.

- Let the patient tell their story in their own words as much as possible.

  At first listen and then take discreet notes as the patient talks.

  When learning to take a history there can be a tendency to ask too many questions in the first two minutes. After asking the first question you should normally allow the patient to talk uninterrupted for up to two minutes.

  Do not worry if the story is not entirely clear or if you do not think the information being given is of diagnostic significance. If you interrupt too early, you run the risk of overlooking an important symptom or anxiety.

  You will be learning about what the patient thinks is important. You have the opportunity to judge how you are going to proceed. Different patients give histories in very different ways. Some patients will need to be encouraged to enlarge on their answers to your questions; with other patients, you may need to ask specific questions and to interrupt in order to prevent too rambling a history. Think consciously about the approach you will adopt. If you need to interrupt the patient, do so clearly and decisively. Most important, do not give the impression you are in a hurry to conclude the discussion as this impression may cause the patient to withhold valuable information you need before commencing your physical examination.

- Try, if feasible, to conduct a conversation rather than an interrogation, following the patient's train of thoughts.

  You will usually need to ask follow-up questions on the main symptoms to obtain a full understanding of what they were and of the chain of events.

- Obtain a full description of the patient's principal complaints.

- Enquire about the sequence of symptoms and events.

  Beware pseudomedical terms, e.g. 'gastric flu' – enquire what happened. Clarify by asking what the patient means.

- Do not ask leading questions.

  A central aim in taking the history is to understand patients' symptoms from their own point of view. It is important not to tarnish the patient's history by your own expectations. For example, do not ask a patient whom you suspect might be thyrotoxic: 'Do you find hot weather uncomfortable?' This invites the answer 'yes' and then a positive answer becomes of little diagnostic value. Ask the open question: 'Do you particularly dislike either hot or cold weather?' (Ball et al. 2014a, b; Bickley and Szilagyi 2013; Coulehan 2006).

- Be sensitive to a patient's mood and nonverbal responses.

  For example, hesitancy in revealing emotional content. Use reflection so that the patient will expand on their discussion.

- Be understanding, receptive, and matter of fact without being sympathetic. Display and express empathy rather than sympathy.

- Avoid showing surprise or reproach.

- Clarify symptoms and obtain a problem list.

- When the patient has finished describing the symptom or symptoms:
  - briefly summarise the symptoms
  - ask whether there are any other main problems (Coulehan 2006)

For example, say, 'You have mentioned two problems: pain on the left side of your tummy, and loose motions over the last six weeks. Before we talk about those in more detail, are there any other problems I should know about?'

Usual Sequence of History

- nature of principal complaints, e.g. chest pain, poor home circumstances
- history of present complaint
- details of current illness
- enquiry of other symptoms (see Functional Enquiry)
- past history
- family history
- personal and social history
- If one's initial enquiries make it apparent that one section is of more importance than usual (e.g. previous relevant illnesses or operation), then relevant enquiries can be brought forward to an earlier stage in the history (e.g. past history after finding principal complaints).

History of Present Illness

- Start your written history with a single sentence summing up what your patient's complaint is. It should be like the banner headline of a newspaper. For example: c/o chest pain for six months.
  (You may choose to state the patient's chief complaint in the patient's own words when documenting.)
- Determine the chronology of the illness by asking:
  - 'How and when did your illness begin?' or
  - 'When did you first notice anything wrong?' or
  - 'When did you last feel completely well?'
- Begin by stating when the patient was last perfectly well. Describe symptoms in chronological order of onset.
  Both the date of onset and the length of time prior to being seen by you should be recorded. Symptoms should never be dated by the day of the week as this later becomes meaningless (Bickley and Szilagyi 2007, 2013; Cox 2010).
- Obtain a detailed description of each symptom by asking:
  - 'Tell me what the pain was like', for example. Make sure you ask about all symptoms, whether they seem relevant or not.
- With all symptoms obtain the following details:
  - duration
  - onset – sudden or gradual
  - what has happened since:
    - constant or periodic
    - frequency
    - getting worse or better
  - precipitating or relieving factors
  - associated symptoms.
- If pain is a symptom also determine the following:
  - site
  - radiation
  - character, e.g. ache, pressure, shooting, stabbing, dull
  - severity, e.g. 'Did it interfere with what you were doing?' 'Does it keep you awake?' 'Have you ever had this type of pain before?' 'Does the pain make you sweat or feel sick to your stomach?'

Avoid technical language when describing a patient's history. Do not say 'the patient complained of melaena', rather: 'the patient complained of passing loose, black, tarry motions'.

Supplementary History

When patients are unable to give an adequate or reliable history, the necessary information must be obtained from friends or relations. A history from a person who has witnessed a sudden event is often helpful.

When the patient does not speak English, arrange for an interpreter to translate for the patient. Bear in mind that numerous authors (Barkauskas et al. 2002; Ball et al. 2014a; Bickley and Szilagyi 2013; Cox 2010; Jarvis 2015; Rhoads and Paterson 2013) indicate that if possible family members and patients' young children should not be used as interpreters. Family members will frequently tell you what they think the patient's problem is rather than what the patient thinks the problem is. Because some questions that you may ask the patient are sensitive in nature, children should not be asked to interpret for their parents (Cox 2010; Lack 2012).

Functional Enquiry

This is a checklist of symptoms not already discovered.

Do not ask questions already covered in establishing the principal symptoms. This list may detect other symptoms.

- Modify your questioning according to the nature of the suspected disease, available time, and circumstances (Lack 2012).

  If during the functional enquiry a positive answer is obtained, full details must be elicited.
  Asterisks (*) denote questions that must nearly always be asked.

General Questions (These May Be Considered as Part of Your Review of Systems.)

- Ask about the following points:
  - *appetite: 'What is your appetite like? Do you feel like eating?'
  - *weight: 'Have you lost or gained weight recently?'
  - *general well-being: 'Do you feel well in yourself?'
  - *feelings of sadness or depression (to rule out feelings of suicide): 'Do you feel sad or depressed?'
  - fatigue: 'Are you more or less tired than you used to be?'
  - fever or chills: 'Have you felt hot or cold? Have you shivered?'
  - night sweats: 'Have you noticed any sweating at night or any other time?'
  - aches or pains
  - rash: 'Have you had any rash recently? Does it itch?'
  - lumps and bumps

Cardiovascular and Respiratory System

- Ask about the following points:
  - *chest pain: 'Have you recently had any pain or discomfort in the chest?'

  The most common causes of chest pain are:
  - *ischaemic heart disease*: severe constricting, central chest pain radiating to the neck, jaw, and left arm; *angina*: pain frequently precipitated by exercise or emotion and relieved by rest; *myocardial infarction*; the pain may come on at rest, be more severe, and last hours

- *pleuritic pain*: sharp, localised pain, usually lateral; worse on inspiration or cough
- *anxiety or panic attacks*: a very common cause of chest pain Enquire about circumstances that bring on an attack.
- *shortness of breath: 'Are you breathless at any time?'

Breathlessness (dyspnoea) and chest pain must be accurately described. The degree of exercise that brings on the symptoms must be noted (e.g. climbing one flight of stairs, after 0.5 km [1/4 mi] walk).

- shortness of breath on lying flat (*orthopnoea*): 'Do you get breathless in bed? What do you do then? Does it get worse or better on sitting up? How many pillows do you use? Can you sleep without them?'
- waking up breathless: 'Do you wake at night with any symptoms? Do you gasp for breath? What do you do then?'

Orthopnoea (breathless when lying flat) and *paroxysmal nocturnal dyspnoea* (waking up breathless, relieved on sitting up) are features of *left heart failure*.

- *ankle swelling

Common in *congestive cardiac failure* (*right heart failure*).

- palpitations: 'Are you aware of your heart beating?'

Palpitations may be:

- single thumps (*ectopics*)
- slow or fast
- regular or irregular

Ask the patient to tap them out.

Paroxysmal tachycardia (sudden attacks of palpitations) usually starts and finishes abruptly.

- *cough: 'Do you have a cough? Is it a dry cough or do you cough up sputum? When do you cough?'
- sputum: 'What colour is your sputum? How much do you cough up?'

Green sputum usually indicates an *acute chest infection*. Clear sputum daily during winter months suggests *chronic bronchitis*. Frothy sputum suggests *left heart failure*.

- *blood in sputum (*haemoptysis*): 'Have you coughed up blood?'

Haemoptysis must be taken very seriously. Causes include:

- carcinoma of bronchus
- pulmonary embolism
- mitral stenosis
- tuberculosis
- bronchiectasis
- blackouts (*syncope*): 'Have you had any blackouts or faints? Did you feel light-headed or did the room go round? Did you lose consciousness? Did you have any warning? Can you remember what happened?'
- *smoking: 'Do you smoke? How many cigarettes do you smoke each day?'

Gastrointestinal System

- Ask about the following points:
  - nausea: 'Are there times when you feel sick?'
  - vomiting: 'Do you vomit? What is it like?'

'Coffee grounds' vomit suggests 'altered' blood such as with a bleeding ulcer.

Old food suggests *pyloric stenosis*.

If blood what colour is it – dark or bright red?

  - difficulty in swallowing (*dysphagia*): 'Do you have difficulty swallowing? Where does it stick?'

For solids: often organic obstruction.

For fluids: often neurological or psychological.

- ○ indigestion: 'Do you have any discomfort in your stomach after eating?'
- ○ abdominal pain: 'Where is the pain? How is it connected to meals or opening your bowels? What relieves the pain?'
- ○ *bowel habit: 'How often do you open your bowels?' or 'How many times do you open your bowels per day?' 'Do you have to open your bowels at night?' (often a sign of true pathology)

If *diarrhoea* is suggested, the number of motions per day and their nature (blood? pus? mucus?) must be established. Frothy, frequent diarrhoea may be suggestive of coeliac disease.

'What are your motions like?' The stools may be pale, bulky, and float (fat in stool – *steatorrhoea*) or tarry from digested blood (*melaena* – usually from upper gastrointestinal tract).

Bright blood on the surface of a motion may be from *haemorrhoids*, whereas blood in a stool may signify *cancer* or *inflammatory bowel disease*.

Question what the patient has eaten. Red stool may indicate the patient has been eating beets, for example.

- ○ jaundice: 'Is your urine dark? Are your stools pale? What tablets have you been taking recently? Have you had any recent injections or transfusions? Have you been abroad recently? How much alcohol do you drink?'

Jaundice may be:

- obstructive (dark urine, pale stools) from:
  - — carcinoma of the head of the pancreas
  - — gallstones
- hepatocellular (dark urine, pale stools may develop) from:
  - — *ethanol* (cirrhosis)
  - — drugs or transfusions (viral hepatitis)
  - — drug reactions or infections (travel abroad, viral hepatitis or amoebae)
- haemolytic (unconjugated bilirubin is bound to albumin and is not secreted in the urine).

Genitourinary System

- Ask about the following points:
  - ○ dysuria: pain on urination – usually burning (often a sign of infection/cystitis)
  - ○ loin pain: 'Any pain in your back?'

  Pain in the loins suggests pyelonephritis.

  - ○ *urine: 'Are your waterworks all right? Do you pass a lot of water at night? Do you have any difficulty passing water? Is there blood in your water?' (suggests haematuria)

  Polyuria and *nocturia* occur in *diabetes*.

  Prostatism results in slow onset of urination, a poor stream, and terminal dribbling.

  - ○ sex: 'Any problems with intercourse or making love?'
  - ○ *menstruation: 'Any problems with your periods? Do you bleed heavily? Do you bleed between periods?'

  Vaginal bleeding between periods or after the menopause raises the possibility of *cervical* or *uterine cancer*.

  Menstrual cycle: Last menstrual period (LMP) and length of bleeding. (Normal cycle is 21–35 days. Normal period is between 5 and 8 days with between 70 and 200 ml of blood loss.) If indicated, ask about intermenstrual bleeding, postmenopausal bleeding or postcoital bleeding.

  - ○ vaginal discharge (if present, ask about colour, consistency, and odour; does it cause itching?)
  - ○ pain on intercourse (*dyspareunia*)

Nervous System

- Ask about the following points:
  - *headache: 'Do you ever have any headaches? Where are they?' (location) 'When do you get headaches?' 'What are they like?' (quality/intensity)

  Headaches often originate from tension and can be either frontal or occipital. Occipital headache on waking in the early morning may be due to *raised intracranial pressure* (e.g. from a *tumour* or *malignant hypertension*). Ask if the headache is associated with flashing lights (*amaurosis fugax*) (Bickley and Szilagyi 2013; Cox 2010).

  - vision: 'Do you have any blurred or double vision?'
  - hearing: ask about tinnitus, deafness, and exposure to noise
  - dizziness: 'Do you have any dizziness or episodes when the world goes round (*vertigo*)?'

  Dizziness with light-headed symptoms, when sudden in onset, may be *cardiac* (enquire about palpitations). When slow, onset may be *vasovagal 'fainting'* or an *internal haemorrhage*.

  Vertigo may be from ear disease *(labyrinthitis/infection, Ménière's disease, Benign Paroxysmal Positional Vertigo [BPPV] 'Ear Crystals' and/or age related)*

  Enquire about deafness, earache, or discharge or *brain-stem dysfunction*.

- unsteady gait: 'Any difficulty walking or running?'
- weakness (consider myelinating encephalophy [ME] or myasthenia gravis)
- numbness or increased sensation: 'Any patches of numbness?'
- pins and needles
- sphincter disturbance: 'Any difficulties holding your water/bowels?' (sign of spinal cord compression; ask about back injury)
- Fits or faints: 'Have you had any funny episodes?' (Syncope – consider cardiac related, e.g. postural orthostatic tachycardia syndrome [POTS] – disautonomia)

  The following details should be sought from the patient:
  - duration
  - frequency and length of attacks
  - time of attacks, e.g. if standing, at night
  - mode of onset and termination
  - premonition or aura, light-headedness, or vertigo
  - biting of tongue, loss of sphincter control, injury, etc.

  Grand mal epilepsy classically produces sudden unconsciousness without any warning and on waking the patient feels drowsy with a headache, has a sore tongue, and has been incontinent.

Mental Health

- Ask about the following points:
  - depression: 'How is your mood? Happy or sad? If depressed, how bad? Have you lost interest in things? Can you still enjoy things? How do you feel about the future?' 'Has anything happened in your life to make you sad or depressed? Do you feel guilty about anything?' If the patient seems depressed: 'Have you ever thought of suicide? How long have you felt like this? Is there a specific problem? Have you felt like this before?'
  - active periods: 'Do you have periods in which you are particularly active?'

  Susceptibility to depression may be a personality trait. In *bipolar affective disease*, swings to *mania* (excess activity, rapid speech, and excitable mood) can recur. Enquire about interest, concentration, irritability, sleep difficulties.

  In schizophrenia active periods are associated with paranoia *(in conjunction with bipolar affective disorder the term is schizoaffective disorder)*

- ○ anxiety: 'Have you worried a lot recently? Do you get anxious? In what situations? Are there any situations you avoid because you feel anxious?' 'Do you worry about your health? Any worries in your job or with your family? Any financial worries?' 'Do you have panic attacks? What happens?'
- ○ sleep: 'Any difficulties sleeping? Do you have difficulty getting to sleep? Do you wake early?'

Difficulties of sleep are commonly associated with depression or anxiety.

Refer to Chapter 12 for more comprehensive information on mental health assessment.

The Eye

- • Ask about the following points:
  - ○ eye pain, photophobia, or redness: 'Have the eyes been red, uncomfortable, or painful?'
  - ○ painful red eye, particularly with photophobia, may be serious and due to:
    iritis (uveitis) – anterior/posterior uveitis must be treated as a medical emergency (it may be related to *ankylosing spondylitis, Reiter's disease, sarcoid, Behçet's disease. Uveitis is also seen in conjunction with ulcerative colitis and Crohn's disease.*)
    scleritis (systemic vasculitis)
    corneal ulcer
    acute glaucoma
  - ○ painless red eye may be:
    episcleritis
    temporary and of no consequence
    systemic vasculitis
  - ○ sticky red eye may be *conjunctivitis* (usually infective)
  - ○ itchy watery eye may be *allergic*, e.g. *hay fever*
  - ○ gritty eye may be dry (sicca or *Sjögren's syndrome*)
  - ○ clarity of vision: 'Has your vision been blurred?'
  - ○ blurring of vision for either near or distance alone may be an error of focus, helped by spectacles
  - ○ blurred vision in general (*serous retinopathy*)
  - ○ loss of central vision (or of top or bottom half) in one eye may be due to a *retinal or optic nerve disorder*
  - ○ transient complete blindness in one eye lasting for minutes – *amaurosis fugax* (fleeting blindness)
    suggests retinal arterial blockage from embolus
    may be from *carotid atheroma* (listen for bruit)
    may have a cardiac source
  - ○ subtle difficulties with vision, difficulty reading – problems at the chiasm, or visual path behind it:
    complete *bitemporal hemianopia* – *tumour* pressure on chiasm
    homonymous
    hemianopia: *posterior cerebral* or *optic radiation lesion*
  - ○ usually *infarct* or *tumour*; rarely complains of 'half vision', but may have difficulty reading
  - ○ Diplopia: 'Have you ever seen double?'
    Diplopia may be due to:
  - ○ *lesion* of the motor cranial nerves III, IV, or VI
  - ○ *3rd-nerve palsy*
    causes double vision in all directions
    often with dilatation of the pupil and ptosis

- ○ *4th-nerve palsy*
  causes doubling looking down and in (as when reading) with images separated horizontally and vertically and tilted (not parallel)
- ○ *6th-nerve palsy*
  causes horizontal, level, and parallel doubling
  worse on looking to the affected side
- ○ *muscular disorder*
  e.g. thyroid related (see below)
  ME (weakness after muscle use, antibodies to nerve end plates)

Refer to Chapter 11 for more comprehensive information on examination of the eye.

Locomotor System

- Ask about the following points:
  - ○ pain, stiffness, or swelling of joints: 'When and how did it start? Have you injured the joint?'
    There are innumerable causes of *arthritis* (painful, swollen, tender joints) and *arthralgia* (painful joints). Patients may incorrectly attribute a problem to some injury.
    Osteoarthritis is a joint 'wearing out' and is often asymmetric, involving weight-bearing joints such as the hip or knee. Exercise makes the joint pain worse.
    Rheumatoid arthritis is a generalised autoimmune disease with symmetrical involvement. In the hands, fusiform swelling of the interphalangeal joints is accompanied by swollen metacarpophalangeal joints. Large joints are often affected. Stiffness is worse after rest, e.g. on waking, and improves with use.
    Gout usually involves a single joint, such as the first metatarsophalangeal joint, but can lead to gross hand involvement (also seen in the elbows and ankles) with asymmetric uric acid lumps (*tophi*) by some joints and in the tips of the ears.
    Septic arthritis is a single, hot, painful joint.
  - ○ functional disability: 'How far can you walk? Can you walk up stairs? Is any particular movement difficult? Can you dress yourself? (Observe how the patient is dressed.) How long does it take?' 'Are you able to work?' 'Can you write?' (In the physical examination observe how the patient walks and their manual dexterity.)

Thyroid Disease

- Ask about the following points:
  - ○ weight change
  - ○ reaction to the weather: 'Do you dislike the hot or cold weather?'
  - ○ irritability: 'Are you more or less irritable compared with a few years ago?'
  - ○ diarrhoea/constipation
  - ○ palpitations
  - ○ dry skin or greasy hair: 'Is your skin dry or greasy? Is your hair dry or greasy?'
  - ○ depression: 'How has your mood been?'
  - ○ croaky voice
    Hypothyroid patients put on weight without increase in appetite; dislike cold weather; have dry skin and thin, dry hair, a puffy face, a croaky voice; are usually calm; and may be depressed.
    Hyperthyroid patients may lose weight despite eating more, dislike hot weather, perspire excessively, have palpitations and a tremor, and may be agitated and tearful. Young people have predominantly nervous and heat intolerance symptoms, whereas old people tend to present with cardiac symptoms. (Exopthalmos may be present.)

Past History

- All previous illnesses or operations, whether apparently important or not, must be included.

  For instance, a casually mentioned attack of influenza or chill may have been a manifestation of an occult infection.
- The importance of a past illness may be gained by finding out how long the patient was in bed or off work (Lack 2012).
- Complications of any previous illnesses should be carefully enquired into and, here, leading questions are sometimes necessary.

General Questions

- Ask about the following:
  - 'Have you had any serious illnesses?'
  - 'Have you had any emotional or nervous problems?'
  - 'Have you had any operations or admissions to hospital?'
  - 'Have you ever:
    - had yellow skin (jaundice), fits (epilepsy), tuberculosis, high blood pressure (hypertension), low blood pressure (hypotension), rheumatic fever, kidney problems, or diabetes?
    - travelled abroad?
    - had allergies?'
  - 'Have any medicines ever upset you?'
    Allergic responses to drugs may include an itchy rash, vomiting, diarrhoea, or severe illness, including jaundice. Many patients claim to be allergic but are not. An accurate description of the supposed allergic episodes is important.
  - Other questions can be included when relevant such as:
    - 'Have you ever had a heart attack?'
  - Additional questions can be asked depending on the patient's previous responses such as:
    - if the patient has high blood pressure, ask about kidney problems, if relatives have hypertension, or whether the patient eats liquorice
    - if a possible heart attack, ask about hypertension, diabetes, diet, smoking, family history of heart disease
    - if the history suggests cardiac failure, you must ask if the patient has had *rheumatic fever*
      Patients have often had examinations for life insurance, disability insurance, or the armed forces.

Family History

The family history gives clues to possible predisposition to illness (e.g. heart attacks) and whether a patient may have reason to be particularly anxious about a certain disease (e.g. mother died of cancer).

Death certificates and patient knowledge are often inaccurate. Patients may be reluctant to talk about relatives' illnesses if they were mental diseases, epilepsy, or cancer (Cox 2010).

It will be useful to construct a genogram of the patient's family history for quick referral.

General Questions

- Ask about the following:
  - 'Are your parents alive? Are they fit and well? What did your parents die from?'
  - 'Have you any brothers or sisters? Are they fit and well?'
  - 'Do you have any children? Are they fit and well?'
  - 'Is there any family history of:
    - heart trouble?
    - diabetes?
    - high blood pressure?'

  These questions can be varied to take account of the patient's chief complaint.

Personal and Social History

You need to find out what kind of person the patient is, what their home circumstances are, and how the illness has affected the patient and family. Your aim is to understand the patient's illness in the context of their personality and home environment.

If in hospital or following day surgery, can the patient convalesce satisfactorily at home and at what stage? What are the consequences of the illness? Will advice, information, and help be needed? An interview with a relative or friend may be very helpful.

General Questions

- Ask about the following:
  - family: 'Is everything all right at home? Do you have any family problems?'
    It may be appropriate to ask: 'Is your relationship with your partner/husband/wife all right? Is sex all right?' Problems may arise from physical or emotional reasons, and the patient may appreciate an opportunity to discuss worries. Note that a patient's sexual preference and sexual orientation may be different.
  - accommodation: 'Where do you live? Is it all right?'
  - job: 'What is your job? Could you tell me exactly what you do? Is it satisfactory? Will your illness affect your work?'
  - hobbies: 'What do you do in your spare time? Do you have any social life?' 'What is your social life like?'
  - alcohol: 'How much alcohol do you drink?'
    Alcoholics usually underestimate their daily consumption. (Normally intake should not exceed 21 units per week for a male and 14 units per week for a female.) It may be helpful to go through a 'drinking day'. If there is a suspicion of a drinking problem, you can ask: 'Do you ever drink in the morning? Do you worry about controlling your drinking? Does it affect your job, home, or social life?'
  - smoking: 'Do you smoke?' Have you ever smoked? Why did you give up? How many cigarettes, cigars, or pipefuls of tobacco do you smoke a day?'
    This is particularly relevant for heart or chest disease, but must always be asked.
    (You may also consider asking about chewing tobacco in relation to mouth cancer.)
  - drugs: 'Do you take any recreational drugs?' If so, 'What do you take?'
  - prescribed medications: 'What pills (tablets) are you taking at the moment? Have you taken any other pills in the last few months?'

  This is an extremely important question. A complete list of all drugs and doses must be obtained including complementary/integrative medicines and vitamins.

- If relevant, ask about any pets, visits abroad, previous or present exposure during working to coal dust, asbestos, etc.

The Patient's Ideas, Concerns, and Expectations

Make sure that you understand the patient's main ideas, concerns, and expectations. Ask for example:

- What do you think is wrong with you?
- What are you expecting to happen to you whilst you are in the surgery, clinic, or hospital?
- Is there something in particular you would like us to do?
- Have you any questions?

  The patient's main concerns may not be your main concerns. The patient may have quite different expectations of the visit to the surgery, the hospital admission, or outpatient appointment from what you assume. If you fail to address the patient's concerns they are likely to be dissatisfied, leading to a difficult practitioner–patient relationship and possible noncompliance (Coulehan 2006; Cox 2010).

Strategy

Having taken the history, you should:

- have some idea of possible diagnoses (in 90–95% of cases the patient will tell you what the problem is whilst you are taking the history)
- have made an assessment of the patient as a person
- know which systems you wish to concentrate on when examining the patient (Swartz 2014).

Further relevant questions may arise from abnormalities found on examination or investigation.

References

Ball, J., Dains, J., Flynn, J. et al. (2014a). *Seidel's Guide to Physical Examination*, 8e. St. Louis: Mosby.

Ball, J., Dains, J., Flynn, J. et al. (2014b). *Student Laboratory Manual to Accompany Seidel's Guide to Physical Examination*, 8e. St. Louis: Mosby.

Barkauskas, V., Baumann, L., and Darling-Fisher, C. (2002). *Health and Physical Assessment*, 3e. London: Mosby.

Bickley, L. and Szilagyi, P. (2007). *Bates' Guide to Physical Examination and History Taking*, 9e. Philadelphia: Lippincott.

Bickley, L. and Szilagyi, P. (2013). *Bates' Guide to Physical Examination and History Taking*, 11e. New York: Wolters Kluwer/Lippincott Williams & Wilkins.

Collins-Bride, G. and Saxe, J. (2013). *Clinical Guidelines for Advanced Practice Nursing - An Interdisciplinary Approach*, 2e. Burlington, MA: Jones and Bartlett Learning.

Coulehan, J. (2006). *The Medical Interview: Mastering Kills for Clinical Practice*, 5e. Philadelphia: F. A. David Company.

Cox, C. (2010). *Physical Assessment for Nurses*, 2e. Oxford: Wiley Blackwell.

Dains, J., Baumann, L., and Scheibel, P. (2012). *Advanced Health Assessment and Clinical Diagnosis in Primary Care*, 4e. St. Louis: Elsevier.

Dains, J., Baumann, L., and Scheibel, P. (2015). *Advanced Health Assessment and Clinical Diagnosis in Primary Care*, 5e. St. Louis: Mosby.

Epstein, O., Perkin, G., de Bono, D., and Cookson, J. (2008). *Clinical Examination*, 4e. London: Mosby.

Hatton, C. and Blackwood, R. (2003). *Lecture Notes on Clinical Skills*, 4e. Oxford: Blackwell Science.

Jackson, P. and Vessey, J. (2010). *Primary Care of the Child with a Chronic Condition*, 5e. London: Mosby.

Japp, A. and Robertson, C. (2013). *Macleod's Clinical Diagnosis*. Edinburgh: Churchill Livingstone, Elsevier.

Jarvis, C. (2008). *Physical Examination and Health Assessment*, 5e. St. Louis: Saunders.

Jarvis, C. (2015). *Physical Examination and Health Assessment*, 7e. Edinburgh: Elsevier.

14

Lack, V. (2012). Consultation skills. In: *Advanced Practice in Healthcare* (ed. C. Cox, M. Hill and V. Lack), 39–55. London: Routledge.

Rhoads, J. and Paterson, S. (2013). *Advanced Health Assessment and Diagnostic Reasoning*, 2e. Burlington: Jones and Bartlett.

Rudolf, M. and Levene, M. (2011). *Paediatrics and Child Health*, 3e. Oxford: Blackwell.

Sawyer, S.S. (2012). *Pediatric Physical Examination and Health Assessment*. London: Jones and Bartlett Learning International.

Seidel, H., Ball, J., Dains, J., and Benedict, G. (2006). *Mosby's Physical Examination Handbook*. St. Louis: Mosby.

Seidel, H., Ball, J., Dains, J., and Benedict, G. (2010). *Mosby's Physical Examination Handbook*, 7e. St. Louis: Mosby-Year Book.

Swartz, M. (2006). *Physical Diagnosis, History and Examination*, 5e. London: W. B. Saunders.

Swartz, M. (2014). *Physical Diagnosis: History and Examination*, With Student Consult Online Access, 7e. London: Elsevier.

Talley, N. and O'Connor, S. (2006). *Clinical Examination: A Systematic Guide to Physical Diagnosis*, 5e. London: Churchill Livingstone.

Talley, N. and O'Connor, S. (2014). *Clinical Examination: A Systematic Guide to Physical Diagnosis*, 7e. London: Churchill Livingstone, Elsevier.

Chapter 2

General Health Assessment

Carol Lynn Cox

Introduction

An initial assessment of the patient will have been made whilst taking the history. As a reminder, the history begins with the subjective component (patient's perspective) of your assessment, which includes a review of systems. The general appearance of the patient will be your first observation (Collins-Bride and Saxe 2013; Coulehan 2006; Hatton and Blackwood 2003; Lack 2012). Subsequently, the order of your physical examination will vary based on the subjective information provided in the patient's history. In an ideal world you would undertake your assessment following the Subjective, Objective, Assessment, and Plan (SOAP) format (Cox 2010). The SOAP format incorporates the subjective (chief complaint or presenting problem) from the patient's perspective, the objective examination you undertake, the assessment from the subjective and objective which is your impression of findings, your differential diagnosis, and finally your plan for the patient such as blood tests, X-rays, or other tests you want to order for the patient as well as instructions for the patient to follow including administration of medications and other treatments.

The system to which the presenting symptoms refer is generally examined first. Otherwise devise your own routine, examining each part of the body in turn, covering all systems as required. An example is:

- general appearance
- alertness, mood, general behaviour
- hands and nails
- skin
- radial pulse
- axillary nodes
- cervical lymph nodes
- facies, eyes, tongue
- jugular venous pulse/distension
- heart
- breasts

Physical Assessment for Nurses and Healthcare Professionals, Third Edition. Edited by Carol Lynn Cox.
© 2019 John Wiley & Sons Ltd. Published 2019 by John Wiley & Sons Ltd.

- respiratory
- abdomen, including femoral pulses
- rectal or pelvic examination
- musculoskeletal
- nervous system including fundi (if not examined with the eyes as noted above).

Whichever part of the body you are examining, always use the same routine*:

1. inspection
2. palpation
3. percussion
4. auscultation.

(*The routine will vary in examination of the abdomen with auscultation following inspection.) (Ball et al. 2014a, b; Barkauskas et al. 2002; Bickley and Szilagyi 2007, 2013; Cox 2010; Dains et al. 2015; Rundio and Lorman 2017)

General Inspection

The beginning of the examination is a careful observation of the patient as a whole. Note the following:

- Does the patient look ill?
  - what age does the patient look?
  - febrile, dehydrated?
  - alert, confused, drowsy?
  - cooperative, happy, sad, resentful?
  - fat, muscular, wasted?
  - in pain or distressed?

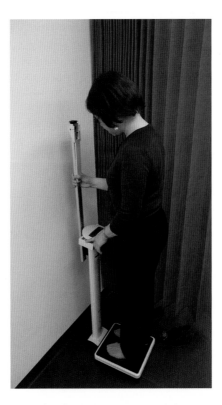

Check your patient's weight

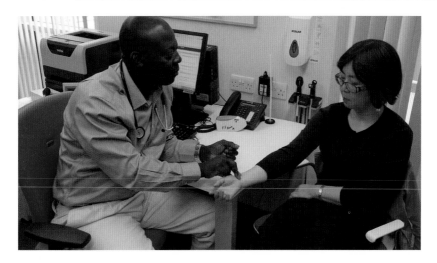

Checking the pulse

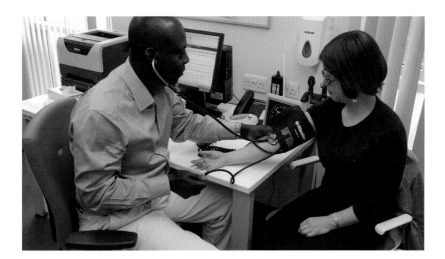

Taking the blood pressure

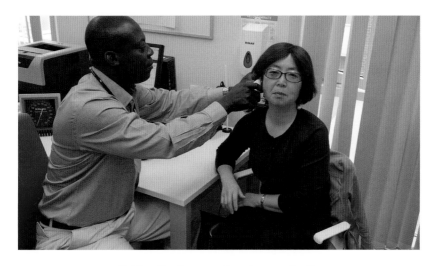

Taking the temperature tympanically

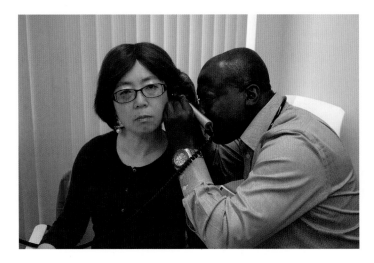

Examining the tympanic membrane with the otoscope. Hold the handle like a pen

Hands

Note the following:

- Temperature:
  - unduly cold hands –? *low cardiac output*
  - unduly warm hands –? *high-output state*, e.g. *thyrotoxicosis*
  - cold and sweaty –? anxiety or other causes of *sympathetic overreactivity*, e.g. *hypoglycaemia*
- Peripheral cyanosis
- Raynaud's
- Nicotine stains
- Nails:
  - bitten
  - leukonychia – white nails
    Can occur in *cirrhosis*.
  - koilonychia – misshapen, concave nails
    Can occur in *iron-deficiency anaemia*.
  - clubbing – loss of angle at base of nail
    Nail clubbing occurs in specific diseases:
    - heart: infectious *endocarditis, cyanotic congenital heart disease*
    - lungs: *carcinoma of the bronchus* (*chronic infection: abscess; bronchiectasis*, e.g. *cystic fibrosis; empyema*); *fibrosing alveolitis* (not chronic bronchitis)
    - liver: *cirrhosis*
    - *Crohn's disease*
    - *congenital*.
  - splinter haemorrhages
    Occur in *infectious endocarditis* but are more common in people doing manual work.
  - pitting – *psoriasis*
  - onycholysis – separation of nail from nail bed; *psoriasis, thyrotoxicosis*
  - paronychia – pustule in lateral nail fold (Bickley and Szilagyi 2013; Collins-Bride and Saxe 2013; Dains et al. 2012, 2015; Epstein et al. 2008; Japp and Robertson 2013; Jarvis 2008).

- Palms:
  - erythema – can be normal, also occurs with *chronic liver disease, pregnancy*
  - Dupuytren's contracture – tethering of skin in palm to flexor tendon of 4th finger; can occur in *cirrhosis* (Barkauskas et al. 2002; Bickley and Szilagyi 2013; Collins-Bride and Saxe 2013; Dains et al. 2012, 2015; Jarvis 2008; Rundio and Lorman 2017; Seidel et al. 2006, 2010; Swartz 2006, 2014; Tally and O'Connor 2006, 2014).
- Joints:
  - symmetrical swellings occur in *rheumatoid arthritis*
  - asymmetrical swellings occur in *gout* and *osteoarthritis* (Bickley and Szilagyi 2013; Collins-Bride and Saxe 2013; Dains et al. 2012, 2015; Jarvis 2008; Rundio and Lorman 2017).

Skin

Inspection of Skin (Refer to Chapter 3 for a full assessment of the skin)

- distribution of any lesions
- examine close up with palpation of skin
- remember mucous membranes, hair, and nails
- Colour:
  - pigmented apart from racial pigmentation or suntan – examine buccal mucosa
  - if appears jaundiced examine sclera
  - if pale examine conjunctivae for anaemia
- Skin texture:
  - ? normal for age (becomes thinner from age 50)
  - thin, e.g. *Cushing's syndrome, hypothyroid, hypopituitary, malnutrition, liver or renal failure*
  - thick, e.g. *acromegaly, androgen excess*
  - dry, e.g. *hypothyroid*
  - tethered or puckered, e.g. *scleroderma* of fingers, attached to underlying breast tumour
- Rash:
  - what is it like? (describe precisely)

Inspection of Lesions

- distribution of lesions:
  - symmetrical or asymmetrical
  - peripheral or mainly on trunk
  - maximal on light-exposed sites
  - pattern of contact with known agents, e.g. shoes, gloves, cosmetics
- number and size of lesions
- look at an early lesion
- discrete or confluent
- pattern of lesions, e.g. linear, annular, serpiginous (like a snake), reticular (like a net), star shaped (melanoma)
- is edge well demarcated? (Edges are well demarcated in syphilis for example.)
- colour (melanomas have atypical pigmentation in the epidermis such as shades of grey, white, red, blue, brown, and black)
- surface, e.g. scaly as in psoriasis; shiny as in thyrotoxicosis or peripheral vascular disease (Bickley and Szilagyi 2013; Collins-Bride and Saxe 2013; Dains et al. 2012, 2015; Jarvis 2008; Rundio and Lorman 2017; Tally and O'Connor 2014).

Palpation of Lesions

- flat, impalpable – *macular*
- raised
  papular: in skin, localised
  plaque: larger, e.g. > 0.5 cm
  nodules: deeper in dermis, persisting more than three days
  wheal: oedema fluid, transient, less than three days
  vesicles: contain fluid
  bullae: large vesicles, e.g. > 0.5 cm
  pustular
- deep in dermis – *nodules*
- temperature
- tender?
- blanches on pressure – most erythematous lesions, e.g. *drug rash, telangiectasia*, dilated capillaries
- does not blanch on pressure
  Purpura or *petechiae* are small discrete microhaemorrhages approximately 1 mm across, red, nontender macules.
  If palpable, suggests *vasculitis*.
  Senile purpura local haemorrhages are from minor traumas in thin skin of hands or forearms. Flat purple/brown lesions.
- hard
  ○ sclerosis, e.g. *scleroderma* of fingers
  ○ infiltration, e.g. *lymphoma* or *cancer*
  ○ scars (Japp and Robertson 2013; Jarvis 2015; Swartz 2014).

Enquire About the Time Course of Any Lesion

- 'How long has it been there?'
- 'Is it fixed in size and position? Does it come and go?'
- 'Is it itchy, sore, tender or has no feeling (anaesthetic)?'
  Knowledge of the differential diagnosis will indicate other questions:
  dermatitis of hand – contact with chemicals or plants, wear and tear;
  ulcer of toe – arterial disease, diabetes mellitus, neuropathy;
  pigmentation and ulcer of lower medial leg – varicose veins.

Common Diseases

Acne	Pilar-sebaceous follicular inflammation – papules and pustules on face and upper trunk, blackheads (*comedones*), cysts.
Basal cell carcinoma (rodent ulcer)	Shiny papule with rolled border and capillaries on surface. Can have a depressed centre or ulcerate.
Bullae	Blisters due to burns, infection of the skin, allergy, or, rarely, autoimmune diseases affecting adhesion within epidermis (*pemphigus*) or at the epidermal–dermal junction (*pemphigoid*).
Café-au-lait patches	Permanent discrete brown macules of varying size and shape. If large and numerous (6 or > 6 café-au-lait spots) requires evaluation – suggests neurofibromatosis.

Drug eruptions	Usually macular, symmetrical distribution. Can be urticaria, eczematous, and various forms, including erythema multiforme or erythema nodosum (see below).
Eczema	*Atopic dermatitis:* dry skin, red, plaques, commonly on the face, antecubital and popliteal fossae, with fine scales, vesicles, and scratch marks secondary to *pruritus* (itching). Often associated with *asthma* and *hay fever*. Family history of atopy. *Contact dermatitis:* may be irritant or allergic. Red, scaly plaques with vesicles in acute stages.
Erythema multiforme	Symmetrical, widespread inflammatory 0.5–1 cm macules/papules, often with central blister. Can be confluent. Usually on hands and feet: *drug reactions* *viral infections* *no apparent cause* *Stevens–Johnson syndrome* – with mucosal desquamation involving genitalia, mouth, and conjunctivae, with fever.
Erythema nodosum	Tender, localised, red, diffusely raised, 2–4 cm nodules in anterior shins. Due to: *streptococcal infection*, e.g. with *rheumatic fever* *primary tuberculosis* and other infections *sarcoid* *inflammatory bowel disease* *drug reactions* *no apparent cause*
Fungus	Red, annular, scaly area of skin. When involving the nails, they become thickened with loss of compact structure.
Herpes infection	Clusters of vesicopustules which crust, recurs at the same site, e.g. lips, buttocks.
Impetigo	Spreading pustules and yellow crusts from staphylococcal infection.
Malignant melanoma	Usually irregular pigmented (grey, white, red, blue, brown, and black), papule or plaque, superficial or thick with irregular edge, enlarging with tendency to bleed.
Psoriasis	Symmetrical eruption: chronic, discrete, red plaques with silvery scales. Gentle scraping easily induces bleeding. Often affects scalp, elbows, and knees (may in severe cases cover the majority of the body). Nails may be pitted. Familial and precipitated by streptococcal sore throats or skin trauma.
Scabies	Mite infection: itching with 2–4 mm tunnels in epidermis, e.g. in webs of fingers, wrists, genitalia.
Squamous cell carcinoma	Warty localised thickening, may ulcerate.
Urticaria	Transient wheal with surrounding erythema. Lasts around 24 hours. Usually due to allergy to food or drugs, e.g. aspirin, or physical, e.g. dermographism, cold.
Vitiligo	Permanent demarcated, depigmented white patches due to autoimmune disease (Rundio and Lorman 2017).

Mouth

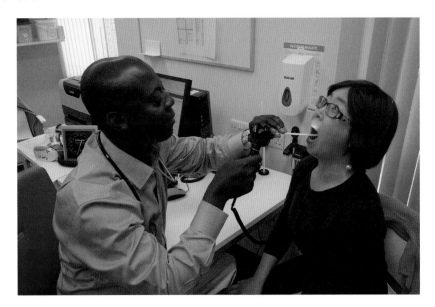

Checking the mouth

- Look at the tongue:
  - cyanosed, moist or dry
    Cyanosis is a reduction in the oxygenation of the blood, with more than $5\,g\,dl^{-1}$ deoxygenated haemoglobin.
    Central cyanosis (blue tongue) denotes a right-to-left shunt (unsaturated blood appearing in systemic circulation):
    — congenital heart disease, e.g. *Fallot's tetralogy*
    — lung disease, e.g. *obstructive airways disease*.
    Peripheral cyanosis (blue fingers, pink tongue) denotes inadequate peripheral circulation.
    A dry tongue can mean salt and water deficiency (often called 'dehydration') but also occurs with mouth-breathing.
- Look at the teeth:
  - caries (exposed dentine), poor dental hygiene, false
- Look at the gums:
  - bleeding, swollen
- Look at the throat:
  - tonsils
  - pharynx: swelling, redness, ulceration
- Smell patient's breath:
  - ketosis
  - alcohol
  - foetor
    constipation, appendicitis
    musty in liver failure

Ketosis is a sweet-smelling breath occurring with *starvation* or *severe diabetes*.
Hepatic foetor is a musty smell in *liver failure* (Bickley and Szilagyi 2013; Collins-Bride and Saxe 2013; Dains et al. 2012, 2015; Jarvis 2008; Rundio and Lorman 2017; Tally and O'Connor 2014).

Eyes
(Refer to Chapter 11 for a full examination of the eyes)

- Look at the eyes:
  - *sclera*, icterus
    The most obvious demonstration of *jaundice* is the yellow sclera.
  - lower lid conjunctiva, anaemia
    Anaemia: If the lower lid is everted, the colour of the mucous membrane can be seen. If these are pale, the haemoglobin is usually $< 9\,g\,dl^{-1}$.
  - eyelids: white/yellow deposit, *xanthelasma* (Xanthelasma may be familial or related to hypercholesteremia.)
  - puffy eyelids
    general oedema, e.g. *nephrotic syndrome*
    thyroid eye disease, hyper or hypo
    myxoedema
  - red eye
    iritis (*uveitis* – anterior/posterior. This must be considered a medical emergency.)
    conjunctivitis
    scleritis or *episcleritis*
    acute *glaucoma* (This must be considered a medical emergency.)
  - white line around cornea, *arcus senilis*
    common and of little significance in the elderly
    suggests *hyperlipidaemia* in younger patients
  - white-band keratopathy-hypercalcaemia
    sarcoid
    parathyroid tumour or *hyperplasia*
    lung oat-cell tumour
    bone secondaries
    vitamin D excess intake
      Hypercalcaemia may give a horizontal band across exposed medial and lateral parts of cornea.
  - white growth of bulbar conjunctival tissue
  - *Pterygium* (Usually occurs from the nasal side towards the centre of the cornea. It may interfere with vision if it covers the pupil.) (Solomer and Bowling 2018)

Examine the Fundi

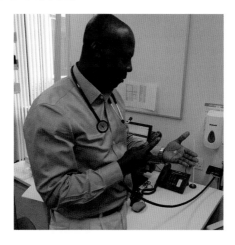

Checking the ophthalmoscope

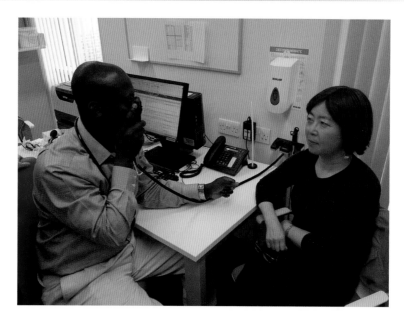

Look for the red reflex

This is often done as part of the neurological system (see Chapter 11) when examining the cranial nerves. It is placed here as features are also covered in the general examination.

- Use ophthalmoscope
  - The patient should be sitting. Remove spectacles from yourself and the patient.
  - Begin by setting the lens dioptre dial at 0 if you do not use spectacles. If you are myopic, you should start with the 'minus' lenses. Set the lens dioptre at −4 to begin, which is indicated as a red number. If you are hyperopic you should use the 'plus' lenses, which are indicated by black numbers. Keep your index finger on the dial to permit easy focusing. Hold the ophthalmoscope about 30 cm from the patient, shine the light into the patient's pupil, identify the red reflex (from the retina), and approach the patient at an angle of 15°. Approach on the same horizontal plane as the equator of the patient's eye. This will bring you straight to the patient's optic disc. After observing the disc examine the peripheral retina fully by following the blood vessels to and back from the four main quadrants.
  - Hold the ophthalmoscope in your right hand in front of your right eye to examine the patient's right eye and your left eye to examine the patient's left eye. Try to hold your breath when using the ophthalmoscope. Do not breathe into the patient's face.
  - If the patient's pupils are small, dilate with 1% tropicamide, 1 drop per eye. Works in 15–20 minutes and lasts two to four hours. Warn the patient that vision will be blurred for approximately four hours. Do **not** dilate if neurological observation of pupils is needed.
  - The patient should be told not to drive, if pupils have been dilated, for at least four to six hours (Cox 2010).
- Look at optic disc
  - normally pink rim with white 'cup' below surface of disc
  - *optic atrophy*
    - disc pale: rim no longer pink
      multiple sclerosis
      after optic neuritis
      optic nerve compression, e.g. tumour

- o papilloedema
  - — disc pink, indistinct margin
  - — cup disappears
  - — dilated retinal veins
    increased cerebral pressure, e.g. tumour
    accelerated hypertension
    optic neuritis, acute stage
- o glaucoma – enlarged cup, diminished rim
- o new vessels – new fronds of vessels coming forwards from disc
     ischaemic diabetic retinopathy
- Look at arteries
  - o arteries narrowed in hypertension, with increased light reflex along top of vessel
       Hypertension grading:

    1. narrow arteries
    2. 'nipping' (narrowing of veins by arteries)
    3. flame-shaped haemorrhages (e.g. hypertension) and cotton-wool spots (e.g. hyperlipidemia; atherosclerosis)
    4. papilloedema.

  - o occlusion artery – pale retina
       occlusion vein – haemorrhages (Kanski 2009; Solomer and Bowling 2018)
- Look at retina
  - o hard exudates (shiny, yellow circumscribed patches of lipid)
       diabetes
  - o cotton-wool spots (soft, fluffy white patches)
       microinfarcts causing local swelling of nerve fibres
       diabetes
       hypertension
       vasculitis
       human immunodeficiency virus (HIV)
  - o small, red dots
       microaneurysms – retinal capillary expansion adjacent to capillary closure
       diabetes
  - o haemorrhages
    - — round 'blots': haemorrhages deep in retina larger than microaneurysms
         diabetes
  - o flame-shaped: superficial haemorrhages along nerve fibres
       hypertension
       gross anaemia
       hyperviscosity
       bleeding tendency
  - o Roth's spots (white-centred haemorrhages)
       microembolic disorder
       subacute bacterial endocarditis
  - o pigmentation
       widespread
          retinitis pigmentosa
       localised
          choroiditis (clumping of pigment into patches)
          drug toxicity, e.g. chloroquine
       tigroid or tabby fundus: normal variant in choroid beneath retina

- peripheral new vessels
  ischaemic *diabetic retinopathy*
  retinal *vein occlusion*
- medullated nerve fibres – normal variant, areas of white nerves radiating from optic disc (see Chapter 11) (Kanski 2009; Solomer and Bowling 2018)

Examine for Palpable Lymph Nodes

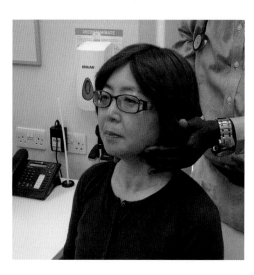

Palpation of lymph nodes

- In the neck:
  - above clavicle (posterior triangle)
  - medial to sternomastoid area (anterior triangle)
  - submandibular (can palpate submandibular gland)
  - occipital
    These glands are best felt by sitting the patient up and examining from behind. A left supraclavicular node can occur from the spread of a gastrointestinal malignancy (Virchow's node).
- In the axillae:
  - abduct arm, insert your hand along lateral side of axilla, and adduct arm, thus placing your fingertips in the apex of the axilla. Palpate gently
- In the epitrochlear region:
  - medial to and above elbow
- In the groins:
  - over inguinal ligament
- In the abdomen:
  - usually very difficult to feel; some claim to have felt para-aortic nodes
    Axillae often have soft, fleshy lymph nodes.
    Groins often have small, shotty nodes.
    Generalised large, rubbery nodes suggest *lymphoma*.
    Localised hard nodes suggest *cancer*.
    Tender nodes suggest *infection*.
- If many nodes are palpable – examine spleen and look for anaemia. *Lymphoma or leukaemia*? (Cox 2010; Talley and O'Connor 2006, 2014).

Lumps

- If there is an unusual lump, inspect first and palpate later:
  - site

  - size (measure in centimetres)
  - shape
  - surface, edge
  - surroundings
  - fixed or mobile
  - consistency, e.g. cystic or solid, soft or hard, fluctuance
  - tender
  - pulsatile
  - auscultation, e.g. thyroid 'hum' from increased vasularity
  - transillumination

    A *cancer* is usually hard, nontender, irregular, fixed to neighbouring tissues, and possibly ulcerating skin.

    A *cyst* may have:
    - fluctuance: pressure across cyst will cause it to bulge in another plane
    - transillumination: a light can be seen through it (usually only if room is darkened).
- Look at neighbouring lymph nodes. May find:
  - spread from cancer
  - inflamed lymph nodes from infection (Swartz 2014)

Heart

Routine Examination

For the full examination refer to Chapter 4, Examination of the Cardiovascular System.

- Inspect precordium
  - observe point of maximum impulse (usually 5th intercostal space [ICS] in an adult)
  - look for heaves
- Palpate precordium
  - heaves or thrusts
  - thrills (palpable murmurs/vibrations)
- Percuss precordium
  - heart will enlarge in congestive heart failure and cardiomegaly
  - apex may shift laterally to the left and be located in the 6th ICS
- Auscultate: S_1, S_2 (? S_3, S_4, clicks, snaps, or murmurs)
  - rate
  - rhythm (regular, regular – irregular)
- Assess jugular venous distension/jugular venous pressure (JVD/JVP) (Cox 2010)

Breasts

If you are a male nurse, arrange for a female chaperone, particularly when the patient is a young adult, shy, or nervous (Cox 2010).

Routine Examination

- Examine the female breasts when you examine the precordium.
- Inspect for asymmetry, obvious lumps, inverted nipples, skin changes.

- Palpate each quadrant of both breasts with the flat of the hand (fingers together, nearly extended with gentle pressure exerted from metacarpophalangeal joints, avoiding pressure on the nipple).
- If there are any possible lumps, proceed to a more complete examination.

Full Breast Examination

When patient has a symptom or a lump has been found:

- Inspect
  - With the patient sitting up ask the patient to raise her hands above her head, put hands on hips, rotate shoulders forwards, and then with hands on hips to lean forwards (so that you can examine under the breast). Look anteriorly and laterally.
  - Inspect for asymmetry or obvious lumps
    - differing size or shape of breasts
    - nipples – symmetry
    - rashes, redness (abscess)
      Breast cancer is suggested by:
    - asymmetry
    - skin tethering or puckering
    - *peau d'orange* (oedema of skin)
    - nipple deviated or inverted.
- Palpate
  - Patient lying flat on one pillow with one arm under her head and other at her side (right arm under head to examine right breast and left arm under head to examine left breast)
  - Examine each breast with flat of hand, each quadrant in turn (ensure that you examine well below each breast and into the tail of Spence)
  - Examine bimanually if large
  - Examine any lump as described in the General Inspection on skin and lymph nodes (this chapter)
    - is lump attached to skin or muscles?
    - examine lymph nodes (axilla, infraclavicular, and supraclavicular)
    - feel liver (Ball et al. 2014a; Cox 2010; Seidel et al. 2006, 2010).

Respiratory

Routine Examination

For the full examination refer to Chapter 5, Examination of the Respiratory System.

- Inspect:
  - symmetry (? flail, tracheal deviation)
  - scars/lesions
  - respiratory rate
  - ? nasal flaring
- Palpate:
  - thoracic integrity
  - lumps/bumps
  - crepitations
  - fremitus
- Percuss:
  - anteriorly
  - posteriorly

- laterally
  - ? dullness on percussion (consolidation or tumour)
- Auscultate:
  - tracheobronchial sounds
  - bronchovesicular sounds
  - vesicular sounds
  - ? adventitious sounds (Ball et al. 2014a; Cox 2010; Dains et al. 2015; Epstein et al. 2008; Jarvis 2015).

Thyroid

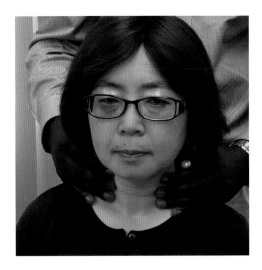

Palpation of the thyroid gland

- Inspect: then give the patient a glass of water and ask them to swallow. Is there a lump? Does it move upwards on swallowing?
- Palpate bimanually: stand behind the patient and palpate with fingers of both hands. Is the thyroid of normal size, shape, and texture? (Avoid the throttling position when examining behind the patient as this may frighten the patient.)
- If a lump is felt:
  - is thyroid multinodular?
  - does lump feel cystic?
    The thyroid is normally soft. If there is a goitre (swelling of thyroid), assess if the swelling is:
    - localised, e.g. *thyroid cyst*, *adenoma*, or *carcinoma*
    - generalised, e.g. *autoimmune thyroiditis*, *thyrotoxicosis*
    - multinodular.
      A swelling does not mean the gland is under- or overactive. In many cases the patient may be euthyroid. The thyroid becomes slightly enlarged in pregnancy.
- Ask patient to swallow – does thyroid rise normally?
- Is thyroid fixed?
- Can you get below the lump? If not, percuss over upper sternum for retrosternal extension
- Are there cervical lymph nodes?
- If possibility of patient being thyrotoxic, look for:
  - warm hands
  - perspiration

- tremor
- tachycardia, sinus rhythm, or atrial fibrillation
- wide, palpable fissure or lid lag
- thyroid 'hum' – bruit (on auscultation)
  Endocrine exophthalmos (may be associated with thyrotoxicosis):
    - conjunctival oedema: *chemosis* (seen by gentle pressure on lower lid, pushing up a fold of conjunctiva when oedema is present)
    - proptosis: eye pushed forwards (look from above down on eyes)
    - deficient upwards gaze and convergence
    - diplopia
    - papilloedema.
- If possibility of patient being *hypothyroid*, look for:
  - dry hair and skin
  - xanthelasma
  - puffy face
  - croaky voice
  - delayed relaxation of supinator or ankle jerks (Ball et al. 2014a; Cox 2010; Dains et al. 2015; Epstein et al. 2008; Jarvis 2015).

Other Endocrine Diseases
Acromegaly
- enlarged soft tissue of hands, feet, face
- coarse features; thick, greasy skin; large tongue (and other organs, e.g. thyroid)
- bitemporal hemianopia (from tumour pressing on optic chiasma)

Hypopituitarism
- no skin pigmentation
- thin skin
- decreased secondary sexual hair or delayed puberty
- short stature (and on X-ray, delayed fusion of epiphyses)
- bitemporal hemianopia if pituitary tumour

Addison's Disease
- increased skin pigmentation, including nonexposed areas, e.g. buccal pigmentation
- postural hypotension
- if female, decreased body hair

Cushing's Syndrome
- truncal obesity; round, red face with hirsutism
- thin skin and bruising, pink striae, hypertension
- proximal muscle weakness

Diabetes
Diabetic complications include:

- skin lesions
  Necrobiosis lipoidica – ischaemia in skin, usually on shins, leading to fatty replacement of dermis, covered by thin skin.
- ischaemic legs
  - diminished foot pulses

- o skin shiny blue, white, or black
- o no hairs, thick nails
- o ulcers
- peripheral neuropathy
  - o absent leg reflexes
  - o diminished sensation
  - o thick skin over unusual pressure points from dropped arch
- autonomic neuropathy
  - o dry skin
- mononeuropathy
  - o lateral popliteal nerve – footdrop
  - o III or VI – diplopia
  - o asymmetrical muscle-wasting of the upper leg
- retinopathy (Ball et al. 2014a; Cox 2010; Dains et al. 2015; Epstein et al. 2008; Jarvis 2015).

Abdominal

The abdomen is divided into four imaginary quadrants with components distributed as shown in Table 2.1.

Routine Examination

For the full examination refer to Chapter 6, Examination of the Abdominal System.

- Inspect:
  - o symmetry (? concave or convex)
  - o scars/lesions (? evidence of liver disease)

Table 2.1   Distribution of components in the four imaginary quadrants of the abdominal system.

Right upper quadrant (RUQ)	Left upper quadrant (LUQ)
Liver	Stomach
Gall bladder	Spleen
Head of pancreas	Body of pancreas
Right kidney	Left kidney
Large intestine	Large intestine
Small intestine	Small intestine
Right lower quadrant (RLQ)	**Left lower quadrant (LLQ)**
Appendix	
Right ovary	Left ovary
Large intestine	Large intestine
Small intestine	Small intestine
Uterus	
Bladder	

- Auscultate:
  - four quadrants
- Palpate:
  - nine quadrants (light and deep palpation)
  - lumps/bumps (? presence of tumour)
- Percuss:
  - nine quadrants
  - tympani
  - ? central dullness and lateral tympani (ovarian tumour)
  - ? central tympani and lateral dullness (ascites – assess for shifting dullness)
  - consider rectal/vaginal examination (Ball et al. 2014a; Cox 2010; Dains et al. 2015; Epstein et al. 2008; Japp and Robertson 2013; Jarvis 2008, 2015; Rhoads and Paterson 2013; Rundio and Lorman 2017).

Musculoskeletal

Normally you would examine the joints briefly when examining neighbouring systems. If a patient specifically complains of joint symptoms or an abnormal posture or joint is noted, a more detailed examination is needed (Cox 2010).

General Habitus

- Note the following:
  - is the patient unduly tall or short? (measure height and span)
  - are all limbs, spine, and skull of normal size and shape?
    - — normal person:
      height = span
      crown to pubis = pubis to heel
    - — long limbs:
      Marfan's syndrome
      eunuchoid during growth
    - — *collapsed vertebrae*:
      span > height
      pubis to heel > crown to pubis
  - is the posture normal?
  - curvature of the spine:
    kyphosis
    lordosis
    scoliosis
    gibbus
  - is the gait normal?
    Observing the patient walking is a vital part of examination of the locomotor system and neurological system.
    Painful gait, transferring weight quickly off a painful limb, bobbing up and down – an abnormal rhythm of gait.
    Painless abnormal gait may be from:
      short leg (bobs up and down with equal-length steps)
      stiff joint (lifts pelvis to prevent foot dragging on ground)
      weak ankle (high stepping gait to avoid toes catching on ground)
      weak knee (locks knee straight before putting foot on the ground)
      weak hip (sways sideways using trunk muscles to lift pelvis and to swing leg through)

uncoordinated gait (arms are swung as counterbalances)
hysterical or malingering causes.

Look for abnormal wear on shoes.

Inspection

Inspect the joints before you touch them.

- Look at:
  - skin
    redness – inflammation
    scars – old injury
    bruising – recent injury
  - soft tissues
    muscle wasting – old injury
    swelling – injury/inflammation
  - bones
    deformity – compare with other side
        varus: bent out from midline (bowleg)
        valgus: bent in towards midline
- Assess whether an isolated joint is affected, or if there is polyarthritis.
- If there is polyarthritis, note if it is symmetrical or asymmetrical.
- Compare any abnormal findings with the other side.
  Arthritis – swollen, hot, tender, painful joint.
  Arthropathy – swollen but not hot and tender.
  Arthralgia – painful, e.g. on movement, without being swollen.
  Swelling may also be due to an effusion, thickening of the periarticular tissues, enlargement of the ends of bones (e.g. *pulmonary osteopathy*), or complete disorganisation of the joint without pain (*Charcot's joint*).

Palpation

- Before you touch any joint ask the patient to tell you if it is painful.
- Feel for:
  - warmth
  - tenderness
    - watch patient's face for signs of discomfort
    - locate signs of tenderness – soft tissue or bone
  - swelling or displacement
  - fluctuation (effusion)
    An inflamed joint is usually generally tender. Localised tenderness may be mechanical in origin, e.g. ligament tear. Joint effusion may occur with an arthritis or local injury.

Movement

Test the range of movement of the joint both actively and passively. This must be done gently.

- Active – how far can the patient move the joint through its range?
  Do not seize limb and move it until patient complains.
- Passive – if range is limited, can you further increase the range of movement?
  Abduction: movement from central axis.
  Adduction: movement to central axis.

is the passive range of movement similar to the active range?

Limitation of the range of movement of a joint may be due to pain, muscle spasms, contracture, inflammation or thickening of the capsules or periarticular structures, effusions into the joint space, bony or cartilaginous outgrowths, or painful conditions not connected with the joint.

- Resisted movement – ask patient to bend joint whilst you resist movement. How much force can be developed?
- Hold your hand round the joint whilst it is moving. A grating or creaking sensation (*crepitus*) may be felt.

Crepitus is usually associated with *osteoarthritis*.

Summary of Signs of Common Illnesses
Osteoarthritis
- 'wear and tear' of a specific joint – usually large joints
- common in elderly or after trauma to joint
- often involves joints of the lower limbs and is asymmetrical
- often in the lumbar or cervical spine
- aches after use, with deep, boring pain at night
- Heberden's nodes – osteophytes on terminal interphalangeal joints

Rheumatoid Arthritis
Characteristically:

- a polyarthritis
- symmetrical, inflamed if active
- involves proximal interphalangeal and metacarpophalangeal joints of hands with ulnar deviation of fingers
- involves any large joint
- muscle wasting from disuse atrophy
- rheumatoid nodules on extensor surface of elbows
- may include other signs, e.g. with splenomegaly it is *Felty's syndrome*

Gout
Characteristically:

- asymmetrical
- inflamed 1st metatarsophalangeal joint (big toe) – *podagra*
- involves any joint in hand, often with tophus – hard round lump of urate by joint
- tophi on ears

Psoriasis
- particularly involves terminal interphalangeal joints, hips, and knees
- often with pitted nails of psoriasis as well as skin lesions

Ankylosing Spondylitis
- painful, stiff spine
- later fixed in flexed position

- hips and other joints can be involved (Ball et al. 2014a; Cox 2010; Dains et al. 2012, 2015; Epstein et al. 2008; Japp and Robertson 2013; Jarvis 2008, 2015; Rhoads and Paterson 2013; Rundio and Lorman 2017).

References

Ball, J., Dains, J., Flynn, J. et al. (2014a). *Seidel's Guide to Physical Examination*, 8e. St. Louis: Mosby.

Ball, J., Dains, J., Flynn, J. et al. (2014b). *Student Laboratory Manual to Accompany Seidel's Guide to Physical Examination*, 8e. St. Louis: Mosby.

Barkauskas, V., Baumann, L., and Darling-Fisher, C. (2002). *Health and Physical Assessment*, 3e. London: Mosby.

Bickley, L. and Szilagyi, P. (2007). *Bates' Guide to Physical Examination and History Taking*, 7e. Philadelphia: Lippincott.

Bickley, L. and Szilagyi, P. (2013). *Bates' Guide to Physical Examination and History Taking*, 11e. New York: Wolters Kluwer/Lippincott Williams & Wilkins.

Collins-Bride, G. and Saxe, J. (2013). *Clinical Guidelines for Advanced Practice Nursing - An Interdisciplinary Approach*, 2e. Burlington, MA: Jones and Bartlett Learning.

Coulehan, J. (2006). *The Medical Interview: Mastering Skills for Clinical Practice*, 5e. Philadelphia: F. A. David Company.

Cox, C. (2010). *Physical Assessment for Nurses*, 2e. Oxford: Wiley Blackwell.

Dains, J., Baumann, L., and Scheibel, P. (2012). *Advanced Health Assessment and Clinical Diagnosis in Primary Care*, 4e. St. Louis: Elsevier.

Dains, J., Baumann, L., and Scheibel, P. (2015). *Advanced Health Assessment and Clinical Diagnosis in Primary Care*, 5e. St. Louis: Mosby.

Epstein, O., Perkin, G., de Bono, D., and Cookson, J. (2008). *Clinical Examination*, 4e. London: Mosby.

Hatton, C. and Blackwood, R. (2003). *Lecture Notes on Clinical Skills*, 4e. Oxford: Blackwell Science.

Japp, A. and Robertson, C. (2013). *Macleod's Clinical Diagnosis*. Edinburgh: Churchill Livingstone, Elsevier.

Jarvis, C. (2008). *Physical Examination and Health Assessment*, 5e. St. Louis: Saunders.

Jarvis, C. (2015). *Physical Examination and Health Assessment*, 7e. Edinburgh: Elsevier.

Kanski, J. (2009). *Clinical Ophthamology, A Synopsis*, 2e. London: Butterworth Heinemann Elsevier.

Lack, V. (2012). Consultation Skills. In: *Advanced Practice in Healthcare* (ed. C. Cox, M. Hill and V. Lack). London: Routledge.

Rhoads, J. and Paterson, S. (2013). *Advanced Health Assessment and Diagnostic Reasoning*, 2e. Burlington: Jones and Bartlett.

Rundio, A. and Lorman, W. (2017). *Lippincott Certification Review: Family Nurse Practitioner & Adult-Gerontology Nurse Practitioner*. London: Wolters Kluwer.

Seidel, H., Ball, J., Dains, J., and Benedict, G. (2006). *Mosby's Physical Examination Handbook*. St. Louis: Mosby.

Seidel, H., Ball, J., Dains, J., and Benedict, G. (2010). *Mosby's Physical Examination Handbook*, 7e. St. Louis: Mosby-Year Book.

Solomer, J. and Bowling, B. (2018). *Kanski's Clinical Ophthalmology, A Systematic Approach*. London: Elsevier.

Swartz, M. (2006). *Physical Diagnosis, History and Examination*, 5e. London: W. B. Saunders.

Swartz, M. (2014). *Physical Diagnosis: History and Examination*, With Student Consult Online Access, 7e. London: Elsevier.

Talley, N. and O'Connor, S. (2006). *Clinical Examination: A Systematic Guide to Physical Diagnosis*, 5e. London: Churchill Livingstone.

Talley, N. and O'Connor, S. (2014). *Clinical Examination: A Systematic Guide to Physical Diagnosis*, 7e. London: Churchill Livingstone, Elsevier.

Chapter 3

Examination of the Skin, Hair, and Nails

Siobhan Hicks

Introduction

Examination of the skin, hair, and nails provides the examiner with substantial information about the patient's overall health. Therefore, this examination constitutes an essential aspect of a physical examination.

Anatomy and Physiology

The Skin

The skin (Figure 3.1) is the largest organ of the body helping to protect against bacteria, regulate body temperature, and permit sensations of touch, heat, and cold. The epidermis is the outermost layer of the skin; it is a semipermeable barrier responsible for producing keratin (a tough waterproof layer) and melanin, which protects the skin from ultraviolet radiation. Disease in the epidermis results in a rash or lesion with abnormal scale, a change in pigmentation, or the loss of structure leading to exudate or erosion.

The dermis contains tough, strong, and resilient connective tissue called collagen and elastin; it also contains hair follicles and sebaceous and sweat glands. Diseases of the dermis tend to result in elevation of the skin for example, as papules, nodules, or atrophy (Ashton et al. 2014).

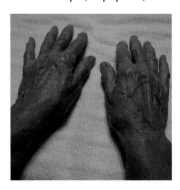

In the older adult the skin is thin and frail

Physical Assessment for Nurses and Healthcare Professionals, Third Edition. Edited by Carol Lynn Cox.
© 2019 John Wiley & Sons Ltd. Published 2019 by John Wiley & Sons Ltd.

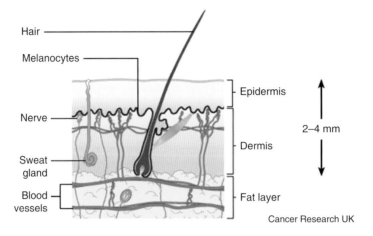

Figure 3.1   The skin.

The Hair

The hair or 'pili' as it is correctly termed is present on all surfaces of the body except for the palms, palmar surfaces of the fingers, the soles of the feet, and plantar surfaces of the feet. The protection hair offers is limited. In particular, hair protects the scalp from the burning rays of the sun and also guards against heat loss from the head. The eyebrows and eyelashes protect the eyes from debris falling into the eyes as does the hair in the nostrils and the external ear canal. Hair root plexuses (touch receptors) associated with hair follicles are activated whenever hair is moved. Therefore, the hair functions in sensing light touch.

Hair is composed of a shaft (superficial portion of the hair), root (shaft that penetrates into the dermis), and follicle (external and internal root sheath). Together the external and internal sheaths comprise the epithelial root sheath. Essentially hair is composed of columns of dead, keratinised cells bonded together by extracellular proteins (Tortora and Derrickson 2013). The dense dermis surrounding the hair follicle is termed the dermal root sheath. The base of the follicle is an onion-shaped structure which is termed the bulb. The blub contains the papilla and the matrix. The papilla nourishes the growing hair follicle whereas the matrix is responsible for the growth of the hair.

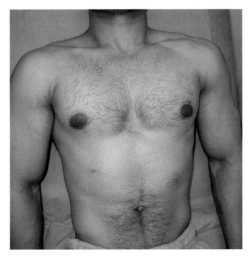

Assess hair distribution

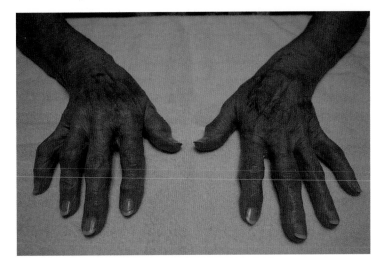

Note bruising in the older adult

The Nails

The nails are densely packed dead, hard keratinised epidermal cells. The nails form a solid covering over the dorsal surface of the distal portions of the fingers and toes. Nails are normally clear in colour. The nail is composed of the nail body, free edge, and root. The nail body is the portion of the nail that is seen along with the free edge, which can be allowed to grow beyond the distal end of each digit. The nail root, on the other hand, is the portion of the nail that is buried in a fold of skin. The nail body normally appears pink in colour because of blood flowing through capillaries in the dermis. The portion of the nail that grows beyond the end of the digits is called the lunula because of its shape and whitish colour. Beneath the free edge is the hyponychium, which is a thickened area of stratum corneum. This secures the nail to the distal tip of the digit. The eponychium (cuticle) is a narrow band of epidermis that adheres to the margins of the nail wall. The nail matrix is the proximal portion of the epithelium which is deep to the nail root. It is in this area that cells divide by mitosis to produce growth.

The growth of hair and nails is determined by the rate of mitosis in cells and is affected by age, health, and nutritional status. Growth also varies depending on the season, time of day, and environmental factors.

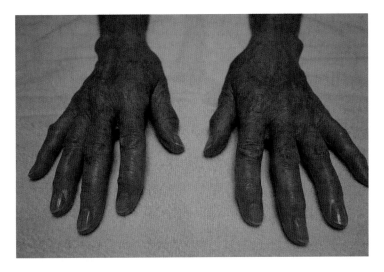

Ridges on the nails are a sign of ageing

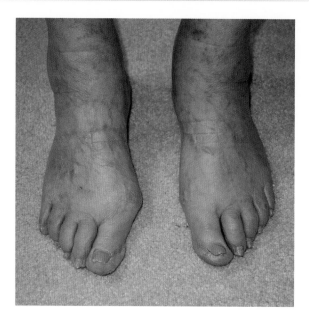

Assess the skin, hair, and nails

Subjective History Taking

Reaching a diagnosis in dermatology can be challenging for both novice and expert practitioners. Experience and pattern recognition combined with appropriate, orderly subjective history taking can provide valuable clues to help you reach your final diagnosis. Using the OLDCART acronym (Onset, Location, Duration, Aggravating, Relieving, and Treatment), proceed methodically and as customary, start with patient demographics. In dermatology history taking, conditions that frequently occur in younger (infectious disease) or older patients (malignancy) may be considered here.

Onset

It is important to differentiate whether the presentation is acute, i.e. lasting less than two weeks, or whether this is a chronic condition that the patient has experienced before. So think and don't hesitate to ask your patient, because they will often know exactly how this recurring complaint looks and feels. Enquire as to whether there has been a change in severity of their chronic condition such as an infective exacerbation of eczema, psoriasis, or an eruption of herpes simplex, or if this is something completely new.

Location

The location of a rash or lesion can point towards the diagnosis; for example, flexural rashes are common in eczema, widespread rashes may indicate drug reaction or a viral infection. Note where the rash started and whether and if it has spread. A typical illustration of this in practice is pityriasis rosea, starting with an isolated 'herald' patch usually on the abdomen or back which proceeds to a more widespread truncal rash over the following 1–20 weeks (DermNetNZ 2014).

Duration

Confirm how long the rash has been evident. Then determine whether is it a recurring problem or something completely new. For example, herpes simplex can be a recurrent complaint and may be tricky to differentiate from impetigo, but a history of recurrent episodes, prodromal pain, and initial vesicles containing clear fluid should help your deci-sion-making process (Ashton et al. 2014).

Characteristics

Itch can be caused by many systemic conditions such as iron deficiency anaemia, lym-phoma, liver disorder, or thyroid disease (Greaves 2005). Alternatively, severe itching at night may be due to eczema, scabies, or ringworm. If the rash is painful, discharging, or offensive, consider a herpes or bacterial infection.

Aggravating

Discuss triggers such as new washing powder, make-up, or soap, which can remove natural oils from the skin resulting in dry, itchy skin that is more sensitive to irritants (Patient 2015b). Suspect a diagnosis of scabies if the patient complains of severe itching that may be worse at night and after a hot bath (NICE CKS 2011). Consider food allergy if symptoms of urticaria develop within 2–24 hours of eating a trigger food (NICE CKS 2011).

Relieving

Find out what the patient has done to help relieve the symptoms. It is essential here to note whether the patient has been using any medicines advised by the pharmacist such as a topical steroid or antifungal ointment or antihistamine tablets. Ask if the patient has used another person's medication or herbal preparations. Elicit the name, strength, and how often the patient has been using the product. This may affect how you subsequently advise or prescribe for the condition. The patient will often present to you once the aforemen-tioned treatments have failed to help. Thus, you must be sure you can either support the patient's self-diagnosis or provide a robust alternative diagnosis and treatment plan.

Treatment

Explore whether the patient has been prescribed any medication in the past that helped with the presenting complaint/problem, especially if it is a recurring condition such as eczema or psoriasis. Check whether the patient has consulted elsewhere and been pre-scribed any medication either recently or in the past. If the patient has, try to obtain the details of what has been prescribed as this may speed your consultation. Do this only if you reach the same diagnosis! Suspect drug-induced rash with any recently prescribed medica-tions because approximately 1 in 15 patients has a reaction to antibiotics, especially penicil-lin and cephalosporins (NHS CHOICES 2014). Investigate recent ingestion or application of a new medication in relation to the presenting complaint/problem. Consider whether this condition needs referral to Accident and Emergency, a general practitioner (GP) with special interest, or consultant dermatologist if there is little or no response to treatment.

Once you have explored the history of the presenting complaint proceed to capture any other information that may be relevant to formulating your diagnosis. Sometimes the patient will be eager to show you the rash at this or an earlier stage; that's okay, but just bear in mind not to jump to any conclusions. Always take a complete history.

Past History

Past/current serious medical conditions and surgical events must be recorded in case they have any bearing on the patient's current complaint/problem or for prescribing decisions. For example a history of atopic conditions such as hay fever and asthma may indicate a predisposition to eczema or recurrent infections or symptoms of nonhealing wounds may be indicative of diabetes.

Family History

There is often a genetic link with eczema or psoriasis. Therefore, a history of atopy in the family is useful when diagnostic atopic eczema is seen in infants for example (DermNetNZ 2012). Check whether anyone else in the household is ill. Contagious diseases such as chickenpox or other viruses may be present in the household or community, especially in day-care nurseries and centres.

Medication

Ask the patient whether any new prescriptions have been taken. When a rash is present, consider whether this could be a drug allergy. Drug reactions can be variable and usually last about 7–14 days (Valeyrie-Allanore et al. 2007). However, when the patient has been taking a drug for more than two months the likelihood of it being the cause of a rash is low (Ashton et al. 2014). Remember to cross-reference/determine whether the medication/ treatment that you would like to prescribe does not interact adversely with present medications the patient is taking or is contraindicated with the patient's current treatment regime or medical condition.

Social History

Verify the patient's occupation, hobbies, and exposure to chemicals. This is especially relevant for patients presenting with hand lesions. For example, contact dermatitis is more prevalent in women and in cleaners (Slodownik and Nixon 2007). Query whether the condition improves when not exposed to the trigger, i.e. when off work. Contemplate a risk of sexually transmitted infection for genital lesions and nonpruritic rash in an adult.

Travel

Before travel provide health promotion advice. If appropriate, discuss the dangers of pre-travel sun bed usage for example, which has been found to be no safer than sun exposure in the long term and can lead to squamous cell carcinoma (SCC) as readily as being exposed to direct sunlight (WHO 2005). Enquire about a history of sun exposure. This is relevant, especially if suspecting skin cancer. The Fitzpatrick Scale (2007) shown in Table 3.1 classifies skin types 1 to V1 from fair to very dark. Those with skin type 1 and 2 are more likely to develop skin cancer (Table 3.1).

Many patients will consult on return from holiday with minor ailments such as insect bites with associated cellulitis or acute otitis externa due to swimmer's ear. It is advised to check the patient's travel history to ascertain whether there may be a risk of the patient having contracted a tropical disease (Lupi et al. 2006).

Table 3.1   Skin types.

Type I	Very sensitive, always burns, never tans
Type II	Very sensitive, always burns, tans minimally
Type III	Sometimes burns, tans gradually
Type IV	Moderately sensitive rarely going red, tans easily going brown
Type V	Minimally sensitive, rarely burns, going brown always, dark brown
Type VI	Never burns, always deeply pigmented, black

Alcohol and Smoking

Increase the risk of some malignancies and have a close association with palmoplantar pustular psoriasis (Hinds and Thomas 2008). This condition may provide the practitioner with another opportunity to discuss health promotion and provide healthy lifestyle advice.

Mental Health

People with severe, chronic, visible, and disfiguring skin diseases may suffer from anxiety, depression, and social isolation. Stress is well known to exacerbate psoriasis flares. Patients with visible skin disease may be prone to depression. A survey of patients with psoriasis revealed that many deliberately avoid swimming or wearing skimpy clothing because they feel that people regard them as untouchable or contagious (Ni and Chiu 2014). The Dermatology Life Quality Index (DLQI) is a series of 10 questions which ask how psoriasis has affected a patient's life in the past seven days (Cardiff University 1994). The score ranges from 0 to 30 with 0 indicating no impact whereas a score above 10 indicates a considerable impact on quality of life. The DLQI does not assess distress. When considering stress, use the Patient Health Questionnaire (PHQ-9) depression module (Patient 2013). This assessment tool/inventory is frequently used in primary care settings.

Review of Systems

Make general enquiries into the patient's general health. Undertake a quick top to toe subjective evaluation of the patient's current health status; noting any systemic symptoms such as fever, lethargy, joint pain, and swelling or weight loss that would need to be examined in more detail. A number of symptoms and skin lesions may be indicators for underlying pathology (Kleyn et al. 2006) and are reflected in Table 3.2.

Objective Examination

Systemic Disease and the Skin, Hair, and Nails

It is important to consider the possibility of underlying disease when patients present with skin, hair, or nail disorders; some signs are obvious, and some are more discreet on inspection. Gather evidence combining subjective and objective knowledge in order find vital clues that may help you reach the correct diagnosis. Table 3.2 outlines some of the more common presentations seen in practice.

Distribution

The region of the body affected by a rash or lesion can provide clues to the diagnosis. Identify the distribution (where it is) and number of lesions. Consider the pattern the rash makes, e.g. a dermatomal rash following nerve roots from the spine is most likely associated with shingles. More examples like this follow and are also shown in Table 3.3.

Nails – paronychia, psoriasis (joint swelling, nail involvement), clubbing (respiratory/cardiac/liver disease), splinter haemorrhage (trauma/ pericarditis), nicotine stains

Hands – palm (palmar erythema), dorsum (scabies, warts, and Reynaud's phenomenon), weight loss (loose skin and jewellery)

Arms – injection marks, psoriasis (plaques), dermatitis (erythema), herpetiformis (vesicles), eczema (lichenification)

Scalp – scaling (psoriasis), thinning (hypothyroid) nits, sebaceous cysts, alopecia

Face – solar keratosis, acne, acne rosacea, lupus (butterfly rash), herpes simplex, cyanosis (peripheral/central), xanthelasma (cardiovascular disease), pallor (anaemia)

Neck – lymph node (infection/malignancy), goitre (thyroid disease)

Table 3.2 Systemic disease.

Disease	Common presentation
Diabetes	Bacterial and fungal infections, itching, neuropathic discolouration, paronychia
Thyroid disorder	Thyrotoxicosis may include warm skin, flushed face and hands; clubbing of nails; fine soft thinned scalp hair; generalised itching. Hypothyroid may result in cold, pale, and dry skin; a yellowish hue to the skin due to carotenaemia; sparse brittle hair; slow growing ridged and brittle nails; goitre; myxoedema resulting in puffy eyelids and hands.
Malignancy	Nonmelanoma skin cancers (squamous and basal cell carcinoma), melanoma, karposi sarcoma, T cell lymphoma
Renal failure	Oedema, pallor secondary to anaemia, loss of body mass, dry skin, itching, bruising
Liver disease	Jaundice, spider naevi, leukonychia, finger clubbing, palmar erythema, rosacea and rhinophyma, scratch marks, loss of axillary hair, and gynaecomastia. Ascites can lead to striae and an umbilical hernia
Crohn's disease/ ulcerative colitis	Crohn's disease; skin tags, fissures, and abscesses around the perineal and perianal region, purple anus; oral swelling and ulcers, cobblestoning of the buccal mucosa, angular cheilitis Ulcerative colitis; erythema nodosum, pyoderma gangrenosum
Malnutrition	Delayed wound healing, loose/dry skin, and loss of muscle mass; evidence of weight loss; loose dentures, rings, and clothing
Hyperlipidemia	Xanthalasmata (yellow fat deposit) of upper and lower eyelids; xanthoma of tendons, achilles, hands, knees
Addison's disease	Hyperpigmentation of the skin, women may have loss of androgen-stimulated hair, such as pubic and underarm hair
Cushing's disease	Thin skin that bruises easily, stretch marks, darkened skin on the abdomen, ankle oedema
Sarcoid	Possible erythema nodosum, with plaques, papules, or nodules.

Table 3.3 Distribution of lesions.

Distribution	Possible diagnosis
Dermatomal	Corresponding with nerve root distribution (shingles)
Extensor	Involving extensor surfaces of limbs (psoriasis)
Flexural	Skin folds (eczema)
Follicular	Individual lesions arise from hair follicles (folliculitis)
Generalised	Widespread distribution possible viral infection (viral exanthema)
Herpetiform	Grouped umbilicated vesicles, herpes simplex, and zoster infections.
Photosensitive	Does not affect skin that is always covered by clothing.
Seborrhoeic	Areas of oily skin (seborrhoea). Scalp, behind ears, eyebrows, nasolabial folds, sternum, and interscapular.
Truncal	Usually on the trunk, rarely affects limbs (pityriasis rosea)

Trunk – acanthosis nigricans (epidermal hyperplasia, stomach cancer), spider naevi (liver disease), stretch marks (pregnancy, systemic disease), scratch marks (scabies), vesicles (shingles), viral infections

Groin – warts, herpes, chancre, discharge, scabies, tinea, hernias, lymph nodes, dermatitis, psoriasis

Legs – erythema nodosum, erythema multiforme, eczema, psoriasis, ulcers, lacerations

Feet – oedema, blisters, poor circulation, ulcers, ischemia, nail disorder including infection, psoriasis and fungal infection, plantar warts

Once you have decided where the rash is distributed, make a note of the number of lesions seen and whether they are isolated (a lesion) or multiple (rash).

Document the size (Table 3.4), shape, border (Table 3.5), and colour of what you see. Some common presentations are shown in the tables. Recognising and describing the primary lesion or rash is an important step towards diagnosis and something practitioners

Table 3.4 Primary lesions.

Macule	Flat lesion < 1 cm, smooth (freckle)
Patch	Flat lesion > 1 cm with colour change (pityriasis rosea)
Papule	Solid lesion < 1 cm that is raised; can be solitary or multiple (acne)
Plaque	Any lesion > 1 cm can be elevated; may have defined or undefined border (psoriasis)
Nodule	An elevated enlarged papule > 1 cm diameter which is palpable (basal cell carcinoma)
Vesicle	Contains clear fluid (herpes simplex)
Pustule	Contains opaque pus (impetigo)
Bulla	Circumscribed elevation of > 1 cm in diameter (bullous pemphigoid)

Table 3.5 The shape and border of lesions.

Appearance	Example in practice
Annular The term 'annular' stems from the Latin word 'annulus', meaning ringed	Ringworm
Gyrate (whirling in a circle)	Urticaria
Linear (a line)	Lichen striatus
Nummular or discoid (coin shaped)	Eczema
Target /iris (like an archery target)	Erythema multiforme
Irregular	Malignant melanoma
Serpiginous	Scabies
Borders	
Well defined	Psoriasis plaques
Poorly defined	The border merges into normal skin, e.g. poorly defined eczema plaques and solar keratosis
Accentuated edge	Tinea corporis or basal cell carcinoma with raised rolled edge

often find challenging, especially when it comes to documenting findings and ruling out differentials. Keeping a list in your mobile/cell phone helps as a reminder of terminology.

Primary lesions: inspect, palpate, and document the appearance of the lesion or rash. Inspect and document shape and border of the lesion or rash.

Colour

The colour of the skin, lesion, or rash provides more signs. Several examples are listed here.

Erythroderma: Affects the whole or nearly the entire body, which is red all over. Intense and usually widespread reddening of the skin occurs because of inflammatory skin disease. It often precedes or is associated with exfoliation when it may also be known as exfoliative dermatitis (ED).

Erythema: Red skin due to increased blood supply which blanches on pressure. There are many types of erythema, including photosensitivity, erythema multiforme, and erythema nodosum.

Purpura: Bleeding into the skin. This may be as petechiae or ecchymoses (bruises). Purpura does not blanch with pressure. Use diascopy to determine this. The 'glass test' to diagnose meningococcal septicaemia for example (pressing a glass slide on the surface of the skin shows the colouration does not blanche) (Figure 3.2).

Carotenaemia: Excessive circulating beta-carotene results in yellow to orange skin colouration. It is most pronounced on palms and soles and, unlike jaundice, it does not affect the cornea.

Hyperpigmentation: May be caused by an excess of melanin or haemosiderin deposits that result in skin colour that is darker than normal, e.g. haemochromatosis.

Hypopigmentation: Loss of normal melanin and results in skin colour that is paler than normal but not completely white, e.g. pityriasis versicolor.

Leukoderma: Known as achromia, which is when the skin is white, e.g. vitiligo.

Infarcts: Black areas of necrotic tissue due to ischaemia.

(DermNetNZ 1997b; Patient 2014)

Secondary Lesions

Secondary lesions define changes that occur to a primary lesion resulting from traumatic injury, e.g. scratching, passing of time, application of lotions or creams, or other external factors. Terms for describing these are shown in Table 3.6.

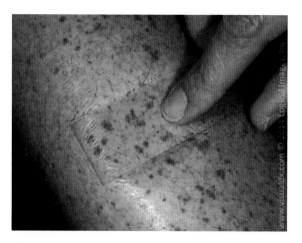

Figure 3.2   Diascopy.

Table 3.6   Secondary lesions.

Scale (Visible exfoliation of the skin)	Desquamation (skin coming off in scales); psoriasiform (large white or silver flakes); lichenoid (apparent scale is tightly adherent to skin surface); keratotic (horny scale); exfoliation (peeling skin); maceration (moist peeling skin); verrucous (warty)
Crust	Dried up exudate containing serous fluid, blood, dead cells
Erosion	Breach in skin due to loss of epidermis but without dermal damage
Ulcer	Loss of epidermis and part of the dermis due to trauma, infection, or vascular insufficiency

In primary care a diagnosis is often made by taking a history and inspection of the rash or lesion. Always examine in good lighting and use a magnifying glass if required. A Wood's lamp if available is useful in differentiating tinea infections including fungal infections of the eye.

Explain to the patient that is essential to examine all the affected body regions even when the patient thinks it is unrelated. This is to exclude serious pathology (Khopkar 2009). (Refer to Table 3.2.)

Think systemically and remember clinical observations. Never forget Vital Signs/Observations (Obs: TPR, BP, and Oxygen Saturation) and any other physical examination necessary, e.g. ears, nose, and throat (ENT) exam if scarlet fever is suspected.

Palpate the surface of the skin with fingertips and document your findings (wear examination gloves when infection is suspected).

- smooth normal skin
- uneven fine scaly/warty
- rough sandpaper solar keratosis, crust

Deep palpation of a lesion is performed by squeezing the lesion between fingers and thumb. Document what you see and feel. Some examples are listed here.

- Normal: feels the same as normal skin
- Soft: easily compressible; feels like lips
- Firm: feels like tip of nose
- Hard: feels like bone (Ashton et al. 2014).

Wood's lamp/light: An ultraviolet light used to show fluorescence in lesions such as tinea capitis and pityriasis versicolor.

Magnifying glass: May be used for signs that are difficult to examine with the naked eye.

Diascopy: The glass test used to differentiate between the petechial rash of meningitis and erythema.

Bacteriology swabs: Can be taken from vesicles, pustules, erosions, or ulcers to identify the causative bacteria.

Mycology: Skin scrapings, nail clippings, and infected hairs are taken to establish or confirm the diagnosis of a fungal infection by microscopy and culture (mycology). Scrapings of a scale are best taken from the edge of the rash by removing the surface skin using a blade or curette and sending the scrapings to the laboratory in a sterile container or a black paper envelope.

Red Flag Presentations in Primary Care

When examining skin lesions, always consider malignancy in nonhealing wounds. This section explores malignant and premalignant lesions and other urgent presentations in primary care.

Nonmelanoma Skin Cancer

Around three-quarters of nonmelanoma skin cancer registrations are basal cell carcinoma (BCC) and less than a quarter are SCC (Cancer Research UK 2012).

Basal Cell Carcinoma

BCCs or rodent ulcers are the most common skin malignancy and are rarely a threat to life (DermNetNZ 1997a, updated 2015). BCCs grow slowly and normally occur on sun exposed skin of the face above the line from the angle of the mouth to the ear. Predisposing factors are xeroderma pigmentosum (a rare skin disorder, high sensitivity to sunlight, premature skin ageing) and other genetic factors. BCCs can vary in size but are commonly nodular (Figure 3.3). Its main features are central dimpling and rolled edges.

Where there is a suspicion that the patient has a basal cell carcinoma, a nonurgent referral should be made to a dermatologist (NICE 2005).

Squamous Cell Carcinoma (SCC)

The 2nd most common cutaneous malignancy is derived from squamous cells in the epidermis. If it metastasises it can be fatal. The most common affected areas are sun-exposed sites such as the face and hands. SCCs are usually slow-growing, tender, scaly, or crusted lumps or nonhealing ulcers. Predisposing factors include actinic keratosis (abnormal skin cell development due to exposure to ultraviolet radiation), Bowen's disease (*in situ* SCC), and viral warts (Figure 3.4).

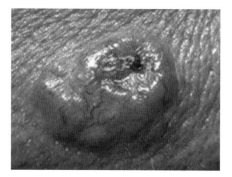

Figure 3.3   Nodular basal cell carcinoma.

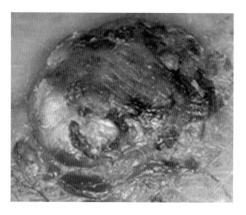

Figure 3.4   Squamous cell carcinoma.

Nonhealing lesions larger than 1 cm with significant induration on palpation, commonly on the face, scalp, or back of hands with a documented expansion over eight weeks, may be squamous cell carcinomas and an urgent referral should be made to a dermatologist (NICE 2005).

Malignant Melanoma

In 2012, there were around 13 500 new cases of malignant melanoma diagnosed in the United Kingdom (UK), which is now the 5th most common cancer diagnosed and rising with 33% of cases occurring in the under 55s. Around 98 400 cases of nonmelanoma skin cancer were registered in 2011 (Cancer Research UK 2012). In the United States of America (USA) in 2016/2017, 91 270 new melanomas were diagnosed (approximately 55 150 in men and 36 120 in women). Approximately 9320 people were expected to die of melanoma (around 5990 men and 3330 women) (American Cancer Society 2018). The causes of malignant melanoma are attributed to lifestyle factors including sunbathing, which is linked to 86% of malignant melanoma cases in the UK and USA. Age, genetics, and preexisting moles and malignant melanomas have a tendency to metastasise to lymph nodes (Figure 3.5).

Tumour thickness is the most important prognostic factor for local, distant recurrence and survival. Patients' five-year survival is related to Breslow thickness, which measures in millimetres (mm) how far the melanoma cells have reached down through the skin from the surface.

- <0.75 mm = 95–99%
- 0.76–1.49 mm = 80–90%
- 1.5–3.99 mm = 60–75%
- 4.0 mm = <50%
- With regional lymphadenopathy 10-year survival is less than 10%

Change is a key element in diagnosing malignant melanoma. For low-suspicion lesions, careful monitoring for change should be undertaken using the seven-point checklist for eight weeks.

Major features of the lesions:

- change in size
- irregular shape
- irregular colour

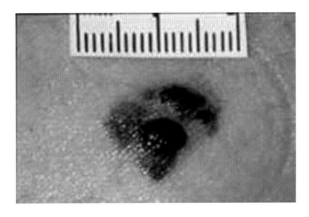

Figure 3.5   Malignant melanoma.

Minor features of the lesions:

- largest diameter 7 mm or more
- inflammation
- oozing
- change in sensation

If there are strong concerns about cancer, any one feature is adequate to prompt *urgent* referral to a dermatologist or other suitable specialist. Excision in primary care should be avoided. *Referral guidelines for suspected cancer: skin cancer* (NICE 2005).

People at Higher Risk

- large numbers of naevi
- tendency to freckle
- atypical naevi
- solar keratosis
- family history of melanoma

Moles

A mole is made of a collection of melanocyte pigment cells, which give the mole its colour. The average adult has between 15 and 40 moles which appear between childhood and up to the age of 40 years. The more sunlight a child is exposed to can increase the number of moles. The number of moles an individual has is to some extent genetically determined.

Health Promotion

Take the opportunity to discuss sunburn prevention by advising patients to use sunscreens with at least sun protection factor (SPF) 15 (the higher the better) and good UVA/B protection, to avoid the sun when it is hottest (between 11 a.m. and 3 p.m.) by spending time in the shade and covering up (like wearing a T-shirt, wide-brimmed hat, and sunglasses) (Cancer Research UK 2012).

Drug Eruptions

Think twice before prescribing any medication as it is a common cause of rash, particularly antibiotics.

Whist verifying the patient's medication history, enquire about anything taken in the last three months including over-the-counter and prescribed medication.

Report a suspected problem ('adverse incident', 'never event') with a medicine or medical device using the Yellow Card Scheme as soon as possible if a medicine causes side effects (MHRA 2015).

Toxic Erythema

The most severe type of drug eruption rash is toxic erythema and is most commonly caused by antibiotics, thiazides, or allopurinol. The rash usually affects the trunk more than the limbs and the patient might have a fever (Figure 3.6).

Treatment consists of discontinuing the drug (it may often take weeks for the rash to resolve) and providing emollients and topical steroids for reduction of symptoms. Up to 3% of patients may require hospital admission (DermNetNZ 2003, updated 2015). Always consider other differential diagnoses such as bacterial or viral reasons which often mimic drug reactions. Remain alert for life-threatening features of adverse drug eruptions such as angioedema and anaphylaxis.

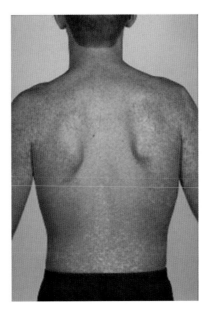

Figure 3.6   Toxic erythema.

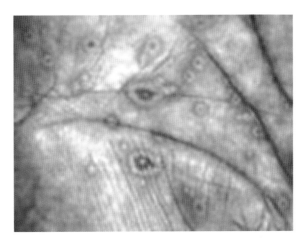

Figure 3.7   Erythema multiforme.

Erythema Multiforme

It means a redness (*erythema*) that is of many (*multi*) shapes (*forme*). The rash of erythema multiforme can be recognised by the presence of spots that look like small targets (bull's eye shaped 'target lesions'). These have a dusky red centre, a paler area around the centre, and a dark red ring round the edge (BAD 2014) (Figure 3.7).

Erythema multiforme is common in the 10- to –40-year-old age group and is usually a mild self-limiting complaint (erythema minor), but occasionally it can affect the oral, conjunctival, genital mucosa surfaces and is then called Stevens–Johnson syndrome (erythema major), which may need hospital admission for supportive treatment. Drug reactions are accountable for 10% of reactions, but 90% of triggers are caused by infection, including streptococcal, herpes simplex virus, hepatitis B, and mycoplasma. Recurrent erythema minor caused by herpes simplex is often treated with oral antivirals (BAD 2014).

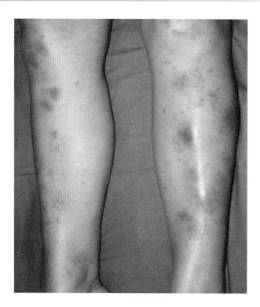

Figure 3.8   Erythema nodosum.

It is usually diagnosed by the way it looks but occasionally skin swabs and biopsy can be taken to exclude other pathology. Treatment includes emollients, topical steroids, and antihistamines.

Erythema Nodosum

This is often thought to be a hypersensitivity reaction or an indicator of infectious or other disease (Shimizu et al. 2012). It presents with tender erythematous nodules (1–5 cm diameter) often on the extensor surfaces of limbs (especially shins). The patient may complain of joint pain and fever that usually resolve in about eight weeks. The ratio of females to males affected is 3:1 and may be associated with sarcoid, drugs, inflammatory bowel disease, malignancy, tuberculosis, strep, or idiopathic (20%) (DermNetNZ 2013) (Figure 3.8).

It is important to exclude serious underlying disease. Investigations may include:

- Throat swab for streptococcus.
- Stool test for campylobacter or salmonella.
- Full blood count/complete blood count, erythrocyte sedimentation rate, and C-reactive protein will be elevated.
- CXR may show bilateral hilar lymphadenopathy in sarcoidosis, unilateral or asymmetrical adenopathy in malignancy, or evidence of pulmonary tuberculosis.
- Intradermal skin tests may be required to exclude tuberculosis.
- Biopsy may be helpful where the diagnosis is in doubt (Schwartz and Nervi 2007).

Erythroderma

Erythroderma is an intense and widespread reddening of the skin associated with exfoliation (ED). It can have a variety of causes including drug eruption, eczema, psoriasis, and lymphoma and can involve nearly all of the skin. Middle-aged and elderly people are usually affected with a male–female ratio of 2:1. Erythroderma is serious; patients require hospitalisation to restore fluid and electrolyte balance, circulatory support, and body temperature management (DermNetNZ 2003, updated 2015) (Figure 3.9).

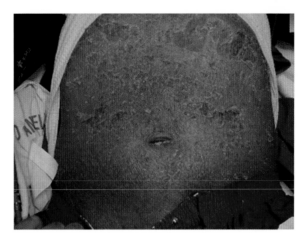

Figure 3.9   Erythroderma.

Common Presentations in Primary Care

The following section addresses common presentations in primary care. Think through how you will assess and differentiate between each case. Remember to take a thorough history using OLDCART and then describe the rash or lesion according to the examples shown in Table 3.6. Decide what the rash or lesion looks and feels like in terms of distribution, colour, shape, and elevation and whether there are there any secondary changes to consider. At that point you can move forwards to rule out any differential diagnosis and formulate a treatment plan.

Eczema

Eczema is a chronic relapsing inflammatory condition with variants affecting different parts of the body. The skin becomes dry, itchy, red, and cracked leading to a chronic condition, commonly affecting the backs of the knees and elbows, the neck, hands, cheeks, and scalp. There are two categories of eczema.

- Endogenous eczema caused by internal trigger factors.
- Exogenous eczemas related to external triggering factors.

History taking should always include standard information, especially noting family history of atopy, any medication changes, prescribed or over the counter, and check concordance with prescribed regimes. Enquire about the possibility of occupational eczema; work clothing may cause sweating and irritation of the skin or a new pet or hobby might be causing a flare. Ask about triggers, in particular diet, or products in contact with the skin used on a daily basis such as washing powder, make-up, or shampoo; new jewellery or shoes can cause contact dermatitis.

Endogenous Eczema

Atopic eczema (Figure 3.10) affects 20% of children in developed countries; about 80% of cases present before the age of five years (Flohr and Mann 2014). Triggers can include infection with *Staphylococcus aureus*, heat and humidity, and abrasive fabrics. Diet has been shown to aggravate atopic eczema in about 50% of children (Werfel et al. 2007).

Seborrhoeic eczema/dermatitis is a harmless scaly rash affecting infants under six months of age. It is demonstrated by yellow waxy scales on the scalp (cradle cap). In adults it affects the scalp, nasolabial folds, eyebrows, chest, and upper back. Males are affected

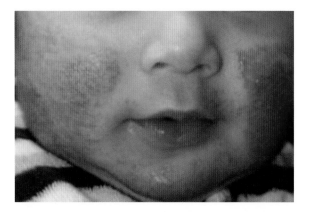

Figure 3.10   Atopic eczema.

rather than females because of the effect of androgen on production of sebum. Peak incidence is in adolescents and young adults and recurs in adults over the age of 50. It is thought to be caused by an inflammatory reaction to a yeast called malassezia spp., which may be a normal skin commensal. Patients with seborrhoeic eczema/dermatitis may have a reduced resistance to this yeast (NICE CKS 2013a).

Discoid (or nummular) eczema. Has a prevalence of 2 per 1000 people and is more common in men than women. Its peak incidence is in ages 50–65. However, in women it can occur between the ages 15–25 predominantly. It is rare in children (Burgin 2012). There may be a past history of atopic eczema or dry skin. It presents with scattered red coin-shaped lesions usually on the lower legs, trunk, and arms. It can be wet with vesicles and exudate or dry with scaling. The discs can be intensely itchy leading to secondary changes from scratching such as crust, scale, and infection. It is often mistaken for tinea corporis because it is round (Ashton et al. 2014).

Pompholyx eczema has multiple triggers such as emotional stress and allergic contact dermatitis and presents with an itchy vesicular eruption of the hands, fingers, and soles of the feet. It can be acute, recurrent or chronic, mild or severe with large bullae, fissures, and nail involvement. It is more common in smokers in spring and summer and in countries with warmer climates (National Eczema Society 2014).

Venous eczema occurs as a consequence of increased venous pressure affected by incompetent valves in superficial or deep veins of the legs. Obesity, age, and spending lots of time standing at work are risk factors. Skin changes are often bilateral. Leakage of blood constituents into the surrounding tissues activate inflammatory cells and fibroblasts leading to the following changes:

- Mild pigmentation from haemosiderin deposition
- Areas of inflammatory change and eczema
- Lipodermatosclerosis – inflammation of the subcutaneous fat causing fibrosis, and hard, tight skin which may be red or brown
- Atrophie blanche – star-shaped, white (ivory), atrophic areas of skin surrounded by reddened areas
- Ulceration and cellulitis of the skin (Barron et al. 2007; Gloviczki et al. 2011).

Investigations can include measuring the ankle brachial pressure index with a Doppler machine if compression stockings are being considered. Provided there is no arterial insufficiency, below-knee compression stockings can be prescribed. The patient can be given general advice including avoiding leg trauma, to elevate legs whilst sitting and to keep as physically active as possible (Beldon 2006; NICE CKS 2012).

Exogenous Eczema

Irritant contact dermatitis and allergic contact dermatitis are inflammatory skin reactions in response to an external stimulus. The hands are primarily affected. Almost 90% of cases are caused by occupational contact (frequently termed contact dermatitis) (NICE CKS 2013b). The occupations at highest risk are florists, hairdressers, cooks, beauty therapists, metal working machine operators, and chemical, rubber, glass and ceramic process operatives. Presentation of symptoms can differ according to whether the condition has been caused by allergy or contact. Differences are described in Table 3.7 and Figure 3.11.

Photodermatosis or photosensitivity affects people who are sensitive to sunlight or fluorescent light. Management includes reducing exposure to sunlight and using adequate sun protection even through windows.

Other complications of eczema include conjunctival irritation due to allergic reaction or an irritant response. Bilateral cataracts can occur in severe atopic dermatitis, usually around 15–25 years of age. Growth retardation may be seen in children with severe eczema, most often due to the eczema rather than its treatment. Oral corticosteroids can also cause short-term growth retardation, so use of these drugs must be closely monitored (NICE CKS 2012).

Table 3.7 Contact and allergic dermatitis.

Typical features of irritant contact dermatitis	Typical features of allergic contact dermatitis
Burning, stinging, and soreness are predominant	Redness, itching, and scaling are predominant
Usual onset within 48 hours; may be immediate	Delayed onset
Rash only in areas of skin exposed to the irritant	Rash may be in areas which have not been in contact with an allergen. However, the distribution of the rash is still helpful in ascertaining the likely allergen
Resolution occurs quickly after removal of the irritant – typically, within four days	Resolution may take longer than irritant contact dermatitis, with or without treatment
Commonly associated with atopic eczema, which increases the risk	Less strong association with atopic eczema
Exposure to friction, soap, detergents, solvents, or wet work make the diagnosis likely	

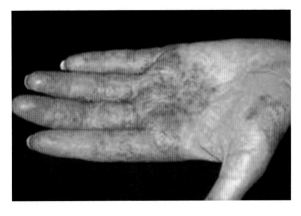

Figure 3.11 Contact dermatitis.

Management of Eczema

The mainstay in treatment of eczema is to provide education and support surrounding the use of emollients and topical steroids. Building a rapport with the patient or carer is of vital importance in order to improve concordance with treatment. Encourage healthcare workers to acknowledge the impact of the condition, paying attention to how key messages are delivered in order to address patients' and carers' treatment beliefs and improve engagement (Santer et al. 2012).

Lifestyle advice involves the following:

- Reassure parents that eczema often improves with time.
- Explain that eczema is a chronic illness characterised by flares, but that these can usually be controlled with appropriate treatment.
- Avoid scratching. Rub the area with fingers to alleviate itching.
- Keep nails short (and use antiscratch mittens in babies with eczema).
- Avoid trigger factors known to exacerbate eczema, such as clothing with synthetic fibres, soaps, or detergents (use emollient substitutes), animals, and heat (keep rooms cool).
- House dust mite avoidance strategies are generally not recommended as they are time consuming and of limited benefit.
- Complementary therapies are not generally recommended. A healthcare professional should be informed if these are used.
- Diet should not be changed unless under specialist advice (NICE 2007).

Emollients

There is a lack of evidence from controlled trials to support the effectiveness of emollients. However, they are almost universally recommended as the first-line treatment for eczema and related dry skin conditions. There is no evidence to support the use of one over another or whether they reduce the need for topical steroids. Therefore, patient preference should guide choice (Grimalt et al. 2007).

Topical Steroids

Historical use of topical corticosteroids has shown them to be an essential part of the management of active atopic eczema. However, studies comparing different topical corticosteroids with each other do not provide sufficient evidence to rank or preference them (Hoare et al. 2000). Therefore, the choice of topical corticosteroid should be made by matching the severity of eczema with known biochemical potency of the drug. Side effects of topical steroids from the very potent and potent group are rare but can include:

- adrenal suppression and Cushing's syndrome
- spreading/worsening of untreated infection
- thinning of the skin
- irreversible striae
- perioral dermatitis
- mild depigmentation.

Topical steroids should be applied sparingly once or twice daily. As a general rule, one fingertip is sufficient to cover an area that is twice that of the flat of an adult hand.

Antihistamines can help reduce the itch/scratch cycle and have a sedating effect, but the level of evidence in support of the benefits of antihistamine treatment is low (Buddenkotte et al. 2010). Tacrolimus and pimecrolimus creams can be prescribed by a consultant dermatologist or GP with special interest but not as a first-line treatment. Wet wrap bandages containing icthamol paste may give relief from pruritis if applied over a corticosteroid.

Table 3.8   Tinea infections.

Scalp	Tinea capitis
Feet	Tinea pedis
Hands	Tinea manuum
Nail	Tinea unguium
Beard	Tinea barbae
Groin	Tinea cruris
Body	Tinea corporis

Shampoos containing ketoconazole and coal tar are usually effective against seborrhoeic eczema, which is associated with yeasts that affect the scalp and face.

Tinea Infections

Tinea infections are fungal infections caused by dermatophytes, a group of fungi that invade and grow in dead keratin and can cause secondary infection on people with eczema. *Epidermophyton, Microsporum*, and *Trichophyton* are most common species (Patient 2015a). They tend to grow outwards on skin, producing a ring-like pattern, hence the term ringworm. Different parts of the body are affected and are classified below (Table 3.8):

Tinea corporis (ringworm) and discoid eczema are often confused. Consider ringworm if the rash has more pink scaly papules or plaques which graduate outwards, healing from the centre and forming a ring. Always consider ringworm in any unilateral or asymmetrical red scaly rash whether or not it is annular in shape. The keratin layer on the surface of the skin is affected in ringworm, so topical antifungal treatment is more effective. Avoid mixed steroid and antifungal treatments if possible because it may exacerbate a fungal infection and eczema responds better to topical steroids alone (Ashton et al. 2014). If a fungal infection is suspected, skin scrapings and hair and nail samples can be sent for mycology.

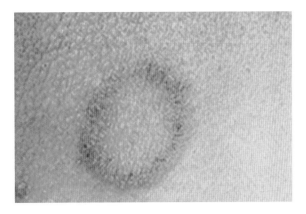

Tinea corporis

Bacterial Infections

Bacterial infection (commonly *S. aureus* and occasionally *Streptococcus pyogenes*) can exacerbate eczema and is in part due to the breaks in the skin from dry, split skin and from scratching the itchy areas. Signs of infection can present with fever, pain, vesicles,

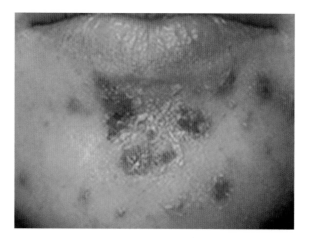

Figure 3.12   Impetigo.

and pustules, oozing and crusting like impetigo. Other bacterial infections include folliculitis and cellulitis. Before prescribing systemic antibiotics, consider the following:

- drug allergy
- renal and hepatic function
- age/sex
- antibiotic resistance.

Become familiar with your local policies, which often limit the use of antibacterials to achieve cost effectiveness consistent with adequate cover and to reduce development of resistant organisms.

Children are mostly affected with impetigo because the organisms gain entry through cuts and grazes. It is very contagious, starting with vesicles that break down to form honey-coloured crusts (Figure 3.12).

Folliculitis is a superficial infection of hair follicles. Pus sits around the protruding hair and there may be erythema at the base. It can be caused or made worse by greasy ointments on the skin, tar preparations, or plasters (Ashton et al. 2014).

Viral Infections

Molloscum contagiosum is most common in children aged one to four years old. It can also affect adults. Risk factors include immunosuppression or steroid treatment (especially topical steroids). It is caused by a virus which can be passed on by skin-to-skin contact or direct contact with fomites. It can take 12–18 months to resolve and is usually self-limiting.

Eczema herpeticum is caused by Herpes simplex virus HV1 and presents with widespread herpetic lesions over the affected skin with clustered areas of worsening painful eczema, punched out erosions, and signs of systemic illness such as fever and lethargy. Referral to secondary care is indicated and treatment involves intravenous, oral and topical antivirals and broad spectrum antibiotics to treat or prevent superinfection (NICE 2007) (Figure 3.13).

Hand, foot, and mouth (HFMD) is a viral illness which commonly causes itchy or painful lesions involving the mouth, hands, and feet but it may also affect the buttocks and genitalia. The most common causes of HFMD are Coxsackievirus A16 (CA16) and enterovirus 71 (EV71). It is normally a mild, self-limiting illness lasting three to six days and no treatment is needed (Patient 2013) (Figure 3.14).

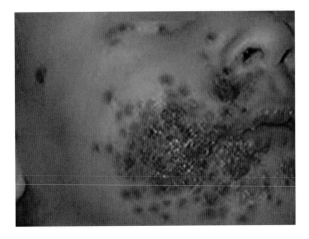

Figure 3.13   Eczema herpeticum.

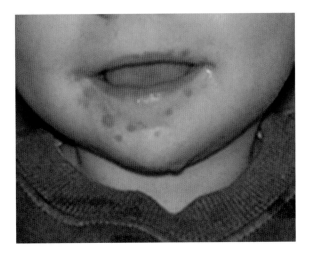

Figure 3.14   Hand, foot, and mouth disease.

Pityriasis Rosea

Pityriasis rosea is an acute, self-limiting skin condition. A primary plaque ('herald patch'), which is often misdiagnosed as ringworm, is followed by a distinctive, generalised itchy rash one to two weeks later that lasts for about two to six weeks. Lesions are oval, dull pink, or tawny and appear in a 'Christmas tree' distribution, usually on the trunk and the upper arms and legs. Check the hands for scabies burrows if the rash is particularly itchy at night (Ashton et al. 2014). Usually no treatment is required other than emollients and antihistamines. (Figure 3.15)

Psoriasis

Psoriasis is a common disorder affecting approximately 2% of the population. Onset is usually in the under 35s and it affects men and women equally. It can relapse and remit throughout life. Joint disease is associated with psoriasis in a significant proportion of patients. Psoriasis has a variety of causes such as inheritance, infection, medication, UV light, alcohol, and stress. As with eczema, there are many forms of psoriasis:

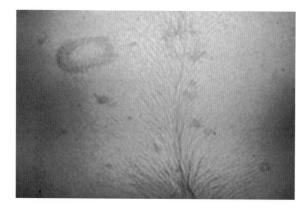

Figure 3.15 Pityriasis rosea.

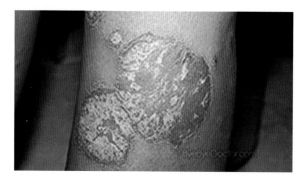

Figure 3.16 Plaque psoriasis.

Chronic plaque psoriasis is the most common form of psoriasis and is illustrated by itchy, well-demarcated circular-to-oval bright red/pink elevated lesions (plaques) with overlying white or silvery scale that are distributed symmetrically over extensor body surfaces and the scalp (Figure 3.16).

Flexural psoriasis affects axillae, below breasts and intertriginous areas.

Guttate psoriasis may follow a streptococcal sore throat and affects young people more frequently. Presentation is an acute symmetrical eruption with drop-like lesions on the trunk and limbs.

Erythrodermic psoriasis begins conventionally but progresses to generalised erythema. It can be triggered in response to withdrawal of a systemic or high-dose topical steroid. It may progress to pustular psoriasis. The usual management is admission to secondary care for treatment.

Pustular psoriasis is a rare but possibly life-threatening form of psoriasis. Small yellow pustules develop on erythematous skin. The onset is rapid and the patient is systemically unwell. Admit urgently (Figure 3.17).

Nail involvement occurs in 50% of cases, with pitting and oncholysis (the nail plate separates from its underlying attachment to nail bed, the nail plate whitens and may detach) (NICE 2014). Nail clippings should be taken to differentiate between suspected fungal nail infection.

Psoriatic arthritis is an inflammatory arthritis affecting the joints and connective tissue. It is a progressive disorder ranging from mild synovitis to severe progressive erosive arthropathy and has an estimated incidence rate of 6.6/100 000 per year. In about 80% of cases the presence of psoriasis precedes the onset of psoriatic arthritis (Habif 2011; NICE 2014).

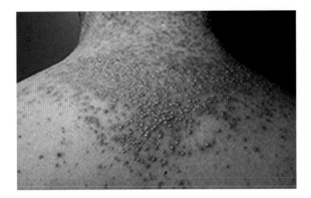

Figure 3.17   Pustular psoriasis.

Management of psoriasis.

- Emollients with or without salicylic acid.
- Dithranol has been proven to work but can stain clothing and is an irritant to surrounding skin.
- Coal tar is smelly, messy, and rarely effective on its own.
- Steroids – Ointments better than creams on thick plaques, as treatment is likely to be long term. Avoid potent steroids.
- Tar/steroid combinations can be helpful (Alphosyl HC).
- Vitamin D3 analogues – First line, e.g. calcipotriol (Dovonex). Calcitriol helps about 65% of cases but can cause irritation especially on face and flexures. Limit dose to < 100 g week (NICE 2014).
- Retanoids – Latest topical therapy for psoriasis.
- Scalp – First descale with cocois ointment, arachis oil, or tar shampoos (Polytar). Then use steroid or calcipotriol scalp applications.
- Other forms and treatments – Guttate psoriasis (topical therapies, may resolve spontaneously, UVB photo therapy may help). Flexural psoriasis (mild steroid and/or tar topical cream. Calcitriol and tacrolimus also used). Pustular psoriasis (potent topical steroids, coal tar paste, PUVA). Injectables such as Cosentyx or Humera are recently becoming the last line of treatment in intractable cases.
- DLQI and PHQ-9 depression module may be required for patients who have emotional distress due to psoriasis.

Case Study of a Four-Year-Old Male Child with a 'Rash on His Face'

Many presentations can be difficult to diagnose in practice because frequently skin presentations can mimic each other. The following case study demonstrates the difficulties and differential diagnoses to consider in practice.

Subjective History
Mohammed age four attended a walk-in centre (primary care centre) with his father who provided the history. The presenting complaint was a 'rash on the face'.

History of Presenting Complaint

The father described he had noticed a rash on Mohammed's chin about three days ago and was concerned that it was weeping and spreading. The child had complained that it was a bit itchy and he had been scratching the area. The father had applied Savlon Cream to the area but was concerned that it was just making it worse. No other treatments had been prescribed or recommended by either GP or pharmacist and his son had never had anything like this before.

Past History

Eczema, tonsillectomy age three years

Medication

Emollient PRN (when necessary)

Allergy

No known drug allergies

Social

Lives with parents and three siblings, council flat, attends day nursery (father says lots of impetigo amongst the children recently), parental smoking.

Family History

Brother has asthma.

Travel

Returned from Bangladesh one week ago.

Up to date with all childhood immunisations

Review of Systems

Well in self. Mild fever. No complaints or pain. No upper respiratory tract disorder. No difficulty breathing. Eating and drinking normally. Normal stool. No dysuria. Dry skin as usual. No other rash.

Objective Examination

O/E, chatty, happy smiling boy, good colour.

Temperature 37.2 C (98.9 F), Pulse 100, Respiratory rate 28, Oxygen saturation 99% on room air.

Generalised dry skin noted over the whole body. Examination of the chin was aided by use of a magnifying glass. Three round lesions noted; approximately 1–2 cm in diameter, inflamed and annular with small vesicles and pustules, the largest of which had formed a yellow crusted area with discharge.

Ear, nose, and throat (ENT) examination NAD (no abnormality detected).

No lymphadenopathy.

Differential Diagnosis

Nonbullous impetigo (also known as impetigo contagiosa or crusted impetigo: the most common form). It presents as vesicles or pustules, which rapidly burst and evolve into gold-crusted plaques, typically 2 cm in diameter. The area around the mouth and nose is most commonly affected.

Herpes simplex virus (HSV-1) Recurrent herpes simplex is preceded by prodromal pain, itching, burning or tingling on the lips, small grouped vesicles that burst crust and heal within 7–10 days.

Varicella (lesions start as pink macular popular rash which develop into vesicles and crusts). Lesions occur in crops and have a widespread distribution.

Scabies (occurs four to six weeks after contact, characterised by intense itching especially at night). The rash is usually papular and scattered over the limbs and trunk but spares the face. Diagnosis is confirmed by finding one or more burrows (linear S shaped papules) usually in finger webs and wrists).

Atopic eczema (in older children it localises in the flexures); extremely itchy with lichenification of the skin.

Insect bites (Itchy papules with a central punctum often in groups or rows). If suspecting bedbugs the lesions will be more evident in the mornings.

Management

A diagnosis of impetigo was concluded taking into account the clinical presentation, the child's age, social (impetigo outbreak at nursery) and travel history (hot climate, not been using emollient recently, plus dry and itchy skin due to eczema).

Impetigo is a common contagious pyogenic infection of the superficial layers of the skin; usually caused by *S. aureus*, and less commonly caused by *St. pyogenes*. Its prevalence is approximately 2.8% in children up to four years and less so in older children (NHS Inform 2018). Nonbullous impetigo is usually asymptomatic apart from some mild itching.

Advice to parents included hygiene measures to prevent cross-infection and to avoid school until the lesions are dry or 48 hours after antibiotics have been started (NHS Inform 2018). Generalised skin care advice was also given such as resuming skin care in terms of emollients and avoiding known triggers for his eczema.

Treatment options for localised infection are topical fusidic acid, topical mupirocin, and retapamulin. A more severe infection may require oral antibiotics (flucloxacillin or clarithromycin/erythromycin if allergic to penicillin) (BNF 2015).

Conclusion

This chapter has been written to aid the diagnosis of an unknown rash or lesion. Remember to take into account the patient's age and medical history. Use a systems (such as OLDCART) approach in subjective history taking. Approach the objective physical examination in a methodical way that will help you collect information in an orderly manner. Pattern recognition and experience will guide you to your conclusions, but in the interim consult experienced colleagues. Ask them to call you to observe when there are interesting cases to view in practice. Do this as often as you can for as many presentations as possible, in varying conditions, especially related to age and skin colours. Finally, listen to your patient. In the majority of cases, the patient will tell you the diagnosis in the initial subjective component of history taking.

References

American Cancer Society (2018) Malignant Melanoma. https://www.cancer.org/cancer/melanoma-skin-cancer/about/key-statistics.html (accessed 16 January 2018).

Ashton, R., Leppard, B., and Cooper, A. (2014). *Differential Diagnosis in Dermatology*, 4e. London: Radcliffe.

Barron, G., Jacob, S., and Kirsner, R. (2007 September). Dermatologic complications of chronic venous disease: medical management and beyond. *Ann. Vasc. Surg.* 21 (5): 652–662.

63

Beldon, P. (2006 Mar). Avoiding allergic contact dermatitis in patients with venous leg ulcers. *Br. J. Community Nurs.* 11 (3): S6. S8, S10–2.

British Medical Association and Royal Pharmaceutical Society 2015 BNF 70 (British National Formulary). https://pharm.reviews/images/statyi/british-national-formulary-2015.pdf (accessed 22 August 2018).

British Association of Dermatologists (2014) Erythema Multiform. http://www.bad.org.uk/shared/get-file.ashx?id=83&itemtype=document (accessed 10 October 2015).

Buddenkotte, J., Maurer, M., and Steinhoff, M. (2010). Histamine and antihistamines in atopic dermatitis. *Adv. Exp. Med. Biol.* 709: 73–80.

Burgin, S. (2012). Nummular eczema, lichen simplex chronicus, and prurigo nodularis. In: *Fitzpatrick's Dermatology in General Medicine*, 8the (ed. L.A. Goldsmith, S.I. Katz, B.A. Gilchrest, et al.), 182–187. New York: McGraw-Hill Medical.

Cancer Research UK (2012) Melanoma Skin Cancer Statistics. http://www.cancerresearchuk.org/health-professional/cancer-statistics/statistics-by-cancer-type/skin-cancer (accessed 1 December 2015).

Cardiff University Department of Dermatology (1994) Dermatology Quality of Life Index. http://sites.cardiff.ac.uk/dermatology/quality-of-life/dermatology-quality-of-life-index-dlqi (accessed 20 December 2015).

DermNetNZ (1997a) (updated 27 December 2015) Basal Cell Carcinoma. http://www.dermnetnz.org/lesions/basal-cell-carcinoma.html (accessed 28 December 2015).

DermNetNZ (1997b) Terminology in Dermatology. http://www.dermnetnz.org/terminology.html (accessed 1 December 2015).

DermNetNZ (2003) Erythroderma. http://www.dermnetnz.org/reactions/erythroderma.html (accessed 21 November 2015).

DermNetNZ (2012) Complications of Atopic Dermatitis. https://www.dermnetnz.org/topics/complications-of-atopic-dermatitis (accessed 1 October 15).

DermNetNZ (2013) All about the Skin. www.dermnetnz.org (accessed 28 August 2013).

DermNetNZ (2014) Pityriasis Rosea. http://www.dermnetnz.org/viral/pityriasis-rosea.html (accessed 13 November 2015).

Flohr, C. and Mann, J. (2014 Jan). New insights into the epidemiology of childhood atopic dermatitis. *Allergy* 69 (1): 3–16. https://doi.org/10.1111/all.12270. Epub 2013 Nov 21.

Gloviczki, P., Comerota, A.J., Dalsing, M.C. et al. (2011 May). The care of patients with varicose veins and associated chronic venous diseases: clinical practice guidelines of the Society for Vascular Surgery and the American Venous Forum. *J. Vasc. Surg.* 53 (5 Suppl): 2S–48S. doi: 10.1016/j.jvs.2011.01.079.

Greaves, M. (2005). Itch in systemic disease: Therapeutic options. *Dermatol. Ther.* 18: 323–327.

Grimalt, R., Menguaud, V., and Cambazard, F. (2007). The steroid-sparing effect of an emollient therapy in infants with atopic dermatitis: a randomized controlled study. *Dermatology* 214 (1): 61–67.

Habif, T. (2011). *Skin Disease: Diagnosis and Treatment*, 3e. St. Louis, MO: Mosby.

Hinds, G. and Thomas, V.D. (2008 Jan). Malignancy and cancer treatment-related hair and nail changes. *Dermatol. Clin.* 26 (1): 59–68. viii.

Hoare, C., Li Wan Po, A., and Williams, H. (2000). Systematic review of treatments for atopic eczema. *Health Technol. Assess.* 4 (37): 1–191.

Khopkar, U. (2009). *Skin Diseases and Sexually Transmitted Infections*, 6e. Mumbai: Bhalani.

Kleyn, C., Lai-Cheong, J., and Bell, H. (2006). Cutaneous manifestations of internal malignancy: diagnosis and management. *Am. J. Clin. Dermatol.* 7 (2): 71–84.

Lupi, O., Madkan, V., and Tyring, S.K. (2006 Apr). Tropical dermatology: bacterial tropical diseases. *J. Am. Acad. Dermatol.* 54 (4): 559–578.

MHRA (2015) Yellow Card Scheme. https://yellowcard.mhra.gov.uk/the-yellow-card-scheme (accessed 1 December 2015).

National Eczema Society 2014 Eczema and Its Management: A Nurse's Guide.

NHS CHOICES (2014) Antibiotics – Side Effects. http://www.nhs.uk/Conditions/Antibiotics-penicillins/Pages/Side-effects.aspx (accessed 1 December 2015).

NHS Inform (2018) Impetigo. https://www.nhsinform.scot/illnesses-and-conditions/infections-and-poisoning/impetigo (accessed 20 August 2018).

Ni, C. and Chiu, M.W. (2014 Apr 17). Psoriasis and comorbidities: links and risks. *Clin. Cosmet. Investig. Dermatol.* 7: 119–132. https://doi.org/10.2147/CCID.S44843. eCollection 2014.

NICE (2005) Referral Guidelines for Suspected Cancer (NICE guideline 27). www.nice.org.uk (accessed 12 December 2012).

NICE (2007) Atopic Eczema. http://cks.nice.org.uk/eczema-atopic (accessed 11 December 2015).

NICE (2011) Scabies. http://cks.nice.org.uk/scabies (accessed 1 December 2015).

NICE (2012) Venous Eczema. http://cks.nice.org.uk/venous-eczema-and-lipodermatosclerosis (accessed 11 December 2015).

NICE (2013a) Seborrhoeic Dermatitis. http://cks.nice.org.uk/seborrhoeic-dermatitis (accessed 20th December 2012).

NICE (2013b) Contact Dermatitis. http://cks.nice.org.uk/dermatitis-contact (accessed 11 November 2015).

NICE. (2014) Psoriasis. http://cks.nice.org.uk/psoriasis (accessed 22 November 2015).

Patient (2013) Patient Health Questionnaire. http://patient.info/doctor/patient-health-questionnaire-phq-9 (accessed 28 December 2015).

Patient (2014) Dermatological History and Examination. http://patient.info/doctor/dermatological-history-and-examination (accessed 1 November 2015).

Patient (2015a) Dermatophytosis. http://patient.info/doctor/dermatophytosis-tinea-infections (accessed 1 January 2016).

Patient (2015b) Eczema Triggers and Irritants. http://patient.info/health/eczema-triggers-and-irritants (accessed 12 December 2015).

Santer, M., Burgess, H., Yardley, L. et al. (2012). Experiences of carers managing childhood eczema and their views on its treatment: a qualitative study. *Br. J. Gen. Pract.* doi:10.3399/bjgp12X636083.

Schwartz, R.A. and Nervi, S.J. (2007 Mar 1). Erythema nodosum: a sign of systemic disease. *Am. Fam. Physician* 75 (5): 695–700.

Shimizu, M., Hamaguchi, Y., Matsushita, T. et al. (2012 Nov 23). Sequentially appearing erythema nodosum, erythema multiforme and Henoch-Schonlein purpura in a patient with Mycoplasma pneumoniae infection: a case report. *J. Med. Case Rep.* 6 (1): 398. doi: 10.1186/1752-1947-6-398.

Slodownik, D. and Nixon, R. (2007). Occupational factors in skin diseases. *Curr. Probl. Dermatol.* 35: 173–189.

The Fitzpatrick Skin Type Classification Scale. (November 2007). *Skin Inc.* https://www.scribd.com/document/275659084/Fitzpatrick-Skin-Type-Classification-Scale (accessed 19 August 2018).

Tortora, G. and Derrickson, B. (2013). *Principles of Anatomy and Physiology*, 14e. Oxford: Wiley and Sons.

Valeyrie-Allanore, L., Sassolas, B., and Roujeau, J.C. (2007). Drug-induced skin, nail and hair disorders. *Drug Saf.* 30 (11): 1011–1030.

Werfel, T., Ballmer-Weber, B., Eigenmann, P.A. et al. (2007 Jul). Eczematous reactions to food in atopic eczema: position paper of the EAACI and GA2LEN. *Allergy* 62 (7): 723–728.

World Health Organization (2005) Exposure to Artificial UV Radiation and Skin Cancer. http://publications.iarc.fr/_publications/media/download/4033/c6dbb6ef039134a92cce28b4bfc7ce5d21ad9a8f.pdf (accessed 3 December 2015).

Chapter 4

Examination of the Cardiovascular System

Carol Lynn Cox and Carrie E. Boyd

Introduction

Examination of the cardiovascular system constitutes an essential aspect in evaluating the patient's health. Functions of the cardiovascular system involve the heart as a pump and the arteries and veins throughout the body in relation to transporting oxygen and nutrients to the tissues and transporting waste products and carbon dioxide from the tissues. Changes in the cardiovascular system affect other systems. The purpose of examining the cardiovascular system is to assess the function of the heart as a pump and arteries and veins throughout the body in transporting oxygen and nutrients to the tissues and transporting waste products and carbon dioxide from the tissues. Your assessment of the cardiovascular system is important because cardiovascular disease is the most prevalent healthcare problem in the United Kingdom. Over 250 000 deaths per year are attributed to cardiovascular disease.

Anatomy and Physiology

The cardiovascular system is composed of the heart and blood vessels (venous and arterial). The heart pumps blood through blood vessels to all body tissues. The heart itself is composed of an epicardium, which is the thin outer layer of the heart, the myocardium, and an endocardium. The myocardium is the muscle tissue that comprises the majority of the heart. It is responsible for the heart's pumping action. The inner layer of the heart is the endocardium. The endocardium is a thin layer of endothelium that overlies a thin layer of connective tissue. The endocardium provides a smooth layer for the chambers of the heart and covers the valves as well as being contiguous with the endothelial lining of the blood vessels that attach to the heart.

The heart has four chambers: two upper chambers called atria which function as entry chambers where blood either unoxygenated (right upper chamber) or oxygenated (left upper chamber) is then transferred to two lower chambers called the ventricles. The right ventricle (RV) gently pumps unoxygenated blood to the lungs where gaseous exchange occurs. The left ventricle (LV) pumps blood to the brain and remainder of the body. The atria have on their anterior surface a pouchlike structure called the auricle, which

Physical Assessment for Nurses and Healthcare Professionals, Third Edition. Edited by Carol Lynn Cox.
© 2019 John Wiley & Sons Ltd. Published 2019 by John Wiley & Sons Ltd.

increases the capacity of the atria to hold blood. On the surface of the heart, a series of grooves called sulci can be found. Sulci contain coronary blood vessels and a variable amount of fat for padding. The sulci mark the external boundaries between the two chambers of the heart. A deep coronary sulcus encircles the majority of the heart and delineates the boundary between the superior atria and the inferior ventricles. The anterior interventricular sulcus is a much shallower groove that delineates the boundary between the RVs and LVs. Finally, the posterior interventricular sulcus delineates the boundary between the ventricles and the posterior part of the heart (Martini et al. 2014; Tortora and Derrickson 2012).

The right atrium receives blood from the superior vena cava, inferior vena cava, and coronary sinus. Between the right and left atrium is a thin divider which is the interatrial septum. Within this septum can be found an oval structure called the fossa ovalis. The fossa ovalis is the remnant of foramen ovale which functioned as an opening between the right and left atria before birth. The foramen ovale normally closes soon after birth.

Unoxygenated blood passes from the right atrium to the RV through a valve called the tricuspid valve. The tricuspid valve has three leaflets. The tricuspid valve is also known as the atrioventricular valve.

The RV comprises most of the anterior surface of the heart. The inside layer of the ventricle has ridges in bundles of cardiac muscle fibres called trabeculae carneae. Some of the trabeculae carneae form part of the conduction system. The RV is separated from the LV by a partition termed the interventricular septum. Blood flows from the RV through the pulmonary valve to the lungs through an artery termed the pulmonary trunk. This trunk divides into the right and left pulmonary arteries. The lungs oxygenate the blood, which then passes through four pulmonary veins into the left atrium (Martini et al. 2014; Tortora and Derrickson 2012).

The left atrium forms the majority of the base of the heart. Oxygenated blood flows from the left atrium through the bicuspid (mitral) valve into the LV. The bicuspid valve has two leaflets (cusps). The bicuspid (mitral valve) is also known as the atrioventricular valve. The passage of blood is primarily passive in nature until the LV is almost entirely full. Then an 'atrial kick' (contraction) occurs passing the last of the oxygenated blood into the ventricle.

The LV forms the apex of the heart and like the RV contains trabeculae carneae. Blood passes from the LV through the aortic valve and the ascending aorta, which then initiates the distribution of blood to the coronary arteries and to the body and brain (Martini et al. 2014; Tortora and Derrickson 2012).

This description of the anatomy and physiology of the heart touches only on the surface of the anatomy and physiology of the heart and does not address the circulatory system. For a complete description of the anatomy and physiology of the heart and circulatory system it is recommended that a comprehensive anatomy and physiology text is consulted.

General Examination

In the narrative that follows, the essential elements associated with examination of the cardiovascular system are presented. Examination normally begins with history taking (subjective assessment), a review of systems (if not reviewed in association with a general physical examination), the objective examination, formation of a differential diagnosis, and diagnosis followed by a plan of treatment (Collins-Bride and Saxe 2013; Cox 2010; Crawford 2014; Jarvis 2008).

- Examine:
  - clubbing of fingernails

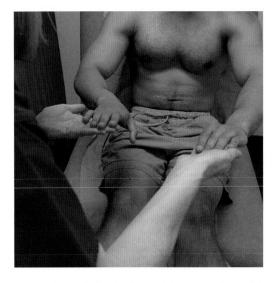

Assess the nails for leukonychia and koilonychia

Clubbing in relation to the heart suggests *cyanotic heart disease*.

- cold hands with blue nails – poor perfusion, peripheral cyanosis
- under the tongue, and at the gum line for central cyanosis (in light skinned patients the colour will be bluish purple, in dark skinned patients the colour will be grey)
- conjunctivae for anaemia
- signs of dyspnoea or distress
  Assess the degree of breathlessness by checking if *dyspnoea* occurs on undressing, talking, at rest, or when lying flat (*orthopnoea*).
- xanthomata:
  - *xanthelasma* (common) –intracutaneous yellow cholesterol deposits occur around the eyes – normal or with *hyperlipidaemia* (Figure 4.1)
  - *xanthoma* (uncommon) (Figure 4.2):
    hypercholesterolaemia – tendon deposits (hands and achilles tendon) or tuberous xanthomata at elbows
- *hypertriglyceridaemia* – eruptive xanthoma, small yellow deposits on buttocks and extensor surfaces, each with a red halo (Ball et al. 2014a, b; Barcauskas et al. 2002; Bickley and Szilagyi 2007, 2013; Cox 2010; Crawford 2014; Dains et al. 2012, 2015; Epstein et al. 2008; Hatton and Blackwood 2003; Japp and Robertson 2013; Jarvis 2015; Seidel et al. 2006, 2010; Swartz 2006, 2014; Talley and O'Connor 2006, 2014).

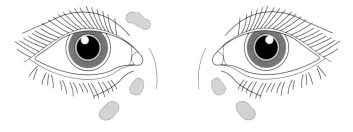

Figure 4.1   Xanthelasma.

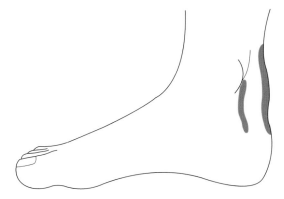

Figure 4.2   Xanthoma.

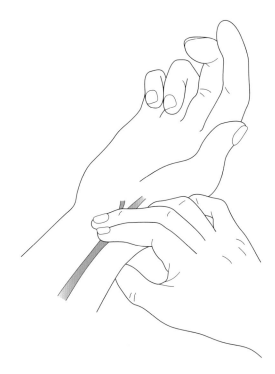

Figure 4.3   Taking a radial pulse.

Palpate the Radial Pulse

Feel the radial pulse just medial to the radius with two forefingers (Figure 4.3).

- Pulse rate:
  Take for one minute (some clinicians will count the pulse for 15 seconds and multiply by four; however, this does not reflect an accurate pulse rate, particularly if the patient has arrhythmias):
- *tachycardia* > 100 beats min^{-1}
- *bradycardia* < 50 beats min^{-1}

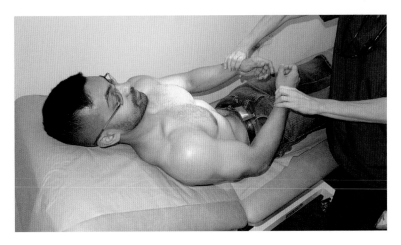

Compare radial pulses

- Rhythm:
  - regular
  normal variation on breathing: *sinus arrhythmia*
- regularly irregular
  pulsus bigeminus, coupled extrasystoles (digoxin toxicity)
  Wenckebach (type I 2nd-degree heart block; the P–R interval lengthens until a P-wave is finally not conducted and the sequence starts again)
- irregularly irregular
  atrial fibrillation
  premature ventricular contractions (PVC), ventricular extrasystoles/ventricular ectopic beats (VE)
  Check apical rate by auscultation whilst palpating the pulse for true heart rate, as ventricular premature beats are not transmitted to radial pulse (Crawford 2014; Fihn et al. 2012; Morse 2017).
- Waveform of the pulse (Figure 4.4):
  - normal (1)
  - slow rising and plateau – moderate or severe *aortic stenosis* (2)
  - collapsing pulse – pulse pressure greater than diastolic pressure, e.g. *aortic incompetence*, elderly *arteriosclerotic* patient or *gross anaemia* (3)
  - bisferiens – moderate *aortic stenosis* with severe *incompetence* (4)
  - pulsus paradoxus – pulse weaker or disappears on inspiration, e.g. *constrictive pericarditis, tamponade, status asthmaticus* (5) (Crawford 2014; Morse 2017).
- Volume:
  - small volume – *low cardiac output (CO)*
  - large volume
  carbon dioxide retention
  thyrotoxicosis (Crawford 2014; Morse 2017).
- Stiffness of the vessel wall:
  - In the elderly, a stiff, strongly pulsating, palpable 5–6 cm radial artery indicates *arteriosclerosis*, a hardening of the walls of the artery that:
  - is common with aging
  - is not atheroma
  - is associated with systolic hypertension.

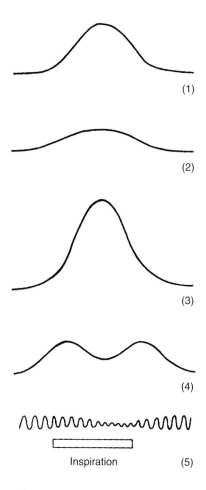

(1)

(2)

(3)

(4)

Inspiration   (5)

Figure 4.4   Waveform of the pulse.

- Pulsus alternans:
  A difference of 20 mmHg systolic blood pressure (BP) between consecutive beats signifies poor left ventricular function. This needs to be measured with a sphygmomanometer (Crawford 2014; Morse 2017; Seidel et al. 2010; Swartz 2014; Talley and O'Connor 2014).

Take the BP

- Wrap the cuff neatly and tightly around either upper arm.
- Gently inflate the cuff until the radial artery is no longer palpable.
- Using the stethoscope, listen over the brachial artery for the pulse to appear as you drop the pressure slowly (3–4 mm s^{-1}) (Figure 4.5).
- Systolic BP: appearance of sounds
  - Korotkoff phase 1
- Diastolic BP: disappearance of sounds
  - Korotkoff phase 5

Use large cuff for large arms (circumference > 30 cm) so that inflatable cuff >1/2 arm circumference.

Beware auscultatory gap with sounds disappearing midsystole. If sounds go to zero, use Korotkoff phase 4.

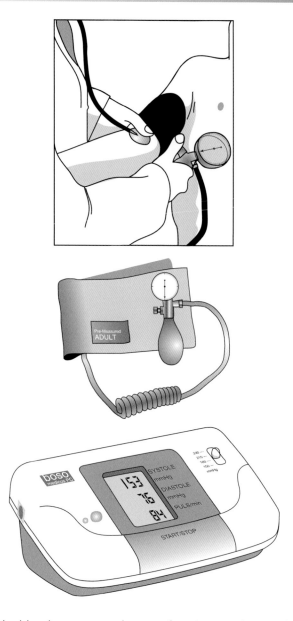

Figure 4.5   Taking the blood pressure and types of equipment that can be used. Reproduced with permission.

In adults, ~ > 140/85 mmHg or more is the current guideline in nondiabetic patients and ~ > 130/80 mmHg in diabetic patients. The patient may be nervous when first examined and the BP may be falsely high. Take it again at the end of the examination.

Wide pulse pressure (e.g. 160/30 mmHg) suggests *aortic incompetence*.

Narrow pulse pressure (e.g. 95/80 mmHg) suggests *aortic stenosis*.

Difference of >20 mmHg systolic between arms suggests *arterial occlusion*, e.g. *dissecting aneurysm* or *atheroma*.

Difference of 10 mmHg is found in 25% of healthy subjects.

The variable pulse from atrial fibrillation means a precise BP cannot easily be obtained (Cox 2010; Dains et al. 2015; Fihn et al. 2012; Jarvis 2015; Morse 2017).

Jugular Venous Pulse (Frequently Called Pressure)

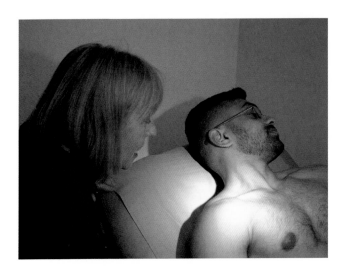

Assess for jugular venous distention

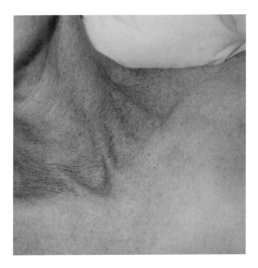

Measuring jugular venous distension

- Observe the height of the jugular venous pulsation (JVP). See Figure 4.6.
  Position the patient lying at approximately 45° to the horizontal with head on pillows. Shine a torch at an angle across the neck.
- Look at the veins in the neck. Use tangential lighting.
  - internal jugular vein not directly visible: pulse diffuse, medial, or deep to sternomastoid
  - external jugular vein: pulse lateral to sternomastoid. Only informative if pulsating
- Assess vertical height in centimetres above the manubriosternal angle, using the pulsating external jugular vein or upper limit of internal jugular pulsation.

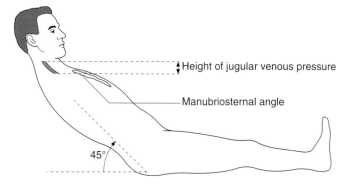

Figure 4.6 Assessing height of JVP.

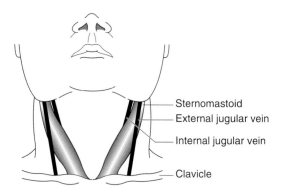

Figure 4.7 The veins of the neck.

The external jugular vein is often more readily visible but may be obstructed by its tortuous course and is less reliable than the internal jugular pulse (Figure 4.7).

The internal jugular vein is sometimes very difficult to see. Its pulsation may be confused with the carotid artery but it:

- has a complex pulsation
- moves on respiration and decreases on inspiration except in tamponade
- cannot be palpated
- can be obliterated by pressure on base of neck
- demonstrates right heart pressure
  The hepatojugular reflux is checked by firm pressure with the flat of the right hand over the liver, whilst watching the JVP.
  Compression on the dilated hepatic veins increases the JVP by 2 cm.
  If the JVP is found to be raised above the manubriosternal angle and pulsating, it implies *right heart failure*. Look for the other signs, i.e. pitting oedema and large tender liver. Sometimes the JVP is so raised it can be missed, except that the ears waggle.
  Dilated neck veins with no pulsation suggest *noncardiac obstruction* (e.g. carcinoma bronchus causing superior caval obstruction or a kinked external jugular vein).
  If venous pressure rises on inspiration (it normally falls), suspect *constrictive pericarditis* or *pericardial effusion* causing *tamponade* (Cox 2010; Crawford 2014) (Figure 4.8).
- Observe the character of JVP. Try to ascertain the waveform of the JVP. It should be a double pulsation consisting of:
  - a-wave atrial contraction – ends synchronous with carotid artery pulse c

    ○ v-wave atrial filling – when the tricuspid valve is closed by ventricular contraction – with and just after carotid pulse

Large a waves are caused by obstruction to flow from the right atrium due to stiffness of the RV from hypertrophy:

    — *pulmonary hypertension*
    — *pulmonary stenosis*
    — *tricuspid stenosis.*

Absent a wave in *atrial fibrillation*.

Large v waves are caused by regurgitation of blood through an *incompetent tricuspid valve* during ventricular contraction.

A sharp y descent occurs in *constrictive pericarditis*.

Cannon waves (giant a waves) occur in *complete heart block* when the right atrium occasionally contracts against a closed tricuspid valve (Cox 2010; Crawford 2014).

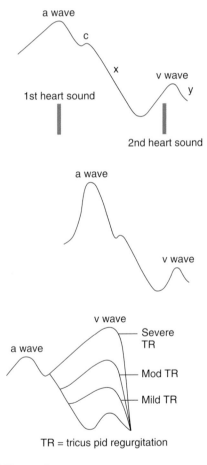

Figure 4.8   Assessing the JVP waveform.

Musset's Sign

- Observe the patient's ability to hold the head still.

Slight rhythmic bobbing of the head in time with the heartbeat may accompany high back pressure caused by aortic insufficiency or aortic aneurysm (Cox 2010).

The Precordium

- Inspect the precordium for abnormal pulsation.
  A large LV may easily be seen on the left side of the chest, sometimes in the axilla.
- Palpate the apex beat (point of maximal impulse = PMI).

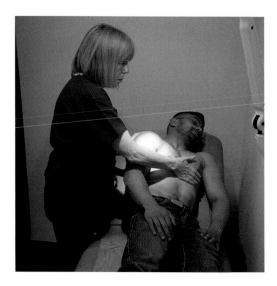

Palpate the PMI point of maximal impulse

- Feel for the point furthest out and down where the pulsation can still be distinctly felt. In the adult this is normally felt in the 5th intercostal space (ICS) midclavicular line (MCL). In the older adult this may shift to the 6th ICS just left of the MCL.
- If you are unable to palpate the PMI, lean the patient forwards and turn the patient onto the left side. (This will slightly shift the heart forwards in the chest so that it is easier to feel.)

(Figure 4.9).

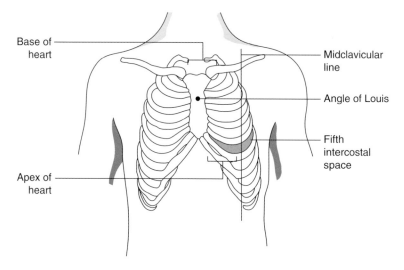

Base of heart
Midclavicular line
Angle of Louis
Fifth intercostal space
Apex of heart

Figure 4.9   Location of PMI at the apex. Reproduced with permission.

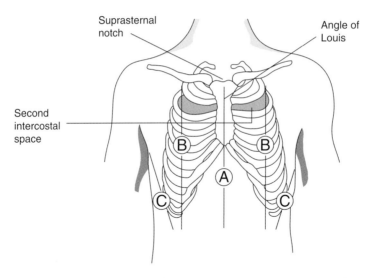

Figure 4.10   (a) Midsternal. (b) Midclavicular. (c) Anterior axillary. Reproduced with permission.

- Measure the position (Figure 4.10).
    - Determine the space, counting down from the 2nd ICS which lies below the 2nd rib (opposite the manubriosternal angle) where the PMI is felt.
    - Measure laterally in centimetres from the midline.
    - Describe the apex beat in relation to the MCL, anterior axillary line, and midaxillary line (Cox 2010).

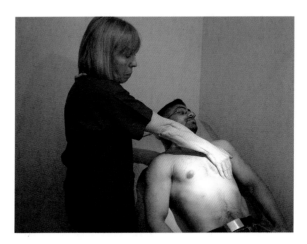

Palpate at the apex for the apex beat

- Assess character:
    Try to judge if an enlarged heart is:
    - feeble (dilated) or
    - stronger than usual (LV or RV hypertrophy or both).
    Thrusting displaced apex beat occurs with volume overload: an active, large stroke volume ventricle, e.g. *mitral* or *aortic incompetence*, *left-to-right shunt* or *cardiomyopathy*.
    Sustained apex beat occurs with pressure overload in *aortic stenosis* and *gross hypertension*. Stroke volume is normal or reduced.
    Tapping apex beat (palpable 1st heart sound) occurs in *mitral stenosis*.

Diffuse pulsation asynchronous with apex beat occurs with a *left ventricular aneurysm* – a dyskinetic apex beat.

Impalpable – obesity, overinflated chest, pericardial effusion (Cox 2010; Bickley and Szilagyi 2013; Talley and O'Connor, 2014).

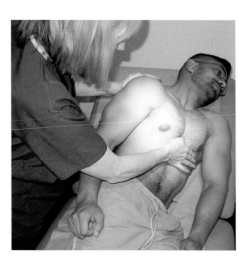

Palpate the apex of the heart

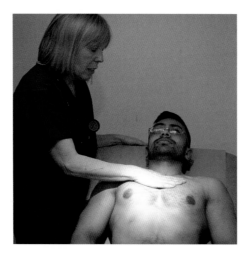

Palpate at the base for heaves, thrusts, and/or thrills

- Palpate firmly the left border of the sternum.
  - Use the flat of your hand.
    - A heave suggests *right ventricular hypertrophy* (Cox 2010).
- Palpate all over the precordium with the flat of hand for thrills (palpable murmurs).

N.B. If by now you have found an abnormality in the cardiovascular system, think of possible causes before you listen.

For example, if LV is forceful:

- ? hypertension – was BP raised?
- ? aortic stenosis or incompetence – was pulse character normal? will there be a murmur?

- ? mitral incompetence – will there be a murmur?
- ? thyrotoxicosis or anaemia

Auscultation

- Listen over the five main areas of the heart and in each area with both the bell and diaphragm of the stethoscope (Figure 4.11).
  The bell will transmit soft sounds (S_3 and S_4) that are lost when the diaphragm is used. The diaphragm transmits loud harsh sounds. Concentrate in order on:
  - heart sounds
  - added sounds
  - murmurs.

  Keep to this order when listening or describing what you have heard, or you will miss or forget important findings.
  The five main areas are (Figure 4.12):

- apex, mitral area in the 5th ICS MCL (and left axilla if there is a murmur) = S_1 (Mitral = M_1)
- tricuspid area in the 4th ICS left sternal border = S_1 (Tricuspid = T_1)

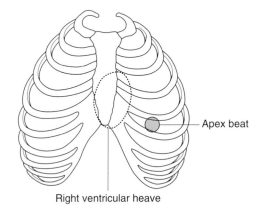

Figure 4.11   Palpation position for right ventricular heave.

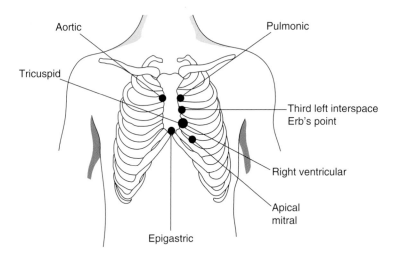

Figure 4.12   Ausculation site landmarks. Reproduced with permission.

- aortic area in the 2nd ICS right of the sternum (and neck if there is a murmur) = S_2 (Aortic = A_2)
- pulmonary area in the 2nd ICS left of the sternum = S_2 (Pulmonic = P_2)
- Erb's point in the 3rd ICS left of the sternum = best location to hear murmurs across chambers

These areas represent where heart sounds and murmurs associated with these valves are best heard. They do not represent the surface markings of the valves.

If you hear little, turn the patient onto the left side, and listen over the apex (having palpated for it).

Note that because the diaphragm filters out low-frequency sounds, the bell should be used for mitral stenosis, which is a low-frequency sound (Brown et al. 2002; Cox 2010).

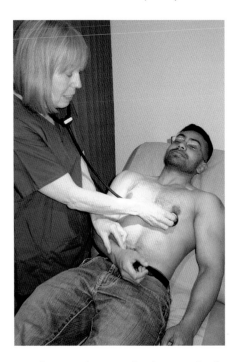

Auscultate at the apex for the mitral valve

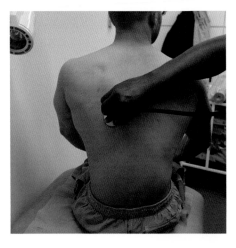

Auscultate below the left scapula to hear the heart

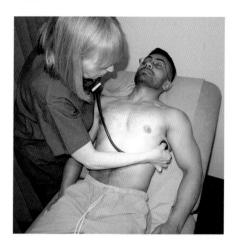

Auscultate for mitral regurgitation (incompetence)

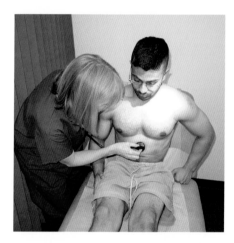

Auscultate for aortic regurgitation (incompetence)

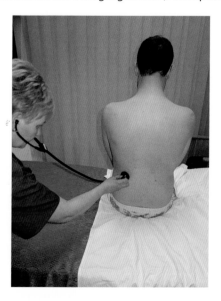

Auscultation of the renal artery

Normal Heart Sounds

I Sudden cessation of mitral and tricuspid flow due to valve closure. (Use both the bell and diaphragm in auscultation.)

- loud in *mitral insufficiency (stenosis)*
- soft in *mitral incompetence, aortic insufficiency (stenosis), left bundle-branch block*
- variable in *complete heart block* and *atrial fibrillation*

II Sudden cessation of aortic and pulmonary flow due to valve closure – usually split (see below). (Use both the bell and diaphragm in auscultation.)

- loud in *hypertension*
- soft in *aortic* or *pulmonary insufficiency (stenosis)* (Heard best with the bell.)
- wide normal split – *right bundle-branch block*
- wide fixed split – *atrial septal defect* (Brown et al. 2002; Cox 2010).

Added Sounds

III First phase–rapid ventricular filling sound in early diastole (S_3). (Heard best with the bell lightly held. Pressure on the bell will extinguish the sound.) (Figure 4.13)

- Common in children and young adults. In these instances it is known as a physiological S_3. It is heard in hyperkinetic states producing an increased CO. Examples include hyperthyroidism, exercise, pregnancy, and anxiety-related tachycardia. It can also be heard in mitral and tricuspid insufficiency, ischaemia, advanced congestive heart failure (CHF), and left to right shunts. When it is heard in middle-aged adults it is considered abnormal. You should suspect *left ventricular heart failure, fibrosed ventricle,* or *constrictive pericarditis*. When it originates in the LV it is best heard at the apex with patient on the left side exhaling. When it originates in the RV it is best heard at Erb's point (Brown et al. 2002; Cox 2010).

IV Second phase – atrial contraction (atrial kick) inducing ventricular filling towards the end of the diastole (S_4). (Heard best with the bell lightly held. Pressure on the bell will extinguish the sound.)

- A physiological S_4 may be heard in middle-aged adults who have thin-walled chests; especially after exercise. It occurs when there is an overload of either the LV or RV when diastolic pressure is increased. In the adult, suspect hyperthyroidism, pulmonary hypertension, aortic or pulmonary insufficiency, myocardial infarction (MI), or heart failure. In the older adult, suspect hypertensive cardiovascular disease, coronary

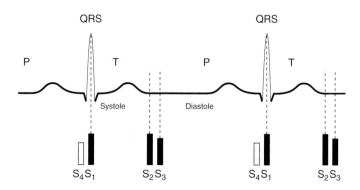

Figure 4.13 Relationship of heart sounds to the electrocardiogram. Reproduced with permission.

artery disease, pulmonary hypertension, aortic or pulmonary insufficiency, myocardial ischaemia, infarction, or congestive heart failure. It may be the first evidence of cardiovascular disease. If it is heard over the left lateral sternal border it is probably RV in origin. If it is heard over the apex it is probably LV in origin (Brown et al. 2002; Cox 2010).

Canter rhythm (often termed gallop) with tachycardia gives the following cadences:

S_3: Frequently indicated as sounding like **Ke**n – **tucky** (k = 1st heart sound). Note that S_3 comes after S_2.

S_4: Frequently indicated as sounding like **Tenne** – **ss**ee (n = 1st heart sound) Note that S_4 comes before S_1 (Brown et al. 2002; Cox 2010).

Clicks and Snaps

- Normally the opening of a heart valve is silent. Ejection clicks arise from abnormal aortic or pulmonary valves when they open. These occur in early systole and may be mistaken as splitting. An opening snap (os) is associated with an abnormal mitral or tricuspid valve and is heard best in diastole (Brown et al. 2002; Cox 2010).

Opening Snap

- Mitral valve normally opens silently after S_2.
- In *mitral insufficiency (stenosis)*, sudden movement of rigid valve makes a snap, after S_2 (Figure 4.14) (Brown et al. 2002; Cox 2010).

Ejection Click

- Aortic valve normally opens silently after S_1.
- In *aortic insufficiency (stenosis* or *sclerosis)*, the valve can open with a click after S_1 (Brown et al. 2002; Cox 2010).

Splitting of Second Heart Sound ($S_2 = a_2p_2$)

Ask patients to take deep breaths in and out. Blood is drawn into the thorax during inspiration and then on to the RV. There is temporarily more blood in the RV than the LV, and the RV takes fractionally longer to empty.

Splitting is best heard during inspiration. If the patient is breathless, do not ask them to hold breath in or out when assessing splitting.

Physiological splitting may occur in children and young people. In older people a delay in closure of p_2 (p_2 comes after a_2) may be associated with right heart failure or pulmonary hypertension.

Paradoxical splitting occurs in *aortic insufficiency (stenosis)* and *left bundle-branch block*.

In both these conditions (Figure 4.15) the LV takes longer to empty, thus delaying a_2 until after p_2. During inspiration p_2 occurs later and the sounds draw closer together (Brown et al. 2002; Cox 2010).

Knock and Rub

A loud low-frequency diastolic noise best known as a knock can be heard in constrictive pericarditis. A pericardial friction rub is a high-pitched frequency noise, heard loudest in systole but frequently present in diastole as well. A rub may vary from hour to hour, and when a significant pericardial effusion occurs the rub will disappear (Brown et al. 2002; Cox 2010).

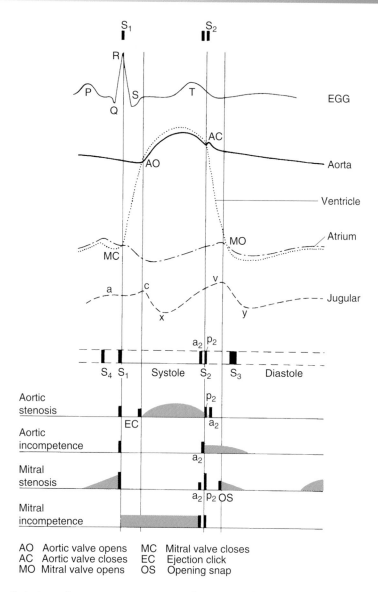

Figure 4.14   Relation of murmurs to pressure changes and valve movements.

Murmurs

Use the diaphragm of the stethoscope for most high-pitched sounds or murmurs (e.g. aortic incompetence) and the bell for low-pitched murmurs (e.g. mitral insufficiency –stenosis). Note the following:

- Timing systolic or diastolic (compare with finger on carotid pulse) (Figure 4.14).
- Site and radiation, e.g.:
  - ○ mitral incompetence → axilla
  - ○ aortic insufficiency (stenosis) → carotids and apex
  - ○ aortic incompetence → sternum (Brown et al. 2002; Cox 2010).
- Character:
  - ○ loud or soft
  - ○ pitch, e.g. squeaking or rumbling, 'scratchy' = pericardial or pleural

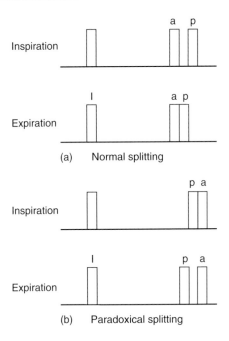

Figure 4.15   (a) Normal and (b) paradoxical splitting.

- ○ length
  - — pansystolic, throughout systole
  - — early diastolic, e.g. aortic or pulmonary incompetence
  - — midsystolic, e.g. aortic insufficiency (stenosis) or flow murmur
  - — middiastolic, e.g. mitral insufficiency (stenosis) (Brown et al. 2002; Cox 2010)
- Relation to posture:
  - ○ sit forwards – aortic incompetence louder
  - ○ lie left side – mitral insufficiency (stenosis) louder
- Relation to respiration:
  - ○ inspiration increases the murmur of a right heart lesion
  - ○ expiration increases the murmur of a left heart lesion
  - ○ variable – pericardial rub
- Relation to exercise:
  - ○ increases the murmur of mitral insufficiency (stenosis) (Brown et al. 2002; Cox 2010)

Optimal Position for Hearing Murmurs (Figure 4.16)

- Mitral insufficiency (stenosis) – the patient lies on left side, arm above head; listen with bell at apex as this is a diastolic murmur. Murmur is louder after exercise, e.g. repeated touching of toes from lying position that increases CO.
- Aortic incompetence (regurgitation) – the patient sits forwards after deep inspiration; listen with diaphragm at lower left sternal edge.

N.B. Murmurs alone do not make the diagnosis. Take other signs into consideration, e.g. arterial or venous pulses, BP, apex, or heart sounds. Also consider the status of the patient when deciding treatment. Does the patient look or state that they feel compromised? Is the patient breathless for example?

- Loudness is often not proportional to severity of disease, and in some situations length of murmur is more important, e.g. mitral insufficiency (stenosis) (Figure 4.17).

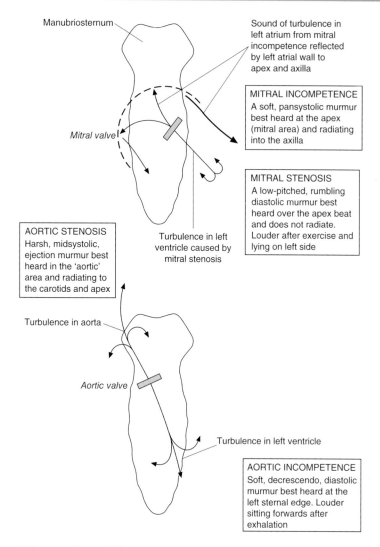

Figure 4.16   Radiation of sound from turbulent blood flow.

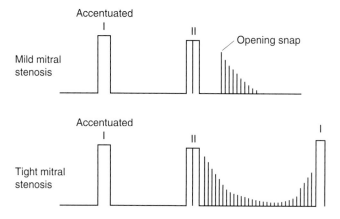

Figure 4.17   Diastolic murmurs in mitral stenosis.

- For completion:
  - auscultate base of lungs for inspiratory and expiratory crackles from left ventricular failure
  - palpate liver – smooth, tender, enlarged in right heart failure
  - palpate peripheral pulses (? stronger in lower extremities than upper)
  - peripheral oedema – ankle/sacral (? right ventricular failure) (Cox 2010).

Summary of Timing of Murmurs
Ejection Systolic Murmur
- *aortic insufficiency (stenosis* or *sclerosis) (same murmur, due to stiffness of valve cusps and aortic walls, with normal pulse pressure); aortic insufficiency (sclerosis)* is present in 50%-of-50-year-olds
- *pulmonary insufficiency (stenosis)*
- *atrial septal defect*
- *Fallot's syndrome* – right outflow tract obstruction

Pansystolic Murmur
- *mitral incompetence (regurgitation)*
- *tricuspid incompetence (regurgitation)*
- *ventricular septal defect*

Late Systolic Murmur
- *mitral valve prolapse – due to incompetence* (Frequently this sound is termed a systolic 'click')
- *hypertrophic cardiomyopathy*
- *coarction aorta* (extending in diastole to a 'machinery murmur')

Early Diastolic Murmur
- *aortic incompetence (regurgitation)*
- *pulmonary incompetence (regurgitation)*
- Graham Steell murmur in *pulmonary hypertension*

Mid–Late Diastolic Murmur
- *mitral insufficiency (stenosis)*
- *tricuspid insufficiency (stenosis)*
- Austin Flint murmur in *aortic incompetence*
- *left atrial myxoma* (variable – can also give other murmurs) (Cox 2010).

Signs of Left and Right Ventricular Failure
Left Heart Failure
- dyspnoea
- basal crackles on inspiration and expiration
- 4th heart sound, or 3rd in older patients
- Sit the patient forwards and listen at the bases of the lungs with the diaphragm of the stethoscope for fine inspiratory and expiratory crackles.
  Fine crackles heard on inspiration only are caused by alveoli opening on inspiration. If a patient has been recumbent for a while, alveoli tend to collapse in the normal lung. On taking a deep breath, fine inspiratory crackles will be heard. This is termed

atelectasis. These do not mean the patient has fluid in the alveoli or pulmonary oedema. Ask the patient to take a deep breath and then cough. The crackles should clear. If crackles are present on inspiration and expiration, this is indicative of fluid in the alveoli. With medium to coarse crackles consider pulmonary oedema and request a chest X-ray for confirmation (Cox 2010).

Right Heart Failure

- raised JVP
- enlarged tender liver (see Chapter 6, Examination of the Abdomen)
- pitting oedema
- With the patient sitting forwards, look for swelling over the sacral area. If there is, push your thumb into the swelling and see if you leave an indentation (pitting oedema). If you do, determine the severity of the oedema in terms of seconds it takes for the pitting to disappear.
- Check both ankles for pitting oedema.
  Oedema (fluid) collects at the most dependent part of the body. A patient who is mostly sitting will have ankle oedema whilst a patient who is lying will have predominantly sacral oedema (Cox 2010).

Functional Result

- Having ascertained the basic pathology (e.g. *MI, aortic insufficiency, stenosis, pericarditis*), make an assessment of the functional result.
  - history: how far can the patient walk, etc.
  - examination: evidence of:
    - cardiac enlargement (hypertrophy or dilatation)
    - heart failure
    - arrhythmias
    - pulmonary hypertension
    - cyanosis
    - endocarditis
- investigations: for example:
  - chest X-ray
  - electrocardiogram (ECG/EKG)
  - treadmill exercise test with ECG/EKG for ischaemia
  - echocardiograph – sonar 'radar' of heart, for muscle and ventricle size, muscle contractility and ejection fraction, valve function
  - 24-hour ECG/EKG tape for arrhythmias (Riley 2002)
  - cardiac catheterization for pressure measurements, blood oxygenation, and angiogram
  - radioactive scan – to image live, ischaemic, or dead cardiac muscle (Cox 2010; Morse 2017).

Summary of Common Illnesses
Mitral Stenosis

- small pulse – fibrillating?
- JVP raised only if heart failure
- RV++ LVo tapping apex
- loud S_1; loud p_2 if pulmonary hypertension

- −os
- middiastolic murmur at apex only (low-pitched rumbling)
  - severity indicated by early os and long murmur
  - best heard with the patient in left lateral position, in expiration with the bell of the stethoscope, particularly after exercise has increased CO
  - presystolic accentuation of murmur (absent if atrial fibrillation and stiff cusps)
- sounds 'ta ta rooofoo T'
- from S_2 os murmur S_1 (Cox 2010; Morse 2017).

Mitral Incompetence

- fibrillating?
- JVP raised only if heart failure
- RV+ LV++ systolic thrill
- soft S_1; loud p_2 if pulmonary hypertension
- pansystolic murmur apex → axilla (Cox 2010; Morse 2017).

Mitral Valve Prolapse

- midsystolic 'click', late systolic murmur
  - posterior cusp – murmur apex → axilla
  - anterior cusp – murmur apex → aortic area

There are three stages (Figure 4.18):

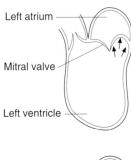

Left atrium

Mitral valve

Left ventricle

Click from billowing of cusp – larger than other cusp – may occur in 10% of females

Heard best on standing

midsystolic click

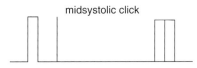

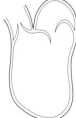

Click/late systolic murmur. After 'click', prolapsing cusp allows regurgitation

midsystolic click

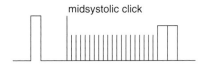

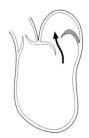

Cusp flails giving pansystolic regurgitation

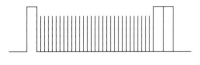

Figure 4.18   Stages of mitral valve prolapse.

Aortic Stenosis
- plateau pulse – narrow pulse pressure
- JVP raised only if heart failure
- LV++ systolic thrill
- soft a_2 with paradoxical split (± ejection click)
- harsh midsystolic murmur, apex and base, radiating to carotids
  - note discrepancy of forceful apex and feeble arterial pulse
- the longer the murmur, the tighter the stenosis; loudness does not necessarily imply severity (Cox 2010; Morse 2017).

Aortic Incompetence
- water-hammer pulse – wide pulse pressure; pulse visible in carotids
- JVP raised only if heart failure
- LV++ with dilatation
- (ejection click)
- early diastolic murmur base → lower sternum (also ejection systolic murmur from increased flow)
  - (sometimes Austin Flint murmur – see below)
  - heard best with patient leaning forwards, in expiration
- the longer the murmur, the more severe the regurgitation (Cox 2010; Morse 2017).

Tricuspid Incompetence
- JVP large v wave
- RV++, no thrill
- soft pansystolic murmur at maximal tricuspid area
- increases on inspiration (Cox 2010; Morse 2017).

Austin Flint Murmur
- middiastolic murmur (like mitral stenosis) in aortic incompetence due to regurgitant stream of blood on anterior cusp mitral valve

Graham Steell Murmur
- pulmonary early diastolic murmur (functional pulmonary incompetence) in mitral stenosis or other causes of pulmonary hypertension

Atrial Septal Defect
- JVP raised only if failure or tricuspid incompetence
- RV++ LVo
- widely fixed split-second sound
- pulmonary systolic murmur (tricuspid diastolic flow murmur) (Cox 2010; Morse 2017).

Ventricular Septal Defect
- RV+ LV+
- pansystolic murmur on left sternal edge (loud if small defect!)

Patent Ductus Arteriosus
- systolic → diastolic 'machinery' or continuous murmur below left clavicle

Metal Prosthetic Valves
- loud clicks with short flow murmur
  - aortic systolic
  - mitral diastolic
- need anticoagulation

Tissue Prosthetic Valves
- porcine xenograft or human homograft
- tend to fibrose after 7–10 years, leading to stenosis and incompetence
- may not require anticoagulation

Pericardial Rub
- scratchy (sounds like two pieces of leather rubbing together), superficial noise heard in systole and diastole
- brought out by stethoscope pressure, and sometimes variable with respiration (Cox 2010; Morse 2017).

Infectious Endocarditis (Diagnosis Made from Blood Cultures)
- febrile, unwell, anaemia
- splinter haemorrhages on nails
- Osler's nodes
- cardiac murmur
- splenomegaly
- haematuria

Rheumatic Fever
- flitting arthralgia
- erythema nodosum or erythema marginatum
- tachycardia
- murmurs
- *Sydenham's chorea* (irregular, uncontrollable jerks of limbs, tongue)

Clues to Diagnosis from Facial Appearance
- *Down's syndrome* from 21 trisomy
  - ventricular septal defect
  - patent ductus arteriosus
- *thyrotoxicosis* – atrial fibrillation
- *myxoedema* from hypothyroid – cardiomyopathy
- dusky, congested face – *superior vena cava obstruction*
- red cheeks in infra-orbital region in mitral facies from mitral stenosis

Clues to Diagnosis from General Appearance
- *Turner's syndrome* from sex chromosomes X0
  - female, short stature, web of neck
  - coarctation of aorta
- Marfan's syndrome
  - tall patient with long, thin fingers
  - aortic regurgitation (Hatton and Blackwood 2003; Cox 2010)

Peripheral Arteries

- Feel all peripheral pulses (Figure 4.19). Lower-limb pulses are usually felt after examining the abdomen.

    Diminished or absent pulses suggest *arterial stenosis* or *occlusion*. The lower-limb pulses are particularly important if there is a history of *intermittent claudication*.

    Auscultation of the carotid and femoral vessels is useful if there is a suspicion these arteries are stenosed. A bruit is heard if the stenosis causes turbulent flow.

    Coarctation of the aorta delays the femoral pulse after the radial pulse.

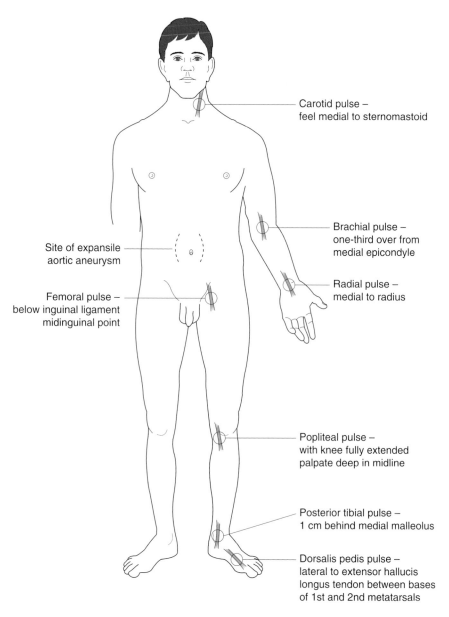

Carotid pulse –
feel medial to sternomastoid

Brachial pulse –
one-third over from
medial epicondyle

Radial pulse –
medial to radius

Site of expansile
aortic aneurysm

Femoral pulse –
below inguinal ligament
midinguinal point

Popliteal pulse –
with knee fully extended
palpate deep in midline

Posterior tibial pulse –
1 cm behind medial malleolus

Dorsalis pedis pulse –
lateral to extensor hallucis
longus tendon between bases
of 1st and 2nd metatarsals

Figure 4.19   Sites of peripheral pulses.

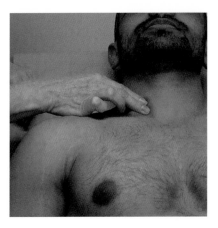

Palpate the carotid pulse

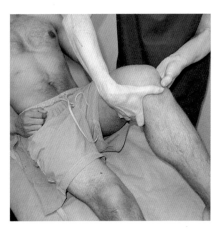

Palpate the popliteal artery

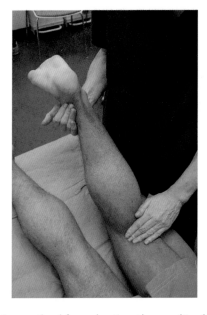

Posterior method for palpating the popliteal artery

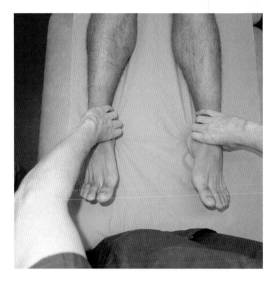

Palpate posterior tibial arteries

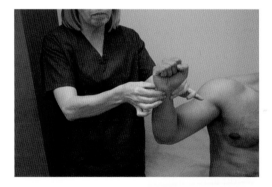

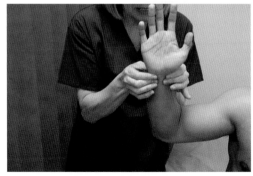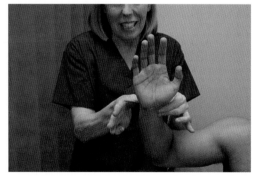

Allen Test

Peripheral Vascular Disease

- white or blue discoloration
- ulcers with little granulation tissue and slow healing (Figure 4.20)
- shiny skin, loss of hairs, thickened dystrophic nails
- absent pulses

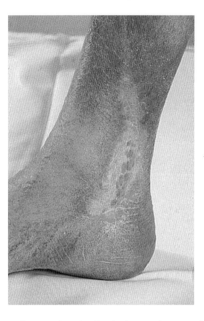

Figure 4.20   Healing varicose ulcer – classic site in lower leg medially with pigmentation from venous stasis.

- Buerger's test of severity of arterial insufficiency
  - loss of autoregulation of blood flow
  - patient lying supine, lift leg up to 45° – positive test: pallor of foot; venous guttering (Cox 2010; Hatton and Blackwood 2003; Morse 2017).
  - hang legs over side of bed: note time to capillary and venous filling; reactive hyperaemia; subsequent cyanosis
  Diabetes, when present, also signs from neuropathy:
- dry skin with thickened epidermis
- callus from increased foot pressure over abnormal sites, e.g. under tarsal heads in midfoot, secondary to motor neuropathy, and change in distribution of weight
- absent ankle reflexes
- decreased sensation

Aortic Aneurysm

- Musset's sign (observe the patient's ability to hold the head still)
- central abdominal pulsation visible or palpable
- need to distinguish from normal, palpable aorta in midline in thin people
  - aortic aneurysm is expansible to each side as well as forwards
  - a systolic bruit may be audible (Figure 4.21)
  - associated with femoral and popliteal artery aneurysms (Hatton and Blackwood 2003; Cox 2010; Morse 2017).

Varicose Veins

- Varicose veins and hernia are examined when the patient is standing, possibly at the end of the whole examination at the same time as the gait.

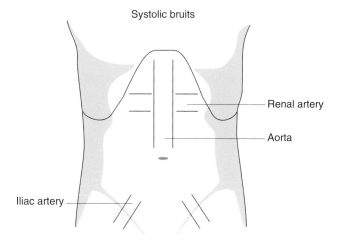

Systolic bruits

Renal artery

Aorta

Iliac artery

Figure 4.21   Site of systolic bruit in aortic aneurysm. Reproduced with permission.

Majority are associated with incompetent valves in the long saphenous vein or short saphenous vein.

Long saphenous – from femoral vein in groin to medial side of lower leg.

Short saphenous – from popliteal fossa to back of calf and lateral malleolus.

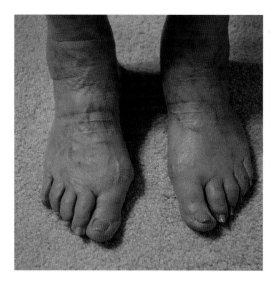

Varicosities and oedema in the ankles and feet

- Observe:
  - swelling
  - pigmentation – indicates chronic venous insufficiency
  - eczema
  - inflammation – suggests thrombophlebitis

- Palpate:
  - soft or hard (thrombosed)
  - tender – thrombophlebitis
  - cough impulse – implies incompetent valves
    Incompetent valves can be confirmed by the Trendelenburg test:
    - Elevate leg to empty veins.
    - Occlude long saphenous vein with a tourniquet around upper thigh.
    - Stand patient up.
    - If veins fill rapidly, this indicates incompetent thigh perforators below the tourniquet.
    - If, after release of tourniquet, veins fill rapidly, this indicates incompetent saphenofemoral junction.

If veins fill immediately on standing, then incompetent valves are in thigh or calf, so do the Perthes test:

- As for Trendelenburg, but on standing let some blood enter veins by temporary release of groin pressure.
- Ask patient to stand up and down on toes.
- Veins become less tense if:
  - muscle pump is satisfactory
- perforating calf veins are patent with competent valves (Hatton and Blackwood 2003; Cox 2010; Morse 2017).

System-Oriented Examination
'Examine the Cardiovascular System'

- hands –? moist, cold clammy, palmar erythema
- nails – leukonychia, splinter haemorrhages, capillary refill
- radial pulse – rate, rhythm, waveform, volume, state of artery
- BP
- eyes – anaemia
- area around eyes – xanthelasma
- mouth – central cyanosis
- JVP – height, waveform
- apex beat – PMI site, character
- auscultate
  - at apex – PMI (with thumb/finger on carotid artery for timing)
    - heart sounds
    - added sounds
    - murmurs
  - in neck over carotid artery – each area of precordium with diaphragm
    - aortic incompetence – lean forwards in full expiration with diaphragm
    - mitral stenosis – lay patient on left side and listen at apex with bell
- listen to the bases of lungs for crackles
- examine for hepatomegaly
- peripheral oedema and peripheral pulses (Ball et al. 2014a, b; Barcauskas et al. 2002; Bickley and Szilagyi 2007, 2013; Cox 2010; Crawford 2014; Dains et al. 2012, 2015; Epstein et al. 2008; Hatton and Blackwood 2003; Japp 2008, 2013; Jarvis 2015;Seidel et al. 2006, 2010; Swartz 2006, 2014; Talley and O'Connor 2006, 2014).

Reference Guide: Intracardiac Values and Pressures

See Table 4.1.

Table 4.1 Intracardiac values and pressures.

Intracardiac values	
Cardiac output (CO)	$4-8\,l\,min^{-1}$
Cardiac index (CI)	$2.4-4.2\,l\,min^{-1}\,m^{-2}$
Stroke volume (SV)	$60-120\,ml$
Stroke volume index (SVI)	$35-70\,ml\,beat^{-1}\,m^{-2}$
Left cardiac work (LCW)/left cardiac work index (LCWI)	$3.4-4.2\,kg\,m\,m^{-2}$
Left ventricular stroke work (LVSW)/	$LVSW = 50-60\,g\text{-}m\,m^{-2}$
left ventricular stroke work index (LVSWI)	
right cardiac work (RCW)/right cardiac work index (RCWI)	$RCW = 0.54-0.66\,km\text{-}m\,m^{-2}$
Right ventricular stroke work (RVSW)/	
right ventricular stroke work index (RVSWI)	$RVSWI = 7.9-9.7\,g\text{-}m\,m^{-2}$
Systemic vascular resistance (SVR)	$900-1600\,dyn\,s^{-1}\,cm^{-5}$
Pulmonary vascular resistance (VR)	$20-120\,dyn\,s^{-1}\,cm^{-5}$
Mixed venous saturation (SvO$_2$)	75%
Delivery of oxygen (DO$_2$)	$900-1100\,ml\,min^{-1}$
Consumption of oxygen (VO$_2$)	$200-290\,ml\,min^{-1}$
Oxygen extraction ratio (OER)	0.22–0.30
Intracardiac pressures	
Central venous pressure (CVP)	$0 - +8\,mmHg$ (right atrial level)
Right ventricle (RV)	$0 - +8\,mmHg$ diastolic
	$+15 - +30\,mmHg$ systolic
Pulmonary capillary wedge pressure (PCWP)	
	$+5 - +15\,mmHg$
Left atrium (LA)	$+4 - +12\,mmHg$
Left ventricle (LV)	$+4 - +12\,mmHg$ diastolic
	$+90 - +140\,mmHg$ systolic
Aorta	$+90 - +140\,mmHg$ systolic
	$+60 - +90\,mmHg$ diastolic
	$+70 - +105\,mmHg$ mean

Case Study of a 62-Year-Old Male with History of Hypertension Presenting with Complaints of Fatigue and Light-Headedness for Past 48 Hours

Presenting Problem/History

A 62-year-old male presents to nurse practitioner with complaints of fatigue and dizziness for past two days. He also states he has had some intermittent chest fluttering. He considers himself to be healthy, is active, and plays tennis twice weekly. He is a nonsmoker. He was diagnosed with high BP five years ago and has been well managed on an angiotensin-converting enzyme (ACEI) inhibitor.

Differential Diagnosis

Anaemia, MI, arrhythmias, hypotension, upper respiratory infection

Assessment Including Labs/Other

Vitals: BP 150/82 T 98.8 RR 18 SAO2 96% Pulse 140 and irregular. No murmurs, gallops, rubs, or extra heart sounds. Lungs are clear to auscultation. 12-lead EKG reveals a narrow complex tachycardia with an irregularly irregular rhythm, with no discernible P waves.

Diagnosis

Atrial fibrillation

Treatment Plan

Transesophageal echocardiogram to rule out embolus formation and thus appropriateness of cardioversion because symptoms present < 48 hours. Concern with cardioversion is the possibility of dislodging a clot in the LV leading to cerebral vascular accident (stroke), thus the recommendation is to convert only for symptoms less than 48 hours. If present more than 48 hours, patient will require anticoagulation for three weeks before cardioversion becomes an option. Labs: thyroid levels, complete metabolic panel, coagulation studies, complete blood count. Beta blocker or nondihydropyridine calcium channel blocker considered drug of choice for long-term rate control in patients with paroxysmal, persistent, or permanent atrial fibrillation. If above medical therapies fail, AV nodal ablation is an alternative option.

Case Study of a 67-Year-Old Obese White Male with Increased Shortness of Breath (SOB), Dyspnoea on Exertion, and Fatigue

Presenting Problem

Complaint of a 'cough that has gotten worse' and 'unable to lie flat to sleep'. History of hypertension (HTN), smoking (80 pack-years), and obesity. No known drug allergies. Has not seen a medical provider in over a year and states 'I often forget to take my blood pressure

medication'. This patient has not had pneumococcal or yearly influenza vaccines. 12-lead ECG reveals atrial fibrillation and chest X-ray shows cardiomegaly with some fluid in bases.
Current medications:
Amlodipine 5 mg QD

Differential Diagnosis
Asthma, CHF, chronic obstructive pulmonary disease (COPD), emphysema, MI, pneumonia

Assessment Including Labs/Other
Ht: 182.88 cm; Wt: 104.5 kg;
Vitals: BP: 174/88, P: 96, T: 37.4 °C, RR: 30, SaO2: 93% on RA
Skin: pale pink; extremities are cool to touch
Cardiovascular: pulses diminished, 1+ bilaterally, and irregular; S_3 gallop; mild JVD; capillary refill > 3 sec; 2+ pitting oedema in lower legs and feet
Respiratory: SOB and dyspnoea with exertion; crackles in bases on inspiration; orthopnoea
Neuro: fatigue; some weakness in extremities
Gastrointestinal/genitourinary (GI/GU): abdomen soft, but slightly distended; no hepatosplenomegaly; decreased appetite

Diagnosis
CHF

Treatment Plan

- Echocardiogram
- Labs (BNP, CMP, CBC, PT/INR, thyroid function tests, LFTs, cholesterol, HgbA1C, ABG, U/A)
- Treat atrial fibrillation
- Medications to start:
  - ACEI and/or angiotensin receptor blocker (ARB; losartan is a medication frequently prescribed as an ARB. It works well in controlling high blood pressure – hypertension.)
  - Diuretic (if potassium wasting, will need K^+ replacement)
  - Beta blocker (metoprolol or carvedilol)
  - Anticoagulation therapy
  - May need a statin if cholesterol/triglycerides are high (Atorvastatin or Simvastatin) and antidiabetic agent (Metformin) if HgbA1C > 6.5%
- Cardiac stress test
- Daily weights
- Monitor daily fluid intake
- Low sodium/cardiac diet
  - Meet with nutritionist
- Smoking cessation
- Avoid alcohol

References

Ball, J., Dains, J., Flynn, J. et al. (2014a). *Seidel's Guide to Physical Examination*, 8e. St. Louis: Mosby.
Ball, J., Dains, J., Flynn, J. et al. (2014b). *Student Laboratory Manual to Accompany Seidel's Guide to Physical Examination*, 8e. St. Louis: Mosby.

Barkauskas, V., Baumann, L., and Darling-Fisher, C. (2002). *Health and Physical Assessment*, 3e. London: Mosby.

Bickley, L. and Szilagyi, P. (2007). *Bates' Guide to Physical Examination and History Taking*, 9e. Philadelphia: Lippincott.

Bickley, L. and Szilagyi, P. (2013). *Bates' Guide to Physical Examination and History Taking*, 11e. New York: Wolters Kluwer/Lippincott Williams & Wilkins.

Brown, E., Collis, W., Leung, T., and Salmon, A. (2002). *Heart Sounds Made Easy*. Edinburgh: Churchill Livingstone.

Collins-Bride, G. and Saxe, J. (2013). *Clinical Guidelines for Advanced Practice Nursing – An Interdisciplinary Approach*, 2e. Burlington, MA: Jones and Bartlett Learning.

Cox, C. (2010). *Physical Assessment for Nurses*, 2e. Oxford: Wiley Blackwell.

Crawford, M. ed. (2014). *Current Diagnosis and Treatment: Cardiology*, 4e. New York: McGraw-Hill Education.

Dains, J., Baumann, L., and Scheibel, P. (2012). *Advanced Health Assessment and Clinical Diagnosis in Primary Care*, 4e. St. Louis: Elsevier.

Dains, J., Baumann, L., and Scheibel, P. (2015). *Advanced Health Assessment and Clinical Diagnosis in Primary Care*, 5e. St. Louis: Mosby.

Epstein, O., Perkin, G., de Bono, D., and Cookson, J. (2008). *Clinical Examination*, 4e. London: Mosby.

Fihn, S., Gardin, M., Abrama, J. et al. (2012). Guideline for the diagnosis and management of patients with stable ischemic heart disease. *J. Am. Coll. Cardiol.* 60 (24): 1–121.

Hatton, C. and Blackwood, R. (2003). *Lecture Notes on Clinical Skills*, 4e. Oxford: Blackwell Science.

Japp, A. and Robertson, C. (2013). *Macleod's Clinical Diagnosis*. Edinburgh: Churchill Livingstone, Elsevier.

Jarvis, C. (2008). *Physical Examination and Health Assessment*, 5e. St. Louis: Saunders.

Jarvis, C. (2015). *Physical Examination and Health Assessment*, 7e. Edinburgh: Elsevier.

Martini, F., Ober, W., Nath, J. et al. (2014). *Visual Anatomy and Physiology*, 2e. San Francisco: Benjamin Cummings.

Morse, C. (2017). Cardiovascular System. In: *Family Nurse Practitioner & Adult-Gerontology Nurse Practitioner* (ed. A. Rundio and W. Lorman), 99–118. New York: Wolters Kluwer.

Riley, J. (2002). Chapter 7: The ECG: its role and practical application. In: *Cardiac Nursing a Comprehensive Guide* (ed. R. Hatchett and D. Thompson). Edinburgh: Churchill Livingstone.

Seidel, H., Ball, J., Dains, J., and Benedict, G. (2006). *Mosby's Physical Examination Handbook*. St. Louis: Mosby.

Seidel, H., Ball, J., Dains, J., and Benedict, G. (2010). *Mosby's Physical Examination Handbook*, 7e. St. Louis: Mosby-Year Book.

Swartz, M. (2006). *Physical Diagnosis, History and Examination*, 5e. London: W. B. Saunders.

Swartz, M. (2014). *Physical Diagnosis: History and Examination*, With Student Consult Online Access, 7e. London: Elsevier.

Talley, N. and O'Connor, S. (2006). *Clinical Examination: a Systematic Guide to Physical Diagnosis*, 5e. London: Churchill Livingstone.

Talley, N. and O'Connor, S. (2014). *Clinical Examination: a Systematic Guide to Physical Diagnosis*, 7e. London: Churchill Livingstone, Elsevier.

Tortora, G. and Derrickson, B. (2012). *Principles of Anatomy and Physiology*, 13e. Oxford: Wiley.

Chapter 5

Examination of the Respiratory System

Carol Lynn Cox and Jessica Ham

Introduction

The respiratory assessment constitutes an essential aspect in evaluating the patient's health. Functions of the respiratory system involve the exchange of oxygen and carbon dioxide in the lungs and tissues and regulation of the acid–base balance. Changes in the respiratory system affect other systems.

Anatomy and Physiology

Anatomy and physiology of the respiratory system are complex. Comprehensive coverage of the anatomy and physiology of the respiratory system in this chapter is not feasible. Therefore, it is recommended the reader access a text which specifically addresses, comprehensively, the anatomy and physiology of the respiratory system. In this section of the chapter, a brief overview of the anatomy and physiology of the respiratory system is presented.

The respiratory system is divided into an upper and lower respiratory system which comprises the basic function of breathing: moving air in and out of the body (Martini et al. 2012). Located outside of the thoracic cavity, the upper respiratory system is composed of the nose, nasal cavity, nasal sinuses, and pharynx, which filter, warm, and humidify air during inspiration and cool and dehumidify air during expiration. These components are composed of cartilage, ligaments, and muscles. Within this system, the larynx produces sound which is termed phonation (Martini et al. 2012). Directly below the trachea and primary bronchi air is conveyed to and from the lungs. The lungs are enclosed in a pleural membrane called the visceral membrane. There is a pleural membrane which also lines the thoracic cavity. This is called the parietal membrane. Enclosed within the visceral membrane, the lungs are seen as paired organs with two lobes on the left and three lobes on the right. Air moves through the lower respiratory tract which is composed of the trachea, bronchi, bronchioles, alveolar ducts, and alveoli. In the alveoli, the gaseous exchange of oxygen and carbon dioxide occurs. Both external and internal respiration permit gaseous exchange termed pulmonary ventilation. Pulmonary ventilation is the exchange of air between the atmosphere and the lungs.

Physical Assessment for Nurses and Healthcare Professionals, Third Edition. Edited by Carol Lynn Cox.
© 2019 John Wiley & Sons Ltd. Published 2019 by John Wiley & Sons Ltd.

This activity consists of pressure changes involving muscle movement, respiratory rate, and volume (Martini et al. 2012). Actual gaseous exchange is dependent on the partial pressures of gases and the diffusion of molecules at the cellular level. Oxygen is transported by binding to haemoglobin. Carbon dioxide is transported in three ways as carbonic acid, bound to haemoglobin, and/or dissolved in plasma. Neurons in the medulla oblongata and pons of the brain along with respiratory reflexes control respiration itself. It should be noted that respiratory function declines with age (Martini et al. 2012). For further information regarding the older adult refer to Chapter 15.

104

General Examination

- Examine the patient for:
  - signs of respiratory distress (tachypnoea, dyspnoea, nasal flaring, use of accessory muscles, cyanosis, patient leans forwards and uses pursed lip breathing, inability to speak without pausing)

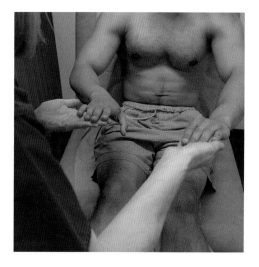

Assess the hands and nails for cyanosis

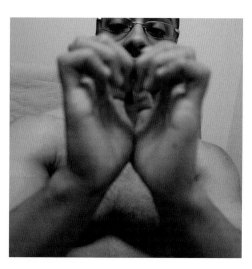

Check for clubbing

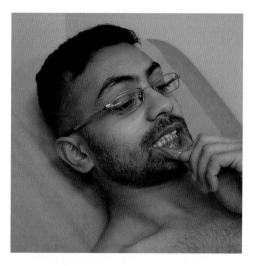

Assess the mucosa for cyanosis

- ○ nicotine on fingers, fingernails, and along the hairline in light haired individuals
- ○ clubbing: respiratory causes include:

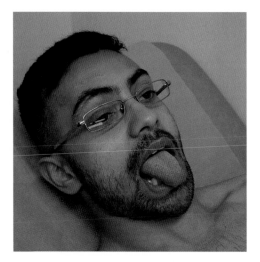

Assess the tongue for cyanosis

- ○ intrathoracic tumours:
  carcinoma of bronchus
  mesothelioma
  cystic fibrosis
- ○ bronchiectasis
- ○ lung abscess
- ○ empyema
- ○ fibrosing alveolitis
- ○ chronic obstructive pulmonary disease (e.g. emphysema)
- ○ mixed venous to arterial shunts
- ○ chronic hepatic fibrosis
- • evidence of respiratory failure:
  - ○ hypoxia: central cyanosis, seen on the lips, tongue (versus peripheral cyanosis seen on the fingers and nail beds)
  - ○ hypercapnia: drowsiness, confusion, papilloedema, warm hands, bounding pulse, dilated veins, coarse tremor/flap
- • respiratory rate: count per minute (note normal or abnormal rate)
- • pattern of respiration:
- • Cheyne–Stokes (causes):
  - ○ alternating hyperventilation and apnoea
  - ○ severe increased intracranial pressure of the brainstem
  - ○ left ventricular failure
  - ○ high altitude
  - ○ congestive heart failure
  - ○ uremia
- • Biot's – ataxic breathing:
  - ○ unpredictable irregularity (respirations may be shallow or deep and are interrupted by periods of apnoea – seen in neurologic disease/disorders)
- • hyperventilation or Kussmaul respiration:
  - ○ increases in both rate and depth (hyperpnoea is an increase in depth only – seen in exercise, anxiety, and metabolic acidosis; Kussmaul is hyperventilation associated with metabolic acidosis)

- tachypnoea:
  - rapid, shallow breathing >24 breaths per minute (seen in restrictive lung disease, pleuritic chest pain, elevated diaphragm, acute illnesses, and pneumonia)
- air trapping:
  - present in pulmonary diseases (as air is trapped in the lungs, respiratory rate rises and breathing becomes shallow)
- positional dyspnoea
  - orthopnoea: inability to lie flat when breathing. The individual must sit or stand in order to breathe deeply or comfortably. (seen in congestive heart failure, severe asthma, emphysema, mitral valve disease, chronic bronchitis, neurologic disease)
  - trepopnoea: dyspnoea when lying on one side but not on the other – lateral recumbent position. (seen in congestive heart failure: patient is more comfortable breathing whilst lying on one side)
  - platypnoea: shortness of breath (breathlessness) that is relieved when lying down and worsens when sitting or standing up. It is the opposite of orthopnoea. (seen in neurologic disease, cirrhosis causing intrapulmonary shunts, hypovolaemia, status post pneumonectomy)
- obstructive airways disease:
  - pursed-lip breathing:
    - expiration against partially closed lips
  - chronic obstructive airways disease to delayed closure of bronchioles
  - use of accessory muscles:
    - sternomastoids
    - strap muscles and platysma muscles
- wheezing (Consider inspiratory versus expiratory.):
  - bronchospasm
  - asthma (crackles and rhonchi)
  - allergy
  - congestive heart failure
  - tumour
  - obstruction (wheezing/respiratory sounds are absent below the obstruction)
  - chronic obstructive pulmonic disease
- stridor: partial obstruction of trachea
  - hoarse voice:
    - abnormal vocal cords
    - or recurrent laryngeal palsy
- cough:
  - haemoptysis (coughing up blood)
  - sputum production (chronic/productive related to chronic bronchitis, bronchiectasis, abscess, bacterial pneumonia, tuberculosis)
  - dry/hacking (viral infection, interstitial lung disease, allergies, tumour)
  - barking (epiglottal disease such as croup)
  - morning ('smoker's cough')
  - nocturnal (postnasal drip, congestive heart failure)
  - when eating or drinking (neuromuscular disease of the upper oesophagus)
- sleep apnoea: characterised by daytime fatigue, sleepiness, disruptive snoring, episodic upper airway obstruction, nocturnal hypoxemia (Ball et al. 2014a, b; Barkauskas et al. 2002; Bickley and Szilagyi 2013; Cox 2010; Hatton and Blackwood 2003; Kacmarck et al. 2017; Swartz 2006, 2014).

First examine the front of the chest fully and then similarly examine the back of the chest.
- Landmarks to locate the lungs (Figures 5.1–5.3):
  - manubrium of the sternum
  - sternal angle (angle of Louis)
  - sternum
  - xiphoid process
  - sternal notch or jugular notch
  - costal angle
  - clavicles
  - scapulae
  - spinous processes
  - acromial processes (Ball et al. 2014a, b; Barkauskas et al. 2002; Bickley and Szilagyi 2013; Cox 2010; Hatton and Blackwood 2003; Japp and Robertson 2013; Jarvis 2008, 2015; Swartz 2006, 2014)
- Demarcation lines of the thorax (Figures 5.4–5.6):
  - used to identify and describe the location/condition of underlying organs/sounds

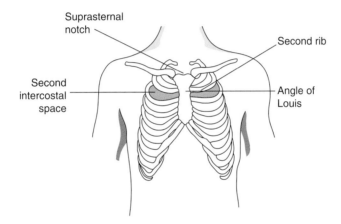

Figure 5.1   Anterior and posterior landmarks to locate the lungs. Reproduced with permission.

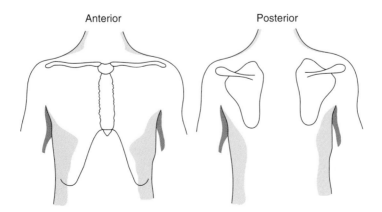

Figure 5.2   Anterior and posterior landmarks to locate the lungs. Reproduced with permission.

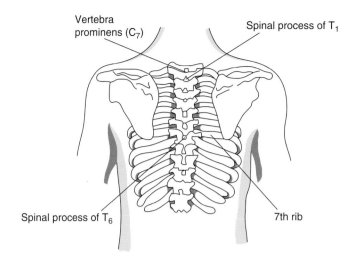

Figure 5.3 Anterior and posterior landmarks to locate the lungs. Reproduced with permission.

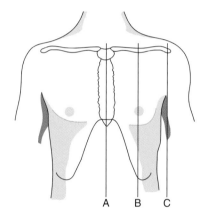

Figure 5.4 Demarcation lines of the thorax. (a) Midsternal line; (b) Midclavicular line; (c) Anterior axillary line (left) or left anterior line. Reproduced with permission.

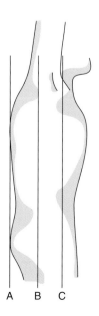

Figure 5.5 Demarcation lines of the thorax. (a) Posterior axillary line; (b) Midaxillary line; (c) Anterior axillary line. Reproduced with permission.

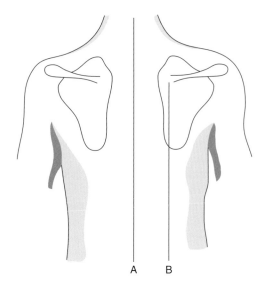

A   B

Figure 5.6   Demarcation lines of the thorax. Reproduced with permission.

Physical Assessment of the Chest

- Examination of the chest

Examination of the chest involves inspection, palpation, percussion, and auscultation. When inspecting, palpating, percussing, and auscultating, the chest terminology for charting a normal examination should reflect:

On inspection – 'breathing without difficulty' or 'normal BBS' (bilateral breath sounds).
On palpation – 'no TTP' (tenderness to palpation).
On percussion – 'clear to percussion bilaterally'.
On auscultation – 'CTAB' (clear to auscultation bilaterally) (Cox 2010).

Inspection of the Chest

- Rest the patient comfortably in the bed or examination couch/table at 45°:
- compare hemithoraces; progress from the neck down
- distended neck, puffy blue face and arms
- superior mediastinal obstruction
- tracheal shift (Cox 2010; Rhoads and Paterson 2013; Seidel et al. 2006, 2010; Talley and O'Connor 2006, 2014; Tallia and Scherger 2013)
- Inspect the shape of the chest:
  - colour, contour, and condition of the skin (ecchymosis, lesions, scars, e.g. from previous surgery)
  - asymmetry: diminution of one side or possible flail
  - lung collapse
  - fibrosis
  - deformity: check spine (Scoliosis: C or S curve often at the level of the thoracic spine; Kyphosis: curvature of the cervical spine forwards – flexion)
  - pectus excavatum: sunken sternum (congenital abnormality)
  - pectus carinatum: 'pigeon breast' (congenital abnormality)
  - barrel chest (increased anterior and posterior diameter)
  - obstructive airways disease

○ barrel chest: lower costal recession on deep inspiration; cricoid cartilage close to sternal notch; chest appears to be fixed in inspiration (Bickley and Szilagyi 2013; Cox 2010; Hatton and Blackwood 2003; Swartz 2006, 2014; Talley and O'Connor 2006, 2014).

Palpation

- Check integrity of the thorax (palpate ribs, clavicles, sternum, and scapulae for abnormalities):
  ○ crepitations (e.g. fracture or unstable sternum; also palpable under the skin in pneumothorax)
  ○ pain (over ribs in fracture versus over intercostal spaces in costochrondritis)
- Check mediastinum position:
  ○ trachea – check position: palpate with a single finger in the midline and determine if it slips preferentially to one side or the other
- Lymph nodes, supraclavicular fossae/axillae – *tuberculosis, lymphoma, cancer of the bronchus*, cancer of the breast, infraclavicular and parasternal
- Apex beat – may be displaced because of enlarged heart and not a shift in the mediastinum
- Unequal movement of chest:
  ○ Look from the end of the examination table/couch or bed.
  ○ Classic method of palpation to discern respiratory excursion:
    — extend your fingers – anchor fingertips far laterally around chest wall whilst your extended thumbs meet in the midline
    — on inspiration, assess whether there is asymmetrical movement of thumbs from midline (movement should be equal 1–2 cm)
  ○ Alternative method of palpation to discern respiratory excursion:
    — lay a hand comfortably on either side of the chest and, using these as a gauge, assess if there is diminution of movement on one side during inspiration

  N.B. Diminution of movement on one side indicates pathology on that side. In older adults respiratory excursion may be minimal to absent as anterior–posterior dimension of the thorax develops and lateral movement diminishes (Bickley and Szilagyi 2013; Cox 2010).

- Palpate intercostal spaces for abnormalities:
  ○ lumps, surgical emphysema
- Tactile fremitus:

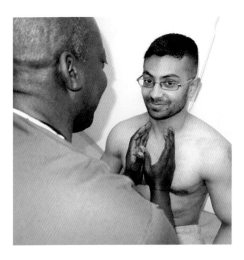

Assess for tactile fremitus

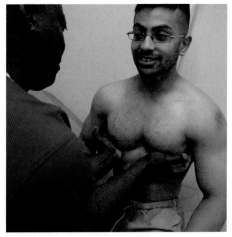

Assess for tactile fremitus. Ask the patient to say '99'. Feel the vibrations

- vocal fremitus (assessed when pathology is suspected) (Cox 2010).

Percussion

- Percuss with the middle finger (hammer finger) of one hand against the middle phalanx of the middle finger of the other, laid flat on the chest. The hammer finger should strike at right angles and the wrist of the hammer finger hand should flick with each strike. See Table 5.1 for discrimination of sounds.
- Percuss both sides of the chest for resonance, at top, middle, and lower segments. Compare sides, and if different also compare the front and back of chest (Figure. 5.7).

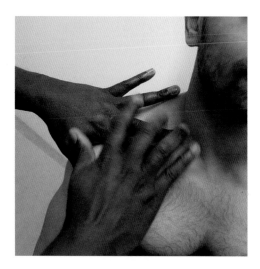

Percussion of the anterior chest

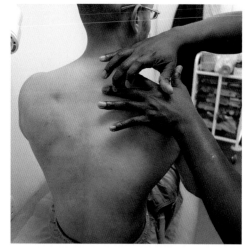

Percussion of the posterior chest

- If a dull area exists, map out its limits by percussing from a resonant to the dull area.
- Percuss the level of the diaphragm from above downwards.
  Increased resonance may occur in:
  - pneumothorax
  - emphysema.
  Decreased resonance may occur in:
  - *effusion:* very dull – sometimes called stony dullness
  - *solid lung*
    - consolidation
    - alveolar collapse
    - abscess
  - neoplasm.

Table 5.1   Discrimination of sounds.

Sound	Relative intensity	Relative pitch	Relative duration
Flatness	Soft	High	Short
Dullness	Medium	Medium	Medium
Resonance	Loud	Low	Long
Hyperresonance	Very loud	Lower	Longer
Tympani	Loud	Hollow	Hollow

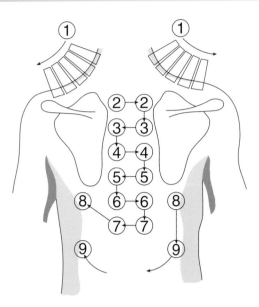

Figure 5.7   Percussion sequence of the chest. Reproduced with permission.

Remember the surface markings of the lungs when percussing. Thus, the lower lobe predominates posteriorly and the upper lobe predominates anteriorly (Figure 5.8) (Bickley and Szilagyi 2013; Cox 2010; Hatton and Blackwood 2003; Swartz 2006, 2014; Talley and O'Connor 2006, 2014).

- Determine diaphragmatic excursion (Figure 5.9) by percussing the level of the diaphragm from above downwards. Start with the patient breathing normally. Percuss downwards from the bottom of the scapula in the intercostal spaces from tympani to dullness. When dullness is heard, mark this space. Ask the patient to take a deep breath and hold it. Percuss from the marked space (tympani) to dullness. Diaphragmatic excursion should be greater on the left than on the right. (Position of the liver diminishes excursion on the right. Position of the heart increases excursion on the left.)
  - *decrease in excursion indicative of diaphragmatic paralysis (seen following cardiothoracic surgery and abdominal surgery or trauma/injury)*

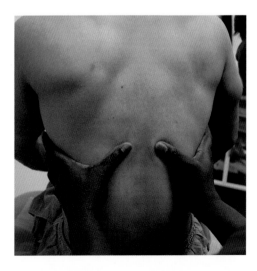

Assess for respiratory excursion

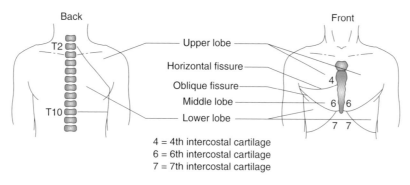

Figure 5.8   Percuss the diaphragm from above downwards. These markings are at full inspiration. Under normal examination conditions the hepatic dullness extends to the 5th intercostal cartilage.

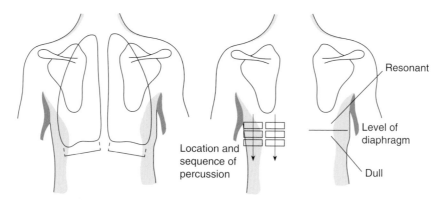

Figure 5.9   Determination of diaphragmatic excursion. Reproduced with permission.

Auscultation

- Before listening, ask patient to cough up any sputum, which may create adventitious sounds.
- Use either the diaphragm or bell of the stethoscope, dependent on the condition/ physique of the patient, and listen starting at the top (apex), middle, and bottom (base) of both sides of the chest, and then in the axilla. Auscultate downwards in approximately 5 cm distances (Figure 5.10).

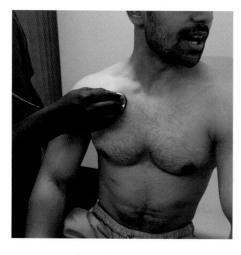

Auscultate the anterior chest

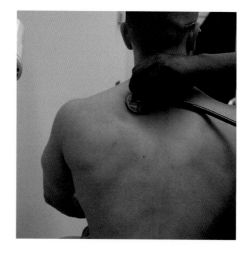

Auscultate the posterior chest. Avoid auscultation over the scapula

Ask the patient to breathe through the mouth moderately deeply. It helps to demonstrate this yourself (Cox 2010).

The bell of the stethoscope is used to hear low-pitched sounds. Hold the bell lightly on the patient's skin. If pressure is put on the bell, a diaphragm will be created and the ability to hear low-pitched sounds will be lost. In cachectic, thin patients, patients with prominent ribs or if the chest is hairy, use of the bell is more effective. Protruding ribs make placement of the stethoscope diaphragm difficult as pressure must be applied to the diaphragm in order to use it effectively (Swartz 2006, 2014).

It is not acceptable to listen to the chest through clothing. The bell/diaphragm must always be in direct contact with the patient's skin.

- Listen for normal breath sounds (Table 5.2), comparing both sides:
  - vesicular: breath sounds heard over most of the lung tissue
  - bronchovesicular: heard near the bronchi (e.g. below the clavicles and between the scapulae, especially on the right)

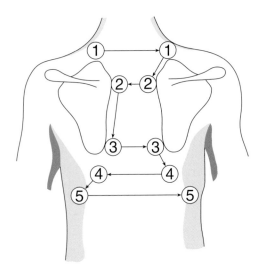

Figure 5.10   Sequence for auscultation. Reproduced with permission.

Table 5.2   Characteristics of sounds.

Breath sound	Duration of inspiration and expiration	Pitch of expiration	Intensity of expiration	Sample location
Vesicular	Inspiration longer than expiration	Low	Soft	Most of lungs
Bronchovesicular	Inspiration and expiration are equal	Medium	Medium	Near bronchi, e.g. below the clavicles and between the scapulae, especially on the right
Bronchial	Expiration longer than inspiration	Medium-high (dependent on location)	Usually high (dependent on location)	Over the lower part of the trachea
Tracheal/tubular	Expiration longer than inspiration	High	High/harsh	Over the upper part of the trachea

- bronchial: patent bronchi plus conducting tissue
- tracheal/tubular: sounds similar to sounds with stethoscope over trachea
- Listen for added sounds (adventitious sounds), and note if inspiratory or expiratory (Figure 5.11)
  - tracheal/tubular or bronchial: sounds heard in an area other than the upper or lower trachea
    - consolidation (usually pneumonia)
    - *neoplasm*
    - *fibrosis*
    - *abscess*

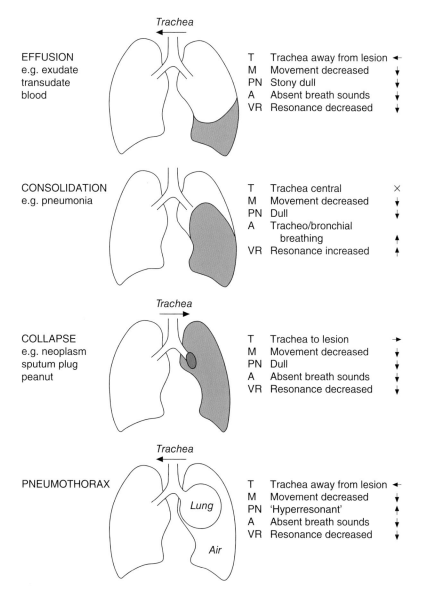

Figure 5.11   Auscultation of adventitious sounds.

- diminution: indicates either no air movement (e.g. obstructed bronchus) or air or fluid preventing sound conduction
  - effusion
  - pneumothorax
  - emphysema (early sign is atelectasis)
  - collapse – obstruction (absent breath sounds)
- crackle (outdated terms include rales, crepitations and creps): caused by either the alveoli popping open on inspiration (indicative of atelectasis) or fluid in the lungs (in which the crackling sound is heard on inspiration and expiration)
  - fine – heart failure, alveolitis, or if late on inspiration indicative of pulmonary fibrosis
  - medium – infection or fluid in the alveoli
  - coarse – air bubbling through fluid in the alveoli and larger bronchioles, e.g. bronchiectasis or pulmonary oedema
- pulmonary fibrosis (delayed crackles on inspiration – late on inspiration)
- wheeze (outdated terms include sibilant rale, musical rale, sonorous rale or low-pitched wheeze): caused by rapid airflow through a constricted airway (Consider whether the wheeze is inspiratory, expiratory, or both.)
  - asthma – note the presence of air trapping
  - chronic obstructive pulmonary disease (COPD) – note the presence of air trapping
  - bronchitis
  - cystic fibrosis
  - pulmonary oedema
  - congestive heart failure
- rhonchus: transient airway plugging caused by mucous secretions
  - bronchitis
- pleural rub: caused by *pleurisy* (inflammation of the pleura due to pneumonia or pulmonary infarction); sounds like two pieces of leather rubbing together
- stridor: high pitched sound on inspiratory caused by turbulent airflow through narrowed trachea (considered a medical emergency in epiglottitis, croup, and allergic reactions) (Bickley and Szilagyi 2013; Collins-Bride and Saxe 2013; Cox 2010; Epstein et al. 2008; Hatton and Blackwood 2003; Swartz 2006, 2014; Talley and O'Connor 2006, 2014).

Vocal Fremitus/Resonance

Should be assessed when pathology is suspected.

Speech creates vibrations that can be evaluated through feeling and hearing. The presence or absence of fremitus can provide useful information about the density of underlying lung tissue and the chest cavity. Conditions that increase density increase the transmission/frequency of tactile fremitus. Conditions that decrease the transmission of sound waves decrease tactile fremitus.

- Ask the patient to repeat '99' whilst you palpate the patient's chest with either the ulnar surface or palms of both of your hands simultaneously in the same general areas as auscultation. The frequency of vibrations is greater over areas of consolidation. Compare both sides.
- You can also auscultate for vocal resonance. Ask the patient to say 'e'.

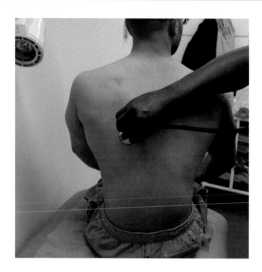

Auscultate for vocal resonance. Ask the patient to say 'e'. Listen for aegophony

- At the surface of an *effusion* the word 'e' takes on a bleating character like a goat, which is called aegophony. If vocal resonance is gross, whispered pectoriloquy can be elicited by asking the patient to whisper: '1, 2, 3' repeatedly. The whispered sound when auscultated will be loud and pronounced rather than soft and muffled (Bickley and Szilagyi 2013; Cox 2010; Hatton and Blackwood 2003; Swartz 2006, 2014; Talley and O'Connor 2006, 2014).

N.B. Vocal fremitus, breath sounds, and vocal resonance all depend on the same criteria and vary together.
To determine further clues check:

- chest movement asymmetry
- mediastinum displacement
- percussion

(Barkauskas et al. 2002; Bickley and Szilagyi 2007; Epstein et al. 2008; Hatton and Blackwood 2003; Jarvis 2008, 2015; Seidel et al. 2006; Swartz 2006, 2014; Talley and O'Connor 2006, 2015; Tallia and Scherger 2013).

Sputum

Examination of the sputum is unpleasant but important. Normally 75–100 ml of sputum is secreted daily by the bronchi.
Describe according to colour, consistency, quantity, presence or absence of blood or pus, and number of times brought up during the day and night.

- Look for:
  - colour (yellow or green suspect mucus; rust colour is from R/T enzyme release from neutrophils which occur in viruses and/or bacteria – suspect infection but this cannot be confirmed without a culture) (Tallia and Scherger 2013)
  - consistency
  - quantity (increased grossly in bronchiectasis)
  - blood (cancer, tuberculosis, embolus).

- Ideally the sputum should be examined under the microscope for:
  - bacteria
  - pus cells
  - eosinophils
  - plugs
  - asbestos (Cox 2010; Epstein et al. 2008).

Functional Result

- Make an assessment of the functional result:
  - history – exertion/exercise: for example, how far can the patient walk and how many stairs can be climbed
  - examination:
    - $Po_2 \downarrow$: central cyanosis
      - confusion
    - $Pco_2 \uparrow$: peripheral signs
      - warm periphery
      - dilated veins
      - bounding pulse
      - flapping tremor
    - central signs
      - drowsy
      - papilloedema
      - small pupils
- Check by arterial blood gases.
- Tests (usually undertaken for COPD):
  - force of expiration: blowing out a lighted match about 15 cm from the mouth and with the mouth wide open is easy as long as the patient's peak flow is above approximately $80\,l\,min^{-1}$ (normal $300–500\,l\,min^{-1}$)
  - expiration time: an assessment of airways obstruction can be made by timing the period of full expiration through wide-open mouth following a deep breath; this should be less than two seconds when normal.
  - chest expansion: expansion from full inspiration to full expiration should be more than 5 cm; reduced if hyperinflation of the chest is due to chronic obstructive airways disease
  - peak flow: a measure of airways obstruction is the peak rate of flow of air out of the lungs; a record is made using a peak flow meter; normal $300–500\,l\,min^{-1}$
  - spirometry: standard test for diagnosis (Cox 2010).

Summary of Common Illnesses
Asthma

- patient distressed, tachypnoeic, unable to talk easily
- wheeze on expiration audible or by auscultation
- overinflated chest with hyperresonance
- if central cyanosis: critically ill, artificial ventilation?
- pulsus paradoxus (variation in systolic pressure during inspiration and expiration and may be normal between attacks)

- often due to atopy
- enquire about exposure to antigens:

  ○ house dust mite
  ○ cats or dogs
  ○ chemical exposure (Cox 2010).

Pneumonia
- inflammatory condition affecting the alveoli

Bronchitis
- inflammation of the bronchi

Bronchiectasis
- chronic condition in which the walls of the bronchi are thickened from inflammation and infection of the bronchi
- abnormal widening and thickening of the bronchi and/or branches
- clubbing
- constant green/yellow phlegm
- coarse crackles over affected area

Obstructive Airways Disease (Chronic)
- also termed COPD (chronic obstructive pulmonary disease)
- barrel chest
- accessory muscles of respiration in use
- hyperresonance
- depressed diaphragm – indrawing lower costal margin on inspiration
- diminished breath sounds:

  ○ blue bloater:
    — central cyanosis
    — signs of carbon dioxide retention
    — obese
    — not dyspnoeic
    — ankle oedema: may or may not have right heart failure
  ○ pink puffer:
    — not cyanosed
    — no carbon dioxide retention
    — thin
    — dyspnoeic
    — no oedema

Allergic Alveolitis
- extrinsic – seen in farmer's lung; mushroom picker's disease; humidifier or air-conditioner lung; bird breeder's or bird fancier's lung. Diagnosed through images and bronchoscopy
- clubbing
- fine, unexplained crackles, widespread over bases (Cox 2010).

System-Oriented Examination
'Examination of the Respiratory System'

Use the techniques of inspection, palpation, percussion, and auscultation in each phase of the examination whilst examining the anterior, posterior, and lateral thorax.

- hands: clubbing, signs of increased carbon dioxide (warm hands, bounding pulse, coarse tremor)
- face: nasal flaring
- tongue: central cyanosis
- trachea: right or left shift
- supraclavicular, infraclavicular and parasternal nodes
- inspection
  - shape of chest contour
  - chest movements
  - respiration rate/rhythm/depth/distress
  - colour and condition of the skin
- palpation
  - interspaces for abnormalities
  - sternum, ribs, clavicles, and scapulae for abnormalities
  - excursion
  - vocal fremitus
- percussion: in 5 cm intervals from apex to base – upper segments (L, R), middle (L, R) and lower segments (L, R)
  - diaphragmatic excursion
- auscultation:
  - breath sounds
  - added sounds (adventitious sounds)
- if COPD:
  - expiration time (Cox 2010; Dains et al. 2012, 2015).

Case Study of a Middle-Aged Man with Shortness of Breath, Cough, and Lower Extremity Oedema

Presenting Problem/History

A 56-year-old homeless man presented to his nurse practitioner (ARNP) with a five-year history of chronic obstructive pulmonary disease. Presenting symptoms included dyspnoea, wheezing, cough, and sputum production. His respiratory rate was increased and there were apparent signs of respiratory distress including circumoral cyanosis. He stated that he could not 'catch his breath' and was 'coughing all the time'. He was shoeless with swollen legs and feet. He stated he 'could not get his shoes on'. Past medical history included asthma since a child, smoking up to two packs of cigarettes a day, alcohol consumption, and drug abuse. He stated that he had 'run out of his inhaler and can't get my shoes on'.

Differential Diagnosis

Chronic obstructive pulmonary disease and cor pulmonale. Additional diagnoses included pneumonia, bronchitis, asthma, and viral upper respiratory infections.

Assessment Including Labs/Other

On inspection the patient was gulping air; pale and clammy to touch. PO_2 was 89. His pulse was 96 beats per min, BP was 156/78 and RR was 28. Temperature was 36.9° C. FEV1/FVC < 65 by spirometer. Assessment of breath sounds included crackles in the bases and expiratory wheezing in the upper lobes. Assessment of the legs showed pitting oedema of > 4 seconds refill.

Diagnosis

COPD, cor pulmonale, asthma, and bronchitis.

Treatment Plan

Bronchodilator (the best agent for long-term treatment in asthma, COPD, and chronic bronchitis), corticosteroid (oral prednisone, which is the most helpful in acute exacerbations), antibiotic (ampicillin – recommended in acute exacerbations when there is increased cyanosis, sputum production, and sputum purulence) and diuretic (furosemide – indicated in the treatment of cor pulmonale and right-sided heart failure). Elevation of the legs, limiting sodium intake, and counselling on the use of medications and potential side effects. Follow-up at the clinic in three days unless condition worsens. If condition worsens, immediate treatment in accident and emergency (A&E/ER).

References

Ball, J., Dains, J., Flynn, J. et al. (2014a). *Seidel's Guide to Physical Examination*, 8e. St. Louis: Mosby.

Ball, J., Dains, J., Flynn, J. et al. (2014b). *Student Laboratory Manual to Accompany Seidel's Guide to Physical Examination*, 8e. St. Louis: Mosby.

Barkauskas, V., Baumann, L., and Darling-Fisher, C. (2002). *Health and Physical Assessment*, 3e. London: Mosby.

Bickley, L. and Szilagyi, P. (2007). *Bates' Guide to Physical Examination and History Taking*, 9e. Philadelphia: Lippincott.

Bickley, L. and Szilagyi, P. (2013). *Bates' Guide to Physical Examination and History Taking*, 11e. New York: Wolters Kluwer/Lippincott Williams & Wilkins.

Collins-Bride, G. and Saxe, J. (2013). *Clinical Guidelines for Advanced Practice Nursing - an Interdisciplinary Approach*, 2e. Burlington, MA: Jones and Bartlett Learning.

Cox, C. (2010). *Physical Assessment for Nurses*, 2e. Oxford: Wiley Blackwell.

Dains, J., Baumann, L., and Scheibel, P. (2012). *Advanced Health Assessment and Clinical Diagnosis in Primary Care*, 4e. St Louis: Elsevier.

Dains, J., Baumann, L., and Scheibel, P. (2015). *Advanced Health Assessment and Clinical Diagnosis in Primary Care*, 5e. St. Louis: Mosby.

Epstein, O., Perkin, G., de Bono, D., and Cookson, J. (2008). *Clinical Examination*, 4e. London: Mosby.

Hatton, C. and Blackwood, R. (2003). *Lecture Notes on Clinical Skills*, 4e. Oxford: Blackwell Science.

Japp, A. and Robertson, C. (2013). *Macleod's Clinical Diagnosis*. Edinburgh: Churchill Livingstone, Elsevier.

Jarvis, C. (2008). *Physical Examination and Health Assessment*, 5e. St. Louis: Saunders.

Jarvis, C. (2015). *Physical Examination and Health Assessment*, 7e. Edinburgh: Elsevier.

Kacmarek, R., Stoller, J., and Heuer, A. (2017). *Egan's Fundamentals of Respiratory Care*, 11e. St. Louis: Mosby.

Martini, F., Nath, J., and Bartholomew, E. (2012). *The Respiratory System in Fundamentals of Anatomy & Physiology*, 9e. San Francisco, California: Pearson Benjamin Cummings.

Rhoads, J. and Paterson, S. (2013). *Advanced Health Assessment and Diagnostic Reasoning*, 2e. Burlington: Jones and Bartlett.

Seidel, H., Ball, J., Dains, J., and Benedict, G. (2006). *Mosby's Physical Examination Handbook*. St. Louis: Mosby.

Seidel, H., Ball, J., Dains, J., and Benedict, G. (2010). *Mosby's Physical Examination Handbook*, 7e. St. Louis: Mosby-Year Book.

Swartz, M. (2006). *Physical Diagnosis, History and Examination*, 5e. London: W. B. Saunders.

Swartz, M. (2014). *Physical Diagnosis: History and Examination*, With Student Consult Online Access, 7e. London: Elsevier.

Talley, N. and O'Connor, S. (2006). *Clinical Examination: A Systematic Guide to Physical Diagnosis*, 5e. London: Churchill Livingstone.

Talley, N. and O'Connor, S. (2014). *Clinical Examination: A Systematic Guide to Physical Diagnosis*, 7e. London: Churchill Livingstone, Elsevier.

Talley, N. and O'Connor, S. (2015). *Clinical Examination*, 8e. Edinburgh: Churchill Livingstone.

Tallia, A. and Scherger, J. (2013). *Swanson's Family Practice Review*, 6e. St Louis: Mosby.

Chapter 6

Examination of the Abdominal System

Anthony McGrath

Introduction

An abdominal assessment constitutes an essential aspect in evaluating the patient's health. Changes in the function of organs within the abdomen affect other systems. This chapter highlights and discusses the anatomy and physiology of the gastrointestinal (GI) tract and also takes you through a detailed physical assessment of the abdominal system. By understanding the role and function of the GI tract you are better placed to understand the signs and symptoms exhibited in abdominal disease as well as having a firmer grasp of the organs you are examining during the examination.

Anatomy and Physiology

The Gastrointestinal Tract

The GI tract is a muscular tube which is controlled by the autonomic nervous system. It is approximately 9 m in length and is made up of the mouth, pharynx, oesophagus, stomach, duodenum, jejunum, small and large intestines, the rectum, and anal canal. Food is digested and absorbed and waste products are then excreted from the tract. As food travels through the tract it is subjected to various digestive fluids and enzymes. The enzymes and fluids are secreted by the salivary glands, stomach, small intestine, pancreas, and liver. It is this secretion of fluids that helps maintain the function of the tract (Martini et al. 2012).

There are four layers:

1. adventitia
2. muscularis
3. submucosa
4. mucosa.

Physical Assessment for Nurses and Healthcare Professionals, Third Edition. Edited by Carol Lynn Cox.
© 2019 John Wiley & Sons Ltd. Published 2019 by John Wiley & Sons Ltd.

Adventitia

The adventitia or outer layer consists of a serous membrane made up of a simple squamous epithelium and a supporting layer of connective tissue. In the abdomen it is called the visceral peritoneum and forms a portion of the peritoneum where it is the largest serous membrane of the body.

The visceral peritoneum covers the external surfaces of most abdominal organs, including the intestine. There is a potential space between the visceral and parietal layers known as the peritoneal cavity. It contains serous fluid. In patients with liver disease serous fluid can enter this cavity; this is referred to as ascites (Japp and Robertson 2013; Jarvis 2015).

Muscularis

In general, throughout the GI tract the muscularis is made up of two layers of smooth muscle, which contract in a wave-like motion. However, this is not the case in the mouth, pharynx, or upper oesophagus, which is made up of skeletal muscle.

Longitudinal and circular fibres make up the two smooth muscle layers. Longitudinal fibres can be found in the outer layer and circular fibres on the inner layer. As these two layers contract food is propelled forwards and mixed with the digestive secretions which help break it down. This motion is referred to as peristalsis. As the muscle constricts and narrows it forces anything in front of the narrowing to move forwards. Within the two layers, blood and lymph vessels as well as the nerve supply to the GI tract can be found. The nerve supply is referred to as the mesenteric or Auerbach's plexus and it consists of both sympathetic and parasympathetic nerves which control GI motility (Martini et al. 2012).

Submucus Layer

The submucus layer is highly vascular and is made up of connective tissue and elastic fibres. It houses the blood vessels, nerves, lymph vessels, and tissue. It also contains the submucosal or Meissner's plexus, which control secretions within the GI tract (Martini et al. 2012).

Mucosa

The mucosa forms the inner lining of the GI tract and is made up of three layers:

1. a layer of epithelium which acts as a protective layer in the mouth and oesophagus and has secretory and absorption function throughout the rest of the tract;
2. the lamina propria which supports the epithelium by binding it to the muscularis and consists of loose connective tissue that contains blood and lymph vessels;
3. the muscularis mucosae layer, which is made up of smooth muscle fibres (Martini et al. 2012).

The Mouth

The digestive process begins in the mouth. When food is placed into the mouth the teeth and tongue work together to reduce the food to small particles.

The Tongue

The tongue is divided into two halves of skeletal muscles both intrinsic and extrinsic and it is covered by a mucus membrane. The extrinsic muscles include the hyoglosssus, styloglossus, and genioglossus, and the intrinsic muscles include the transversus linguae, longitudinalis superior, longitudinalis inferior, and verticalis linguae (Martini et al. 2012).

The extrinsic muscles enable the tongue to move from side to side as well in and out. The intrinsic muscles help form the size and shape of the tongue. The underside of the tongue is divided in the midline by the lingual frenulum and at the base of the tongue it is attached to the hyoid bone. The superior surface and sides of the tongue consist of papillae, which contain nerve endings that are concerned with taste, called taste buds (Martini et al. 2012; Tortora and Derrickson 2012).

There are three types of papillae on the tongue:

1. circumvallate papillae (vallate papillae)
2. fungiform papillae
3. filiform papillae.

Circumvallate papillae, the largest of the papillae, are found near the base of the tongue and are arranged in an inverted V shape. Fungiform papillae are usually located along the tip and the edges of the tongue. Filiform papillae are the smallest and are usually found laid out in parallel rows along the anterior two-thirds of the tongue.

When food enters the mouth it becomes moistened with saliva, which consists of water, lingual lipase, bicarbonate, lysozyme, and the enzyme salivary amylase, which initiates starch digestion. Nerve endings in the mouth relay information to the brain via the glossopharyngeal and vagus nerves, which control the swallowing mechanism.

Moistened and reduced food is then passed into the stomach via the oesophagus, which is a muscular tube measuring approximately 25 cm. At the opening to the stomach the oesophagus narrows and forms the gastro-oesophageal or cardiac sphincter. This sphincter relaxes during swallowing to allow food to pass into the stomach and then closes again to prevent regurgitation of gastric contents back into the oesophagus (Martini et al. 2012; Tortora and Derrickson 2012).

The Stomach

The principal function of the stomach is the digestion of proteins and further maceration of food whilst mixing it with a colourless liquid that contains hydrochloric acid, pepsin, and, in infants, rennin, which is secreted from the gastric mucosa. The mixing process is assisted by peristaltic waves that occur every 15–25 seconds. Hydrochloric acid is necessary for the conversion of pepsinogen to active pepsin. Pepsin is responsible for the digestion of proteins. It does this by breaking down amino acids into peptides. This process reduces the food into a liquid called chyme before it moves on to the duodenum. The amount of chyme passing into the duodenum is controlled by what can be processed by the small intestine. This control is achieved in three ways, first by reducing the level and intensity of the peristaltic contractions, second by the enterogastric reflex, and third by the secretion of hormones. The enterogastric reflex inhibits gastric secretion and motility and it is controlled by nerve impulses that travel to the medulla from the duodenum. The hormones secretin, cholecystokinin, and gastric inhibiting peptide (GIP) are released in response to the contents of chyme (Martini et al. 2012; Tortora and Derrickson 2012).

The Pancreas

The pancreas is attached to the duodenum and it can be found lying posterior to the greater curvature of the stomach. As chyme enters the duodenum secretin is released, which stimulates the pancreas to secrete its juices. These juices then pass through the ducts and into the duodenum. They aid in the digestive process by neutralising the acid content of chyme (Martini et al. 2012; Tortora and Derrickson 2012).

The Liver

The liver is the largest organ of the body and is designed to maintain the body's chemical and metabolic homeostasis. It weighs about 1.5 kg and can be found in the right hypochondrium. It extends into the epigastric region. The liver consists of four lobes: the right, left, caudate, and quadrate lobes. The falciform ligament divides the liver into right and left lobes. Two small caudate and quadrate lobes are squeezed between the right and left lobes on the visceral surface. The liver is wrapped in a tough fibrous capsule that is covered by layer of visceral peritoneum. The liver's 'portal' circulation is made up of veins that drain blood from the stomach, spleen, pancreas, and gall bladder. Venous blood from the GI organs flow to the liver before returning to the heart. This allows blood rich in nutrients and other substances to be processed by the liver. This unique process facilitates the liver in sorting out the various substances before releasing them into the general circulation (Martini et al. 2012; Tortora and Derrickson 2012).

In the case of ingestion of toxic substances, the liver works to detoxify them, thus rendering them harmless to the body. The liver consists of hepatocytes which form a series of irregular plates arranged like a spoke of a wheel. Digested nutrients are absorbed into the mesenteric veins which in turn drain into the portal vein. This then drains into the sinusoids before emptying into the central vein. The lining of the sinusoids consists of endothelial cells and a large number of Kupffer cells, which are specialised macrophages that defend against unwanted microbes that have managed to bypass the body's first line of defences in the bowel. Blood enters the sinusoids from small branches of the portal vein and the hepatic artery. As blood flows through the hepatocytes they absorb solutes from plasma and secret plasma proteins (Martini et al. 2012; Tortora and Derrickson 2012).

Blood then leaves the sinusoids and enters central veins, which in turn merge to form the hepatic vein which then empties its contents into vena cava. Pressures in the portal system are usually around 10 mmHg or less. If pressure increases because of damage or a clot, portal hypertension occurs. If the flow is obstructed a backlog occurs. Then the veins in the portal system can become overfilled and engorged. This can be seen when a patient suffers from cirrhosis. Because of the obstruction caused by liver damage, pressures build up in the portal system causing portal hypertension. This usually occurs in the oesophagus, which can lead to its blood vessels bursting, resulting in a massive haemorrhage. Patients will vomit large amounts of blood that require emergency treatment to control if the patient is to survive (Martini et al. 2012; Tortora and Derrickson 2012).

The Gall Bladder

The gall bladder is pear shaped. It consists of a fundus, body, and neck and is located in the fossa that divides into the right and quadrate lobes. Its function is to concentrate and store bile. Bile is produced in the liver and then passes from the hepatic ducts into the cystic duct prior to entering the gall bladder for storage. When fatty foods are detected in the duodenum the hormone cholecystokinin is secreted. This causes the gall bladder to contract thus pushing bile into the duodenum to emulsify the fatty food (Martini et al. 2012; Tortora and Derrickson 2012).

The Duodenum, Jejunum, Ileum, and Caecum (Small Intestine)

The main function of the small intestine is digestion and absorption as it coils through the central and lower aspects of the abdominal cavity. It joins the large intestine at the ileocaecal valve. It is approximately 6.5 m long and has a diameter of approximately 2.5 cm. The nerve supply for the small bowel is both sympathetic and parasympathetic. Walls of the small intestine consist of the same four layers as the rest of the GI system. However, both the mucosal and submucosal layers are modified. The mucosal layer consists of glands which are lined with glandular epithelium. These glands secrete intestinal juices. The submucosa in the duodenum contains glands that secrete alkaline mucus, which is designed to protect the small intestine walls from the acid contained in chyme. It also stops the enzymes from digesting its walls. Throughout the small intestine's length, the epithelium is made up of simple columnar epithelium which contains both goblet and absorptive cells. The absorptive cells contain fingerlike projections known as microvilli which allow the small intestine to cope with large volumes of digested nutrients by increasing the overall surface area. There are approximately 20–40 villi per mm^2. These cells enclose a network of blood and lymphatic capillaries. The surface area of the small intestine is further increased by the presence of the circular folds which are approximately 10 mm high. As chyme moves through the small intestine it twists around the folds, which further assists the digestive and absorptive process as it is broken into small molecules that can be transported across the epithelium and into the bloodstream. Within the small intestine chyme moves at approximately 1 cm per min and can remain in the small intestine for up to eight hours. Digestion is completed in the small intestine with the aid of juices from the liver and pancreas. Waste matter is then transported to the large intestine for disposal. The superior mesenteric artery supplies the whole of the small intestine. Venous blood is drained by the superior mesenteric vein that links with other veins to form the hepatic portal vein (Martini et al. 2012; Tortora and Derrickson 2012).

The small intestine also plays a critical role in water and acid–base balance as it absorbs water and electrolytes (sodium, chloride, potassium) and glucose, amino acids, and fatty acid from chyme. Throughout the small intestine there are numerous lymph nodes contained in the mucus membrane that occur at irregular intervals. The nodes are either solitary lymphatic follicles or aggregated lymphatic follicles (Peyer's patches) that occur in groups (Martini et al. 2012; Tortora and Derrickson 2012).

The Duodenum

The duodenum is approximately 25 cm in length and curves around the head of the pancreas. In the midsection of the duodenum there is an opening from both the pancreas and the common bile duct. This opening is controlled by the sphincter of Oddi (Martini et al. 2012; Tortora and Derrickson 2012).

The Jejunum

This is approximately 2.5 m in length and extends to the ileum.

The Ileum

This is the terminal part of the small intestine, which terminates at the ileocaecal valve. It measures about 3.5 m in length. The ileum will usually empty approximately 1.5 l of fluid (chyme) into the large intestine daily.

The Caecum

The small intestine terminates at the posteromedial aspect of the caecum. The caecum is fixed to the right side near the iliac crest. At the opening to the caecum there is a fold of mucus membrane known as the ileocaecal valve, which allows the passage of materials from the small intestine into the large intestine and prevents the reflux of contents from the colon back into the ileum. The caecum is dilated and has been described as a blind pouch approximately 6 cm in width and 8 cm in length. It is continuous with the ascending colon superiorly and has a blind end inferiorly. Attached to the caecum is a coiled tube called the vermiform appendix that is closed at one end. It is usually 8–13 cm in length although this can vary from 2.5 to 23 cm and has the same structure as the walls of the colon; however, it contains more lymphatic tissue than other structures in the intestine (Martini et al. 2012; Tortora and Derrickson 2012).

The Large Intestine (Colon)

The large intestine is so called because of its ability to distend. It is divided into four sections: the ascending colon, transverse colon, descending colon, and sigmoid colon.

Its main function is to absorb water and to expel waste products from the body. The large intestine is approximately 1.5 m in length and extends from the ileum to the anus. Its diameter decreases gradually from the caecum where it is approximately 7 cm to the sigmoid where it is approximately 2.5 cm in diameter. The large intestine houses a variety of bacteria. These bacteria live happily in the bowel and play an important part in digestion as they synthesise a number of vitamins such as vitamin K and some B vitamins. They are also responsible for breaking down bilirubin into urobilinogen. This causes faeces to have their characteristic brown colour.

Blood supply to the large intestine is mainly by the superior and inferior mesenteric arteries. The internal iliac arteries supply the rectum and anus. Venous drainage is mainly via the superior and inferior mesenteric veins, whereas the rectum and anus are drained by the internal iliac veins. Nerves supplying the large intestine are via the sympathetic and parasympathetic nerves. The external anal sphincter is under voluntary control and is supplied by motor nerves from the spinal cord (Martini et al. 2012; Tortora and Derrickson 2012).

Ascending Colon

The ascending colon is approximately 15 cm long and joins the caecum at the ileocaecal junction. The ascending colon is covered with peritoneum anteriorly and on both sides; however, its posterior surface is devoid of peritoneum. It ascends on the right side of the abdomen to the level of the liver where it bends acutely to the left. It is at this point that it forms the right colic or hepatic flexure to become the transverse colon (Martini et al. 2012; Tortora and Derrickson 2012).

Transverse Colon

The transverse colon is a loop measuring approximately 45 cm long that continues from the left hepatic flexure across to the left side of the abdomen to the left colic flexure. It passes in front of the stomach and duodenum and then curves beneath the lower part of the spleen on the left side as the left colic or splenic flexure where it then passes acutely downwards as the descending colon (Martini et al. 2012; Tortora and Derrickson 2012).

Descending Colon

The descending colon passes downwards on the left side of the abdomen to the level of the iliac crest. It is approximately 25 cm in length. The descending colon is narrower and more dorsally situated than the ascending colon (Tortora and Derrickson 2012; Martini et al. 2012).

Sigmoid Colon

The sigmoid colon begins near the iliac crest and is approximately 36 cm long and ends at the centre of the midsacrum, where it becomes the rectum at about the level of the 3rd sacral vertebra. It is mobile and is completely covered by peritoneum and attached to the pelvic walls in an inverted V shape.

Rectum

The rectum is approximately 13 cm in length. It lies in the posterior aspect of the pelvis and ends 2–3 cm anterioinferiorly to the tip of the coccyx where it bends downwards to form the anal canal. When faeces reach the rectum the stretch receptors contained in the rectal wall transmit signals to the brain informing it of the presence of faeces (Martini et al. 2012; Tortora and Derrickson 2012).

Anal Canal

The anal canal is the terminal segment of the large intestine. It is approximately 4 cm in length; opening to the exterior as the anus. The mucus membrane of the anal canal is arranged in longitudinal folds that contain a network of arteries and veins. The anus remains closed at rest. The anal canal corresponds anteriorly to the bulb of the penis and in the female the lower vagina and posteriorly it is related to the coccyx. The internal anal sphincter is composed of smooth muscle and is slightly higher than the external sphincter. It is about 2.5 cm long and can be palpated during rectal examination. It controls the upper two thirds of the canal. The external sphincter is made up of skeletal muscle and is normally closed except during elimination of faeces. Its nerve supply is from the perineal branch of the 4th sacral nerve and the inferior rectal nerves (Martini et al. 2012; Tortora and Derrickson 2012).

General Examination

Before commencing your abdominal examination, introduce yourself to the patient as this will allow you to establish a rapport and allow you to identify the patient to be examined. Ensure you maintain privacy and the patient's dignity by screening the examination couch/table/bed by closing the curtains and/or the door. You should ensure that the patient can be assessed in good light as this will allow you a better opportunity to note any abnormalities (Amico and Barbarito 2016; McGrath 2010). In order to conduct a detailed assessment of the patient they will need to be exposed from their nipples to their knees. Therefore, it is important that you maintain their dignity by covering them with a sheet as much as possible. Inform the patient of what you are going to do and obtain their consent prior to commencing the examination. Stand on the patient's right as this will enable you to easily determine the span of the liver (Amico and Barbarito 2016; Ball et al. 2014a, b; Bickley and Szilagyi 2013; McGrath 2010; Ranson et al. 2014; Thomas and Monaghan 2014).

Your history should have alerted you to any specific problems that you will need to explore further such as dyspepsia, vomiting, dysphagia, pain, bleeding, or an altered bowel habit. The symptoms and signs noted in GI disease usually reflect disorders in the main abdominal organs (McGrath 2010).

Abdominal Pain

Pain is probably one of the most significant symptoms in abdominal problems and whilst it will vary greatly depending on the cause, by carefully considering the nature of pain you can gain some insight as to what may be wrong with the patient. Visceral pain is caused by increased tension on the splanchnic nerves contained in the muscular wall. It is common in obstructive lesions and it is sometimes colicky in type. Referred pain is usually caused by the abdominal viscera being irritated by an inflamed organ or a neoplasm. Peritoneal pain is associated with a deep tenderness and often with muscular rigidity. As part of your assessment you need to consider the character of the pain. Is it just a mild discomfort or is it severe? Ask what aggravates or relives the pain. Ask about duration, whether it comes on after or before meals. Pain that is of short duration is more likely due to an obstructive cause. Ask about any associated symptoms such as nausea and vomiting, sweating, or a temperature (Ball et al. 2014a, b; Bickley and Szilagyi 2013; Dains et al. 2012, 2015; Douglas et al. 2013; Japp and Robertson 2013; Ranson et al. 2014; Talley and O'Connor 2013; Thomas and Monaghan 2014).

Before you begin your examination, it is important for the patient to be relaxed as much as possible as tense muscles will hinder your examination. Ensure that the room is warm. Ask the patient to empty their bladder. This has a twofold effect: (i) it will make them more comfortable and (ii) it allows you the opportunity to test the urine. Ask the patient to lie flat, arms loosely by their sides and their head resting on a pillow, as this will allow the abdominal muscles to relax. By propping another pillow under the patient's knees, the patient is made more comfortable (McGrath 2010). Do not allow the patient to place their hands above their heads as this action stretches and tightens the abdominal wall making examination more difficult (Ball et al. 2014a, b; Bickley and Szilagyi 2013; Douglas et al. 2013; Epstein et al. 2008; Japp and Robertson 2013; Jarvis 2015; McGrath 2010; Ranson et al. 2014; Thomas and Monaghan 2014).

Your examination should follow a straightforward format.

- Inspection

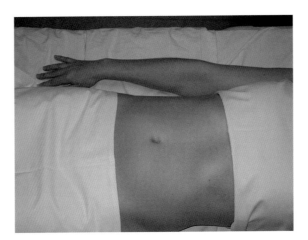

Inspect the abdomen

- Auscultation (Note that in examination of the abdomen it is important to auscultate before percussing and palpating as percussion and palpation can alter bowel sounds.)

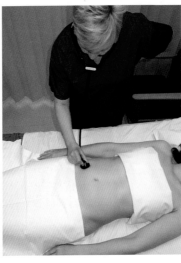 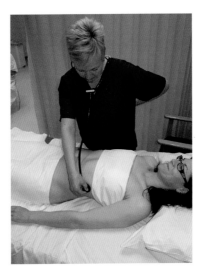

Auscultate the abdomen in four quadrants   Auscultate the spleen

- Percussion

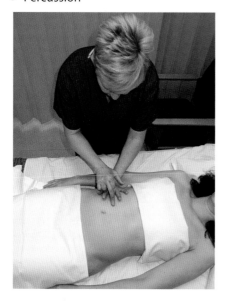

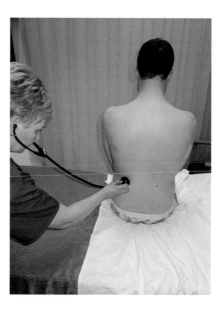

Percuss the abdomen in nine quadrants

Auscultation of the renal artery

- Palpation

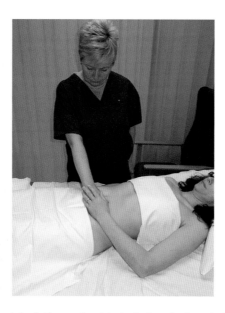

With 'ticklish patients' ask the patient to help by placing their hand over yours

Inspection

Conduct a systematic inspection of the patient. This involves a generalised inspection followed by a more detailed inspection. Any abnormalities detected on inspection will provide you with clues to any underlying pathology which can be investigated further during auscultation, percussion, and palpation. Before you begin your inspection take and record the patient's pulse and note its rate and regularity. A tachycardia may suggest infection or internal bleeding whereas atrial fibrillation may be linked to emboli lodging in the mesenteric arteries which in turn can lead to bowel ischaemia and the patient presenting with severe abdominal pain (Ball et al. 2014a, b; Bickley and Szilagyi 2013; Douglas et al. 2013; Epstein et al. 2008; Japp and Robertson 2013; Jarvis 2015; Ranson et al. 2014; Talley and O'Connor 2013; Thomas and Monaghan 2014).

To begin your inspection ask yourself does the patient look well or do they look ill? Stand at the foot of the couch/table/bed as this will allow you to gain an overview of the symmetry and shape of the abdomen. The normal abdomen is concave and symmetrical. It will rise and fall in line with respiration. Look for signs of peristalsis. Note the skin colour and condition. Is the skin jaundiced, dry, or bruised or does it have scratch marks?

During your inspection note the presence of any surgical scars as these may provide information regarding previous pathology. If the patient has striae (stretch marks), note the colour. If silvery in appearance this can be due to the patient previously losing weight or a result of pregnancy. Striae that are purplish/pink and wider may be indicative of Cushing's syndrome which is caused by the excessive secretion of cortisol (Bickley and Szilagyi 2013; Douglas et al. 2013; Jarvis 2015; McGrath 2010; Ranson et al. 2014; Talley and O'Connor 2013; Thomas and Monaghan 2014).

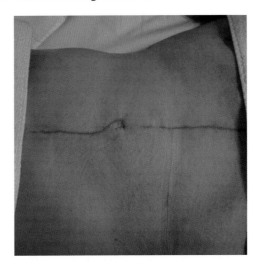

Assess the condition of healing incisions

Now squat down so that you can view the abdomen tangentially. You will need to do this from both sides. It is important that you do this in good light. In this position you can more easily pick out subtle changes of shadow and contour. Asymmetrical movement may indicate the presence of a mass.

Now inspect the patient's face and then work your way down the body. If the patient is jaundiced this is best seen in the sclera and in the oral mucosa. Whilst inspecting the eyes note the presence of Kayser-Fleischer rings. These are brownish-greenish rings which are visible at the periphery of the cornea. They are caused by copper deposits and a sign of Wilson's disease. Now look at the conjunctivae for signs of anaemia.

Whilst inspecting the face note the presence of brown freckles 1–5 mm in diameter on lips or buccal mucosa which may indicate Peutz–Jeghers syndrome. The freckles can also be seen on fingers; another feature of this syndrome is polyps in the small bowel that can give rise to abdominal pain, bleed, or intussusception or become malignant (Ball et al. 2014a, b; Bickley and Szilagyi 2013; Dains et al. 2015; Douglas et al. 2013; Jarvis 2015; Ranson et al. 2014; Talley and O'Connor 2013; Thomas and Monaghan 2014).

Note the presence of telangiectasia (Figure 6.1), which are small, widened blood vessels on the skin. They are usually harmless and have been associated with sun exposure. However, they are also linked with poor flow to the vessels and may be caused by alcohol abuse, pregnancy, and aging. They can also be found in the intestines, which can bleed.

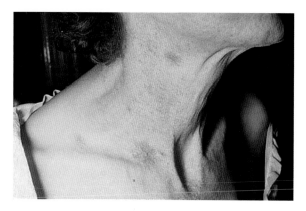

Figure 6.1   Spider naevi in cirrhosis – telangiectasia radiating from central arteriole.

Now with a pen torch (pen light) inspect around and inside the mouth. A dry tongue may be indicative of 'dehydration' or mouth-breathing. If the patient appears dehydrated, check for Maxwell's sign (lift fold of skin on forehead above the nose between the eyebrows). The skin fold remains raised in patients who are dehydrated. Look at the lips – are they cracked or sore? Reddish brown cracks radiating from the corners of the mouth are indicative of angular stomatitis, which is caused by vitamin B6, B12, folate, and iron deficiency (Bickley and Szilagyi 2013; Japp and Robertson 2013; Jarvis 2015; McGrath 2010; Ranson et al. 2014; Talley and O'Connor 2013; Thomas and Monaghan 2014).

Note the colour of the lips and mouth. If you note any cyanosis it is important to determine if it is peripheral or central. Simply ask the patient to stick out their tongue. If the tongue is a normal colour and moist, then the patient has peripheral cyanosis. You need to warm them up. However, if the tongue and mucosa are discoloured (blue to purple in colour) it may be indicative of central cyanosis or chronic liver disease from pulmonary arteriovenous shunting (Ball et al. 2014a, b; Bickley and Szilagyi 2013; Douglas et al. 2013; Jarvis 2015; Ranson et al. 2014; Talley and O'Connor 2013; Thomas and Monaghan 2014).

Whilst the patient is sticking out their tongue, note the presence of a red tongue and whether it has creamy white curdlike patches as this is indicative of candidiasis. However, if you do note white coloured lesions on the tongue or in the mouth this may be due to leukoplakia, which is a premalignant condition. The presence of glossitis which presents as a smooth red tongue is indicative of B12, folate, and iron deficiency. Note that in patients with B12 or folate deficiency the tongue is painful whereas in iron deficiency the patient experiences no pain (McGrath 2010).

Note any breath odours as these can be indicative of underlying problems. A faecal smell may be linked to obstruction, whereas patients with hepatic failure may have a sickly sweet odour on their breath. The presence of an alcohol smell may indicate the need to explore for liver problems (Ball et al. 2014a, b; Bickley and Szilagyi 2013; Thomas and Monaghan 2014).

As you are looking into the mouth note any gingivitis or ulcers. In patients with Crohn's disease ulcers may be seen at the corners of the mouth or they may be caused by ill-fitting dentures. Poor dental hygiene may also lead to gingivitis. Furring of the tongue can occur in patients who smoke, are taking antibiotics, or have GI problems (Thomas and Monaghan 2014).

As you inspect the neck note the presence of any enlarged nodes in the left supraclavicular fossa which may indicate a malignancy in the GI tract. A hard node felt behind the left sternoclavicular joint may be a Virchow's node and suggests an abdominal neoplasm spread by lymphatics via the thoracic duct (Figure 6.2). A large left supraclavicular node in association with carcinoma of the stomach is known as Troisier's sign (Bickley and Szilagyi 2013; Douglas et al. 2013; Jarvis 2015; Thomas and Monaghan 2014).

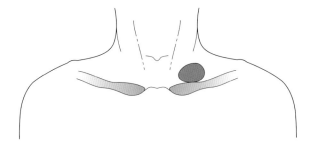

Figure 6.2   Virchow's node.

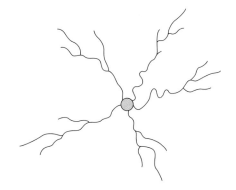

Figure 6.3   Spider naevus: a small collection of capillaries fed by a central arteriole.

Now look at the chest. Is there the normal distribution of hair? Males with liver disease may present with gynaecomastia. Also in males, poor hair distribution over the trunk is linked with patients with alcoholic liver disease. Patients with liver disease may also present with a loss of axillary and chest hair. However, please bear in mind the current fashion of removing body hair. Note the presence of spider naevi which are dilated blood vessels and are linked to pregnancy, malnutrition, and liver disease (Figure 6.3). In pregnancy they usually appear between the 2nd and 3rd trimesters and usually disappear following the birth. However, the presence of more than five of them is considered abnormal and may be linked to cirrhosis (Bickley and Szilagyi 2013; Douglas et al. 2013; Jarvis 2015; Thomas and Monaghan 2014).

Normally, the abdomen is concave and symmetrical and moves gently with respiration. However, if the abdomen is distended this may be due to one of the 5 Fs: flatus, faeces, fetus, fat, or fluid. Localised swellings may indicate the enlargement of an abdominal or pelvic organ. If you note a swelling, try to determine if it moves with or is independent of respiration. Bulging around scars may indicate the presence of an incisional hernia (Bickley and Szilagyi 2013; Douglas et al. 2013; Jarvis 2015; Thomas and Monaghan 2014).

As you inspect the abdomen note the presence of any dilated or engorged veins in the abdominal wall. Veins are rarely prominent in healthy individuals. If you can see them it is important to determine whether it is abnormal or not. You can do this by determining the flow of blood within the vein. This is done by placing two fingers onto the vein (Figure 6.4). By doing this you are applying pressure and preventing the flow of blood. Now slide one finger along the vein thus creating a gap between your two fingers. By doing this you empty the vein. Now lift the finger you slid away from the other finger and observe if the vein refills and if so from which direction. If the blood flow below the umbilicus flows up towards the umbilicus it may be due to inferior vena cava obstruction. If the flow of blood is downwards away from the umbilicus this may be due to portal vein hypertension (Bickley and Szilagyi 2013; Douglas et al. 2013; Epstein et al. 2008; Jarvis 2015; McGrath 2010; Thomas and Monaghan 2014).

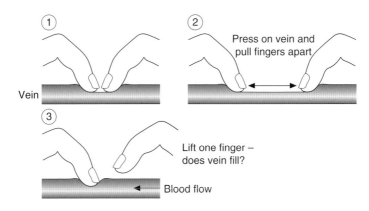

Figure 6.4 William Harvey's method of checking vein filling.

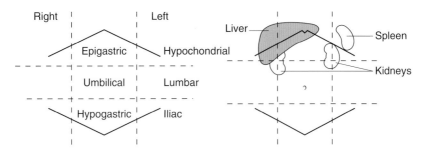

Figure 6.5 Nine abdominal quadrants and location of organs in epigastric, hypochondrial, and lumbar regions.

If there is visible peristalsis this is not usually normal. However, it may be visible in very thin patients. Demonstrative (hyperactive) peristalsis can be indicative of pyloric obstruction or obstruction of the distal small intestine. If you think it is a possible pyloric obstruction you will need to test for a succession splash. To do this, first make sure that the patient has been nil by mouth for at least three hours. Once this has been established gently shake the patient's abdomen by holding either side of the pelvis. If you hear a splashing noise either with the naked ear or with the chest piece of a stereoscope placed just above the umbilicus, this is a positive sign. The patient is likely to have a pyloric obstruction (Bickley and Szilagyi 2013; Douglas et al. 2013; Jarvis 2015; McGrath 2010; Thomas and Monaghan 2014) (Figure 6.5).

Note the presence of an expansile pulsation in the epigastric region as this may be caused by an aortic aneurysm. If your patient is aged 60 years or more, smokes, and has hypertension you may wish to consider this if you note a pulsation in the abdomen (McGrath 2010).

Note any discoloration on the abdominal wall. A bluish discoloration or ecchymosis in either the flank (Grey Turner's sign) or around the periumbilical area (Cullen's sign) is caused by the seepage of blood-stained ascetic fluid into the subcutaneous tissue and is seen in acute haemorrhagic pancreatitis or a retroperitoneal haemorrhage. Whilst looking at the umbilicus note the presence of a hernia. The umbilicus is normally located within 1 cm of the midpoint between the xiphoid and the symphysis pubis. It you note any deviation of more than 1 cm you will need to palpate this area as it may be displaced by an underlying mass (Bickley and Szilagyi 2013; Jarvis 2015; Thomas and Monaghan 2014).

Inspect the patient's hands to look for signs of palmar erythema. Although it can be a normal finding it is usually found in pregnancy and in chronic liver disease. When inspecting the nails note any pitting, ribbing, and brittleness, which are linked to malabsorption syndromes. The presence of koilonychia (spoon-shaped spongy nails) are indicative of iron deficiency anaemia. Leukonychia or white nails occurs in liver failure or hypoalbuminaemia.

A Dupuytren's contracture is a visible and palpable thickening and contraction of the palmar fascia. It causes a permanent flexion and is generally associated with alcohol abuse; however, it can also be found in manual workers. Look at the fingers and note any clubbing, which is caused by inflammatory bowel disease or coeliac disease. Ask the patient to hold their arms outstretched with their wrists dorsiflexed for a minimum of 20 seconds to elicit whether they have a liver flap (asterixis). A liver flap is an irregular coarse tremor that occurs in liver failure (Bickley and Szilagyi 2013; Jarvis 2015; Thomas and Monaghan 2014).

As you inspect the arms note any bruising or scratch marks as excessive bruising may indicate a clotting abnormality and scratch marks suggest that the patient has pruritus, which is symptom of cholestatic jaundice (McGrath 2010).

Auscultation

Auscultation will provide information about bowel motility. Therefore, it is important to listen to the bowel before performing palpation or percussion as they can alter the frequency of bowel sounds. Bowel sounds are caused by intestinal peristalsis moving gas and fluid through the bowel. Place the diaphragm of the stereoscope on the abdomen. Listen over the abdomen for about 10–15 seconds. If sounds are difficult to hear listen for up to seven minutes. Normal bowel sound can be heard as gurgles and clicks. Borborygmi are prolonged gurgling sounds, the sounds you hear when your stomach rumbles (Bickley and Szilagyi 2013; Jarvis 2015; Thomas and Monaghan 2014).

In progressive bowel obstruction large amounts of fluid and gas accumulate and hyperactive 'tinkling' bowel sounds can be heard. This is an ominous sign of impending bowel paralysis. Paralytic ileus or generalised peritonitis gives complete absence of bowel sounds. Listen for hepatic bruits in patients with liver disease. A soft and distant bruit heard over an enlarged liver is always abnormal and may indicate primary liver cell cancer, alcoholic hepatitis, or acquired arteriovenous shunts from biopsy or trauma (Bickley and Szilagyi 2013; Jarvis 2015; Thomas and Monaghan 2014).

Arterial Bruits

If appropriate from the history or examination (e.g. the patient has high blood pressure), listen for bruits over the renal, iliac, and femoral arteries (Figure 6.6). Renal arteries are sometimes best heard over the back. Renal artery stenosis may be the cause of hypertension. Patients with intermittent claudication may have flow bruits over the femoral arteries from narrowing, e.g. atheroma (McGrath 2010).

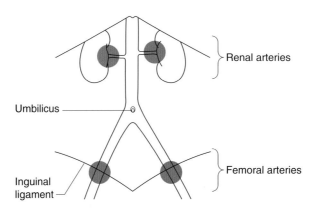

Figure 6.6   Auscultation sites for arterial bruits.

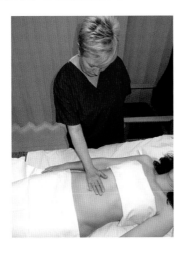

Light palpation of the epigastric area

Palpation

Before you feel or palpate the patient's abdomen ask 'Is your abdomen painful anywhere?' Get the patient to point to where the pain is worst. Ask whether the pain radiates anywhere and its onset and duration. Ensure your hands are warm. Tell the patient to inform you if it hurts when you begin to palpate. In order to elicit the most information it is important that you palpate in two stages: first, light palpation as this will allow you to identify any tenderness and second, deep palpation which will allow for the detection of deeper masses. It also allows for any masses previously found to be defined.

To begin lightly palpate 1–3 cm in depth in each quadrant, starting away from the site of pain or tenderness. Your hand should be flat on the patient's abdomen. Palpate each abdominal quadrant in turn using the palmar surface of the fingers as this will allow you to mould your hand to the shape of the abdominal wall. Be gentle. As you palpate look at the patient's face to see if palpation is hurting the patient or causing any discomfort. Note any tenderness which may be superficial, deep, or rebound. Rebound tenderness will be exhibited when inflamed viscera in peritonitis move against the parietal peritoneum. Note any guarding, which is a voluntary muscle spasm to protect from pain. The patient may lie on their side with knees flexed to prevent stretching of the abdominal wall. In peritonitis, for example, stretching of the abdominal wall causes the patient to experience pain (McGrath 2010).

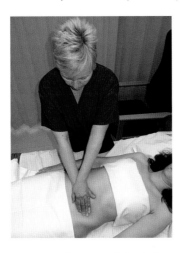

Deep palpation of the left
lumbar area

Now perform deeper palpation. Press deeply 4–6 cm and evenly into the abdominal wall. Muscle rigidity along with distention is suggestive of peritonitis. As you palpate the abdomen note any masses and if a mass is found, describe the site, size, shape, consistency (e.g. faeces may be indented by pressure), fixation, or mobility. Does it move on respiration? Note if it is tender or pulsatile, which is the transmitted pulsation from the aorta or pulsatile swelling. Note if it is dull to percussion. This is particularly important to determine if bowel is in front of mass. Note if the mass is present after defecation or micturition.

Liver and Gall Bladder

Now palpate for the liver edge (Figure 6.7). Start about 10 cm below the costal margin and work up towards the ribs. You can use your fingertips or two hands or if you prefer the radial side of your index finger on one hand. Ask the patient to take a deep breath. As the patient takes a deep breath press your fingers inwards and upwards. At the height of the patient's inspiration slightly relax your inward pressure whilst maintaining the upward pressure. The liver should descend and as it does so, the liver edge should slide under your fingers. In healthy individuals the liver edge can usually be palpated just below the costal margin. Describe position of liver edge in centimetres below the costal margin of the midclavicular line. Liver enlargement is described as mild, moderate, or massive. If enlarged, feel the shape of liver edge to determine whether the edge is firm or hard, regular/irregular, tender, or pulsatile (in tricuspid incompetence). If the liver is large remember to palpate for the spleen as the presence of a palpable spleen suggests cirrhosis with portal hypertension. Percuss the upper and lower borders of liver after palpation to confirm findings (Bickley and Szilagyi 2013; Jarvis 2015; McGrath 2010; Thomas and Monaghan 2014).

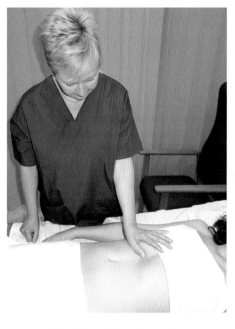

Palpation of the liver edge

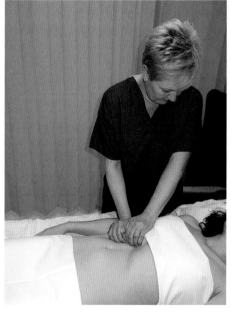

Palpation of the liver edge by 'hooking'

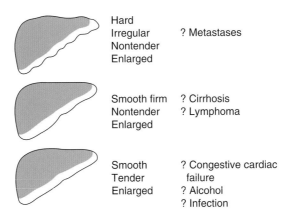

Hard
Irregular   ? Metastases
Nontender
Enlarged

Smooth firm   ? Cirrhosis
Nontender   ? Lymphoma
Enlarged

Smooth   ? Congestive cardiac
Tender   failure
Enlarged   ? Alcohol
               ? Infection

Figure 6.7 Examination of the liver.

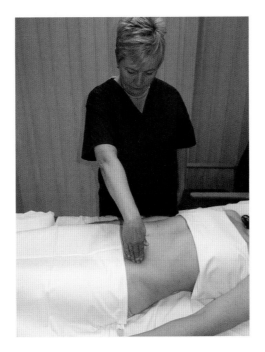

Assess for rebound tenderness

Conclude your liver palpation by feeling for the gall bladder. The fundus can normally be found where the rectus muscle intersects with the costal margin (tip of 9th costal cartilage). Ask the patient to take a deep breath and using the tips of your fingers, apply firm pressure. If the gall bladder is inflamed the patient will exhibit tenderness, guarding, and intense pain as your fingers make contact with the gall bladder (Murphy's sign). If your patient has jaundice and the gall bladder is palpable then the cause is most likely to be a malignancy (Courvoisier's law).

Spleen

The normal spleen cannot be felt and becomes palpable only when it has doubled/trebled in size (Figure 6.8). Ask the patient to take deep breaths, as air-filled lungs push the spleen down so it can be palpated. Roll the patient onto their right side with his left arm

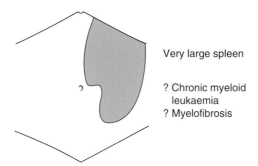

Very large spleen

? Chronic myeloid
  leukaemia
? Myelofibrosis

Figure 6.8 Splenic enlargement.

hanging loosely in front as your examining hand is gently worked up towards the left costal margin. If the spleen is not palpable, percuss area for splenic dullness. The spleen can be enlarged to the hypogastrium. Common causes of splenomegaly include portal hypotension, malaria, haemolytic anaemia, and leukaemia. If you can feel the spleen it is important to note the size and shape (Can you feel the splenic notch?); whether you can feel above it or whether it moves on respiration. You will describe your findings as you do for the liver (Bickley and Szilagyi 2013; Jarvis 2015; McGrath 2010; Thomas and Monaghan 2014).

Groin

Now palpate the spermatic cord, lymph nodes, and arteries that occupy the groin. Swellings here are usually caused by hernias or enlarged lymph nodes. Palpate the groin to detect enlarged lymph nodes. Most people have small, shotty nodes. Most enlarged tender nodes arise from infection in the legs or feet. However, in some Afro-Caribbean men this is normal. If large nodes are felt, palpate the spleen carefully (reticulosis or leukaemia) (McGrath 2010).

Hernia

When checking for the presence of a hernia examine the patient standing and ask them to cough. An enlargement of a swelling in the groin is highly suggestive of a hernia. With an indirect (oblique) inguinal hernia the swelling can be reduced to the internal inguinal ring by applying pressure on the contents of hernial sac and then controlled by pressure over the internal ring when the patient is asked to cough. When your hand is removed, the impulse passes medially towards the external ring and is palpable above the pubic tubercle. In patients with a direct inguinal hernia the impulse is felt in a forward direction mainly above the groin crease medial to the femoral artery. Swelling is not controlled by pressure over the internal ring (Bickley and Szilagyi 2013; Jarvis 2015; McGrath 2010; Thomas and Monaghan 2014).

Kidneys and Bladder

The kidneys are difficult to feel. Deep bimanual palpation is required to explore them. This is achieved by placing one hand under the back and the other on the front of the loin. Ask the patient to take deep breaths as you ballot the kidney. As they do so push up with left hand in the renal angle and feel kidney anteriorly with right hand (this is termed 'cupping'). Getting the patient to take a deep breath will bring the kidneys between your hands.

A common sign of infection is tenderness over the kidneys. The presence of a large kidney may indicate a tumour (e.g. polycystic disease or hydronephrosis). To assess further for kidney tenderness, you can check for costal-vertebral angle tenderness. Ask the patient to sit forwards and place the palm of your hand over the renal angle. Then using the ulnar surface of your other hand, make a fist and strike your hand placed on the patient's renal angle with moderate force. Perform on each kidney in turn and assess the patient's reaction. This should not cause any pain unless there is some inflammation of the kidney (McGrath 2010).

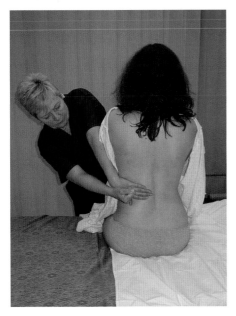 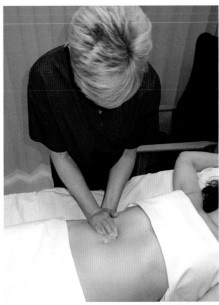

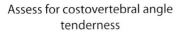

Assess for costovertebral angle   Cupping of the right kidney
tenderness

Palpate for the bladder in the hypogastric area and if a mass is found, percuss to confirm the presence of fluid. If the patient is suffering from urinary retention a full bladder may be felt above the pubic symphysis. As you palpate the patient will feel uncomfortable and will want to pass urine. Therefore ensure your patient has emptied their bladder before you perform this manoeuvre.

Aorta

Palpate in the midline above the umbilicus for a pulsatile mass. If easily palpated, suspect aortic aneurysm and proceed to ultrasonography in males over 60 and women over 65 years. As you inspect the patient note any bobbing of the head with each pulsation of the aorta (de Musset's sign). De Musset's sign is indicative of coarctation of the aorta. Refer to Chapter 4, Examination of the Cardiovascular System, for more information regarding this sign.

Percussion

It is important to percuss all four quadrants for dullness and tympany (Figure 6.9). Good percussion technique will allow you to assess the amount and distribution of gas in the abdomen. It will also allow you to determine the size of the liver and spleen.

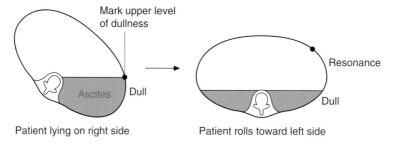

Figure 6.9 Shifting dullness.

Dull sounds are normal over solid organs; however, any dull sound is abnormal is the middle of the abdomen. If dullness is noted in areas other than over a solid organ note the presence of ascites and consider a possible cause such as a mass (e.g. large ovarian cyst). Percuss over liver, spleen, and kidneys and percuss over any suspected mass. The midline of the abdomen should be resonant. If not, think of gastric neoplasm, omental secondaries, enlarged bladder, ovarian cyst, pregnancy. If you note a generalised swelling or distention of the abdomen lay the patient on one side and mark the upper level of dullness. Roll the patient flat and see if the level shifts. If it does, this is referred to as shifting dullness. Note that in ascites there is central tympani and lateral dullness. In ovarian tumour, there is central dullness and lateral tympani as the gas-filled bowel is pushed laterally (McGrath 2010).

Examination of Genitals

Ask in a sensitive way before you proceed. For example, 'I should briefly examine you down below. Is that all right?' In the male, palpate the scrotum for the testes and epididymis. It is rarely necessary to examine the penis unless the patient complains of a rash, discharge, or ulceration. However, tender and enlarged testes may occur with orchitis or torsion of the testis. A large, soft swelling which transilluminates suggests hydrocele or an epididymal cyst. A hydrocele surrounds the testis; an epididymal cyst lies behind the testis. A large, hard, painless testis suggests cancer. On inspection of the penis if you note the presence of balanitis (inflamed glans of penis) this should remind you to check for diabetes (McGrath 2010).

Digital Rectum Examination

- Tell the patient at each stage what you are going to do.
- Lay the patient on the left side with knees flexed to the chest.
- Say: 'I am going to put a finger into your back passage.'
- Inspect the anus for lumps, haemorrhoids, fissures, ulcers, inflammation, excoriation, and discolouration. A bluish discolouration of perineal skin may be indicative of Crohn's disease.
- With lubricant on the examination glove, press your fingertip against the anal verge then gently slip your forefinger into the anal canal and then into the rectum. Feel the tone of the sphincter by asking the patient to squeeze your finger with their anal muscles; then check the size and character of the prostate and any lateral masses. If appropriate, proceed to proctoscopy.
- Test stool on your glove for occult blood.

Per Vaginam Examination

- Tell the patient at each stage what you are going to do.
- Lay the patient on her left side as for per rectum examination (although some nurses prefer the patient lying on her back with hips flexed and knees abducted. Note that this position is difficult for the older adult to maintain and uncomfortable.)
- Inspect the external genitalia.
- With lubricant on the examination glove insert one finger into vagina and then a 2nd finger if there is room. (If a smear must be taken, this should be done before bimanual palpation is undertaken.)
- Palpate the cervix (check for cervical excitation, which is present in pelvic inflammatory disease).
- Examine for the position and enlargement of the uterus, tenderness of appendages and masses.
- Check for discharge by observing the glove.

143

Summary of Common Illnesses
Cirrhosis

- leukonychia
- clubbing
- palmar erythema
- spider naevi
- jaundice
- firm liver

Portal Hypertension

- splenomegaly
- ascites
- caput medusa

Hepatic Encephalopathy

- liver flap
- drowsy
- constructional apraxia (cannot draw five-pointed star)
- musty fetor

'Dehydration' (Water and Salt Loss)

- dry skin
- veins collapsed
- diminished skin turgor – pinched fold of skin on forehead remains raised (Maxwell's sign)
- tongue dry
- eyes sunken
- blood pressure low with postural drop

Intestinal Obstruction

- patient 'dehydrated' if they have been vomiting
- abdomen centrally swelling
- visible peristalsis
- not tender (unless inflammation or some other pathology)
- resonant to percussion
- high-pitched 'tinkling' bowel sounds

Pyloric Stenosis
- otherwise like intestinal obstruction
- may have 'succussion splash' on shaking abdomen
- upper abdomen swelling

Appendicitis
- slight fever
- deep tenderness right iliac fossa or per rectum-
- otherwise little to find unless has spread to peritonitis

Peritonitis
- lies still
- abdomen:
- does not move on respiration
- rigid on palpation (guarding)
- tender, particularly on removing fingers rapidly (rebound tenderness)
- absent bowel sounds
- tender right hypochondrium, particularly on breathing in (Murphy's sign – tender gall bladder descends on inspiration to touch your palpating hand)

Jaundice and Palpable Gall Bladder
- obstruction is not due to gallstones but from another obstruction such as neoplasm of the pancreas (Courvoisier's law); gallstones have usually caused a fibrosed gall bladder which cannot dilate from back pressure from gallstones in common bile duct

Enlarged Spleen
- infective, e.g. septicaemia or subacute bacterial endocarditis
- portal hypertension, e.g. cirrhosis
- lymphoma
- leukaemia and other haematological diseases
- autoimmune, e.g. systemic lupus, Felty's syndrome

Case Study of Young Female with Acute Appendicitis

Presenting Problem/History

A 19-year-old clinically obese female presented in the emergency department with a four-day history of abdominal pain which has now localised to the right iliac fossa. The patient stated that the pain was constant and that it was aggravated by moving or coughing. She also complained of feeling nauseous and exhibited a low-grade pyrexia. There was no history of any previous bowel or urinary symptoms. The patient had all her childhood vaccinations and had not travelled overseas in the past two years. There was no family history of note. Furthermore, the patient was not taking any medication other than some over the counter painkillers which she took when she first experienced the pain.

Differential Diagnosis
It is important to rule out any other causes of abdominal pain which include constipation, inflammatory bowel disease, acute cholecystitis, perforated ulcer, diverticulitis, gastroenteritis, GI obstruction, pancreatitis, urinary tract infection, renal calculi, pelvic inflammatory disease, ectopic pregnancy, and ovarian cyst.

Assessment Including Labs/Other

On carrying out a physical examination the patient was found to have a soft abdomen with tenderness and guarding in the right iliac fossa. There was no rebound tenderness and Rovsing's sign was negative in that when the left lower quadrant was palpated no increase in pain was felt in the right lower quadrant. A urinalysis did not show any abnormalities and a pregnancy test was negative. Blood results showed a mild leukocytosis of 12.8×10^9/l (range, 4.00–11.00 10^9/l) with a neutrophilia of 10.6×10^9/l (range. 2.0–7.5 $\times 10^9$/l). Chest and abdominal X-rays were unremarkable. An ultrasound showed a small amount of free fluid in the right lower quadrant, which was suggestive but not conclusive of acute appendicitis. The Alvarado scoring system was used and scored a 7/10.

Diagnosis
Acute appendicitis

Treatment Plan
The patient was admitted to the surgical ward and prescribed a course of antibiotics. The plan was to initially treat conservatively and to observe the patient closely. Intravenous fluids commenced and opiate analgesia was administered.

The patient was reviewed two days following admission to the surgical ward and whilst her blood values had improved the patient still demonstrated a low-grade pyrexia. Abdominal pain was increasing with subsequent increased administration of opiates. It was decided to take her to the operating room to undergo a laparoscopic appendectomy. Following surgery, the patient had an unremarkable recovery and was discharged home.

Case Study of a 48-Year-Old Man with a Peptic Ulcer

Presenting Problem/History
A 48-year-old married man presented to his general practitioner (primary care provider) with a two-day history of upper abdominal pain and the passing of foul smelling black stools. He described the pain as gnawing. He did not have any nausea or vomiting and his appetite remained the same. He stated that the abdominal pain was partly relieved by drinking milk or taking yoghurt. He had not noted any weight loss and apart from the black stool his bowel habit had not altered. He smoked up to 40 cigarettes a day and had a weekly alcohol consumption of approx. 70 units. He had no previous medical or family history of note. He stated that he occasionally takes nonsteroidal anti-inflammatory drugs (NSAIDs) to relieve a hangover.

Differential Diagnosis

The following conditions will need to be considered as the patient has been taking NSAIDs and he has upper abdominal pain with some of the signs of liver disease as well as a history of excessive alcohol consumption and smoking.

Gastritis, peptic ulceration, upper GI neoplasia, hepatitis, oesophageal varices, or oesophagitis

Assessment Including Labs/Other

On inspection the patient was pale and sweaty and appeared unwell. His pulse was 116 beats per min and his BP was 90/58. His temperature was 36.9C/98.4F. His sclera had a hint of jaundice. There was no flapping tremor noted; however, there were spider naevi on his chest wall. He had no scratch marks on his skin. His abdomen was not distended and there was no evidence of any ascites. There were no veins visible on his abdomen. He had no jugular venous distension and he had normal breath and heart sounds. His neurological examination was normal. On palpation he was found to be tender in the right hypochondria and his liver was palpable 4 cm below the costal margin. A digital rectal examination revealed melaena stool. His bloods AST 300 (range 10–40 iu/L), GGT 244 (range 6–32 iu/L^{-1}), ALT 100 iu/L (range 5–40 iu l^{-1}), Bilirubin 95 μmol/L^{-1} (range 0–17 μmol/L^{-1}), MCV 90 fl (range 83–96 fL).

Diagnosis

Despite having a history of excessive alcohol consumption as well some of the symptoms associated with liver disease, i.e. jaundice, hepatomegaly, spider naevi, and elevated liver function test levels it was not determined that the patient had liver disease. As the patient had melaena an upper GI bleed was considered the most likely cause. Although patients with varices may present with melaena, variceal haemorrhage is usually associated with melaena and haematemesis. Another cause of bleeding is oesophagitis; however, this usually presents with heartburn and odynophagia, and neoplasms are usually associated with significant weight loss and vomiting. The patient's history of intermittent ingestion of NSAIDs would suggest gastritis and erosions may cause upper GI bleeding. This would need to be ruled out. However, the most likely cause for the bleeding is peptic ulcer as the patient had concurrent upper abdominal pain.

Treatment Plan

The patient was referred to the gastroenterology team at the local hospital and admitted to a medical ward and commenced on IV fluids to correct his hypovolaemia. An upper GI gastroscopy was performed which confirmed the presence of a single peptic ulcer in the antrum. Samples taken during the endoscopy showed the presence of *Helicobacter pylori*. The patient was prescribed proton pump inhibitors and two antibiotics and given advice regarding his alcohol consumption and smoking. He was referred back to his general practitioner for follow-up on his liver problems and a strong recommendation that he stop drinking.

References

Amico, D. and Barbarito, C. ed. (2016). *Health and Physical Assessment in Nursing*. New Jersey: Prentice Hall.

Ball, J., Dains, J., Flynn, J. et al. (2014a). *Seidel's Guide to Physical Examination*, 8e. St. Louis: Mosby.

Ball, J., Dains, J., Flynn, J. et al. (2014b). *Student Laboratory Manual to Accompany Seidel's Guide to Physical Examination*, 8e. St. Louis: Mosby.

Bickley, L. and Szilagyi, P. (2013). *Bates' Guide to Physical Examination and History Taking*, 11e. New York: Lippincott, Williams and Wilkins.

Dains, J., Baumann, L., and Scheibel, P. (2012). *Advanced Health Assessment and Clinical Diagnosis in Primary Care*, 4e. St Louis: Elsevier.

Dains, J., Baumann, L., and Scheibel, P. (2015). *Advanced Health Assessment and Clinical Diagnosis in Primary Care*, 5e. St. Louis: Mosby.

Douglas, G., Nichol, F., and Robertson, C. ed. (2013). *Macleod's Clinical Examination*. Edinburgh: Churchill Livingston.

Epstein, O., Perkin, G., de Bono, D., and Cookson, J. (2008). *Clinical Examination*, 4e. London: Mosby.

Japp, A. and Robertson, C. (2013). *Macleod's Clinical Diagnosis*. Edinburgh: Churchill Livingstone, Elsevier.

Jarvis, C. (2015). *Physical Examination and Health Assessment*, 7e. Edinburgh: Elsevier.

Martini, F., Nath, J., and Bartholomew, E. (2012). *The Abdominal System in Fundamentals of Anatomy & Physiology*, 9e. San Francisco, California: Pearson Benjamin Cummings.

McGrath, A. (2010). Examination of the Abdomen. In: *Physical Assessment for Nurses*, 2e (ed. C. McGrath), 101–112. Oxford: Wiley Blackwell.

Ranson, M., Braithwaite, W., and Abbott, H. ed. (2014). *Clinical Examination Skills for Healthcare Professionals*. Cumbria: MK Publishing.

Talley, N. and O'Connor, S. (2013). *Clinical Examination: A Systematic Guide to Physical Diagnosis*, 7e. Oxford: Blackwell Science.

Thomas, J. and Monaghan, T. ed. (2014). *Oxford Handbook of Clinical Examination and Practical Skills*, 2e. Oxford: Oxford University Press.

Tortora, G. and Derrickson, B. (2012). *Principles of Anatomy and Physiology*, 13e. Oxford: Wiley.

Chapter 7

Examination of the Male Genitalia

Michael Babcock, Carol Lynn Cox, and Anthony McGrath

Introduction

Research indicates that patients may become embarrassed when discussing their genitals so it is important to try to put them at ease (Collins-Bride and Saxe 2013; Dains et al. 2012, 2015). It is essential that the sexual history and examination should be undertaken in a sensitive manner. Reassure the patient that the information shared will remain confidential. This will help encourage the patient to be more open and honest with you. The questions asked may be perceived by the patient as intrusive. The patient may feel that your questioning has no bearing on the symptoms or problem that they have. Take time and give clear explanations as to why you are asking certain questions. If you use careful questioning and tact, patients are more likely to provide you with answers that will assist in reaching a diagnosis. It is useful to begin by stating something like 'I am now going to ask you some questions about your sexual health and practices'. Try to determine the patient's risk of acquiring a sexually transmitted infection (STI). Depending on the problem you may wish to begin by asking general questions about sexual function, sexual history, duration of their relationships, and timing of their last sexual encounter. Ask whether it with a regular or casual partner, the contraceptive methods used, the number of sexual partners that they have had, and their sexual orientation. Ask about having sex with men and women or both. Ask if their partner has any symptoms. You can then ask about any previous STIs and any previous treatments that they may have had. If he previously had an STI, ask the patient about the symptoms he had. Ask about any previous sexual health check-ups. Ask about the use of injected drugs. Ask if the patient has had any vaccinations against hepatitis A or B. Ask if they have been tested for HIV, hepatitis, or syphilis (Ball et al. 2014a, b; Bickley and Szilagyi 2013; Dains et al. 2012, 2015; Japp and Robertson 2013; Jarvis 2015; Rhoads and Paterson 2013). See Figure 7.1 for a depiction of the male reproductive system.

Physical Assessment for Nurses and Healthcare Professionals, Third Edition. Edited by Carol Lynn Cox.
© 2019 John Wiley & Sons Ltd. Published 2019 by John Wiley & Sons Ltd.

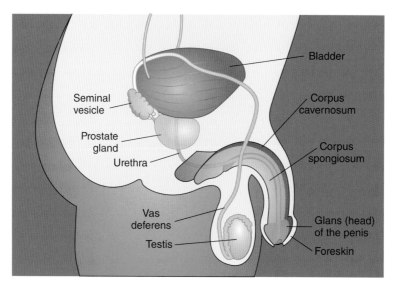

Figure 7.1   The male reproductive system.

General Examination
Important Symptoms to Consider

- urethral discharge
- warts
- ulceration
- testicular pain
- swelling
- ulceration
- rashes
- inflammation
- frequency and urgency
- hesitancy
- haematuria
- nocturia
- impotence
- loss of sexual desire
- infertility
- incontinence
- oliguria
- dysuria (Bickley and Szilagyi 2013; Dains et al. 2012, 2015; Seidel et al. 2010, Swartz 2014; Talley and O'Connor 2014)

Erectile Function

If the presenting problem is erectile dysfunction (ED) ask the following questions:

- Are you suffering from stress – in work or relationships?
- Are you afraid that sexual intercourse may cause cardiac problems?
- Do you drink alcohol? How much? How often?

- What medications do you take? Over the counter? Prescription and/or illicit drugs?
- Do you smoke? How much (number of cigarettes/packs per day)? How often? (Smoking, like alcohol, is a risk factor for ED.)

Note the distribution and amount of body hair, note size of testes as testosterone levels may be reduced.

Possible Sexually Transmitted Infection

- To assess the possibility of an STI ask questions about any discharge or dripping from the penis.
- If the patient has a penile discharge try to ascertain the amount, colour, and consistency.
- Ask if they have any other symptoms such as a temperature, rash, or pain.
- Tell the patient that STI's can affect any opening that comes into contact with sexual organs.
- Ask the patient about oral sex and anal sex and if he answers yes ask about the presence of sore throats, rectal bleeding, pain, itching, or diarrhoea.
- Ask about the presence of any sores, warts, swelling on the penis, or swelling in the scrotum/testicles.
- Ask if the patient has any concerns about HIV infection (Bickley and Szilagyi 2013; Dains et al. 2012, 2015; Japp and Robertson 2013; Jarvis 2015; Tallia and Scherger 2013).

Examination of the Male Genitalia

The patient may lie down or you can ask him to stand whilst you carry out your inspection. Ask in a sensitive way before you proceed, e.g. 'I need to briefly examine you down below. Is that all right?' Then begin your examination by inspecting the penis and groin area. Some examiners recommend that the patient hold his penis during inspection rather than the examiner holding it.

Inspection

- Note the size, colour, shape, and the presence or absence of a prepuce (foreskin). The size of the penis is usually dependent on the patient's age and overall development.
- Note any abnormal curvatures.
- Examine penis – retract the prepuce (foreskin) to expose glans – it may be useful to get the patient to do this for you. Note the presence of any chancres, ulceration, or erythema and the presence of smegma, which is a cheesy white substance that accumulates normally under the foreskin.
- Examine and inspect the glans; look for the presence of warts, ulcers, nodules, or the signs of any inflammation. Examine the external urethral meatus. If you are a female examiner, ask the patient to squeeze it open gently in an anterior–posterior direction to open the external urethral meatus to inspect for discharge (normally you will find none). If you are a male examiner you will find it easier to do this yourself unless the patient expresses concerns regarding you doing this.
- Balanitis (inflamed glans of penis) should remind the examiner to check for diabetes.
- If any discharge is noted, take a swab and send it for microbiology examination.
- Inspect the skin around the groin for any excoriation or inflammation. Note the presence of any nits or lice – these can usually be found at the base of the pubic hairs.
- Lift up the scrotum to inspect the posterior surface.
- Note any obvious hernia.

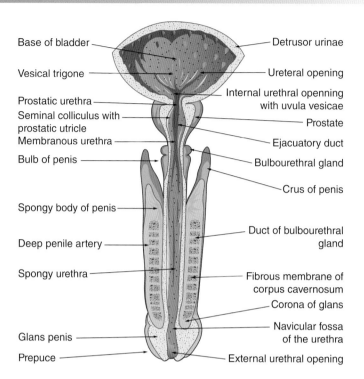

Base of bladder
Vesical trigone
Prostatic urethra
Seminal colliculus with prostatic utricle
Membranous urethra
Bulb of penis
Spongy body of penis
Deep penile artery
Spongy urethra
Glans penis
Prepuce

Detrusor urinae
Ureteral opening
Internal urethral openning with uvula vesicae
Prostate
Ejacuatory duct
Bulbourethral gland
Crus of penis
Duct of bulbourethral gland
Fibrous membrane of corpus cavernosum
Corona of glans
Navicular fossa of the urethra
External urethral opening

Figure 7.2   Longitudinal section of the penis and its relationship to the bladder and urethra.

- Examine scrotal swellings – Transilluminate to discern the presence of fluid.
- A poorly developed scrotum on one or both sides may suggest cryptorchidism (Cox 2010; Swartz 2014; Talley and O'Connor 2014).

See Figure 7.2.

Abnormalities of the Penis

- Priapism (persistent, usually painful, erection of the penis)
- Hypospadias or epispadias (birth defects where the urethra and urethral groove are malformed)
- Phimosis (tight prepuce that cannot be retracted over the glans). Note that this is normal in babies
- Paraphimosis (a tight prepuce that once retracted cannot be returned and oedema may occur) is common following the insertion of a catheter and the healthcare professional does not return the prepuce over the glans (Bickley and Szilagyi 2013; Dains et al. 2012, 2015; Japp and Robertson 2013; Jarvis 2015; Rundio 2017; Seidel et al. 2010; Swartz 2014; Talley and O'Connor 2014).

Abnormalities of the Scrotum

- Cryptorchidism (undescended testis)
- Inguinal hernia
- Cystic swelling
- Varicocele (Occurs in about 8% of male population. It will feel like a bag of worms). Occurs because of varicosity of the veins of the pampiniform plexus.

- Epididymal cyst
- Hydrocele
- Scrotal swelling (common scrotal swellings include inguinal hernias, scrotal oedema, and hydroceles). Tender painful swellings may indicate acute orchitis, acute epididymitis, and torsion of the spermatic cord. Swelling in the scrotum can be evaluated by transillumination (Bickley and Szilagyi 2013; Dains et al. 2012, 2015; Japp and Robertson 2013; Jarvis 2015; Rundio 2017; Seidel et al. 2010; Swartz 2014; Talley and O'Connor 2014).

Look for Signs of Syphilis – Primary, Secondary, and Tertiary
- Chancre (painless hard ulcer) seen in primary syphilis
- Skin rash, with brown sores about the size of a penny, the rash may cover the whole body or appear only in a few areas. It is almost always on the palms of the hands and soles of the feet and may be seen in secondary syphilis.
- Mild pyrexia, fatigue, headache, sore throat, patchy hair loss, and swollen lymph glands throughout the body. These symptoms may be very mild and, like the chancre of primary syphilis, will disappear without treatment.
- In tertiary syphilis, the brain, nervous system, heart, eyes, bones, joints can be affected. This stage can last for years and may result in mental illness, blindness, other neurological problems, heart disease, and death (Bickley and Szilagyi 2013; Dains et al. 2012, 2015; Japp and Robertson 2013; Jarvis 2015; Seidel et al. 2010; Swartz 2014; Talley and O'Connor 2014).

Look for Signs of Gonorrhoea
- painful urination
- yellowish urethral discharge
- painful discharge of bloody pus from the rectum (Rectal gonorrhoea)
- throat infection can occur as a result of oral sex with infected partner

(Note that disseminated gonorrhoea can cause purulent arthritis – often of the knee joint.)

Look for Signs of Herpes
- Painful blisters or bumps in the genital or rectal area that crust over, form a scab, and heal.
- Patient complains of itching, burning, or tingling sensation in the genitals.
- Inguinal lymphadenopathy (swollen, tender lymph nodes).
- Headache.
- Muscle ache.
- Pyrexia.
- Penis discharge.
- Infection of the urethra causing a burning sensation.
- During urination (Bickley and Szilagyi 2013; Dains et al. 2012, 2015; Japp and Robertson 2013; Jarvis 2015; Rundio 2017; Seidel et al. 2010; Swartz 2014; Talley and O'Connor 2014).

Look for Signs of HPV Infection
- Genital warts (condylomata acuminata) usually appear as small bumps or groups of bumps. They can be raised or flat, single or multiple, small or large, and sometimes cauliflower shaped.

Look for Signs of Chlamydia
- no symptoms in 70–80% of cases
- lower abdominal pain and burning pain during urination
- mucopurulent discharge from the penis
- tenderness or pain in the testicles
- burning and itching around the meatus
- rectal pain, discharge, or bleeding in patients who engage in anal sex

Palpation
Groin
- The spermatic cord, lymph nodes, and arteries occupy the groin.
- Swellings here are usually caused by hernias or enlarged lymph nodes.
- Palpate the groin to detect enlarged lymph nodes.
- Most people have small, shotty nodes. Most enlarged tender nodes arise from infection in the legs or feet. However, in some Afro-Caribbean men this is normal.
- If large nodes, palpate spleen carefully (*reticulosis* or *leukaemia*) (Bickley and Szilagyi 2013; Dains et al. 2012, 2015; Japp and Robertson 2013; Jarvis 2015; Rundio 2017; Seidel et al. 2010; Swartz 2014; Talley and O'Connor 2014).

Hernia
When checking for the presence of hernia examine the patient standing and ask him to cough – enlargement of a groin swelling suggests a hernia (Figure 7.3).

- indirect (oblique) inguinal hernia: swelling reduced to internal inguinal ring by pressure on contents of hernial sac and then controlled by pressure over the internal ring when patient asked to cough; if your hand is then removed, impulse passes medially towards external ring and is palpable above the pubic tubercle
- direct inguinal hernia: impulse in a forward direction mainly above groin crease medial to femoral artery and swelling not controlled by pressure over internal ring
- femoral hernia: swelling fills out the groin crease medial to the femoral artery (Bickley and Szilagyi 2013; Dains et al. 2012, 2015; Japp and Robertson 2013; Jarvis 2015; Rundio 2017; Seidel et al. 2010; Swartz 2014; Talley and O'Connor 2014).

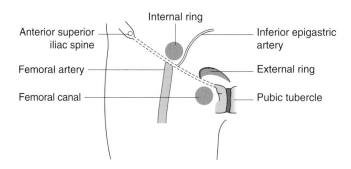

Figure 7.3   Checking for hernia.

Penis
Palpate the whole length of the penis to the perineum, and note the state of the dorsal vein. Note any hardened or tender areas. Hardness may indicate a urethral stricture or cancer whereas tenderness may indicate an infection.

Scrotum

- Ask 'Is your scrotum painful anywhere? Tell me if I hurt you'.
- Warm your hands, and remember to use gentle pressure.
- Palpate the scrotum for the testes and epididymis.
- Palpate each testes and epididymis with your thumb and 1st two fingers.
- Observe the patients face.
- *Note the size, shape, and consistency of each testis. Note any tenderness.*
- Tender and enlarged testes may occur with *orchitis* or *torsion of the testis. Multiple torturous veins may indicate a varicocele.*
- A large, soft swelling which transilluminates suggests *hydrocele* or an *epididymal cyst.* A hydrocele surrounds the testis; an epididymal cyst lies behind the testis.
- A large, hard, painless testis suggests testicular cancer, a potentially curable cancer with a peak incidence between the ages of 15 and 35 years.

Prostate Gland

Lay the patient on the left side with knees flexed to the chest or if he can, ask the patient to bend over the examination table.

Inspect anus for lumps, haemorrhoids, fissures, ulcers, inflammation, excoriation, and warts.

Explain to the patient that you will need to place your finger into his rectum to examine the prostate. This procedure may be uncomfortable but should not be painful. Say: 'I am going to put a finger into your back passage'.

With lubricant on glove, press your fingertip against the anal verge then gently slip forefinger into anal canal and then into the rectum. Inform the patient that he may feel the urge to pass urine but he will not. It helps to have the patient push whilst you insert your finger. Palpate the prostate gland on the anterior rectal wall. Check the size and character of the prostate. It should feel smooth and rubbery and be approximately the size of a walnut. Note any nodules or tenderness. A swollen tender prostate may indicate acute prostatitis whereas an enlarged smooth but firm prostate may indicate benign prostatic hypertrophy. Hard roughened areas are suggestive of cancer (Figure 7.4).

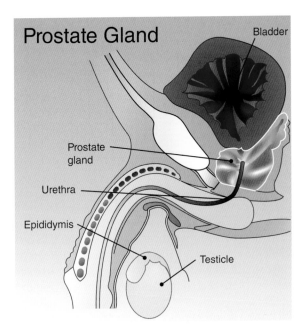

Figure 7.4 The prostate. *Source:* Courtesy of MedicineNet, Inc.

Case Study of a 54-Year-Old Obese Male with Erectile Dysfunction

Presenting Problem/History

A 54-year-old obese male presents to the primary care clinic asking for a prescription for sildenafil (Viagra). He has recently relocated to the area because of a job transfer. He is unmarried and has not been seen in the clinic before. He indicates that the only medication he has been taking is isosorbide mononitrate (Monoket). He says he has type II diabetes which is controlled by diet.

Subjective

(Note a review of systems [ROS] for ED should include depression and anxiety. Also consider whether the patient uses tobacco products. Does he have true ED or does he just have decreased libido?)

The patient indicates his overall health is fine. Family history reflects his father and mother had diabetes, suffered strokes, and died at the ages of 60 and 65. Siblings (Unremarkable except for one brother who also has diabetes.). A ROS reflects Integumentary (No complaint); Head and Neck (No complaint); Eyes, Ears, Nose, and Throat (No complaint); Cardiac (Chest pain on exertion); Respiratory (Shortness of breath with ambulation lasting more than five minutes); Abdominal (Complaints of bloating and heartburn); Genitourinary (Complaints of nocturia and erectile dysfunction); Musculoskeletal (Complaints of pain in both knees and back); Neurological (No complaints); Endocrine (Diabetes).

Objective

Observations reflect: T 98.6 F/37 C; BP 150/87; P 86; O2 Sat 99; HT 5'10"; WT 269; BMI 38.6 (Severely Obese).

Physical examination: H&N (WNL); EENT (WNL); Chest (Resp – BBS, Clear A&P) (CVS – Cardiac – S1 S2 no rubs, splits, or murmurs; apex 5th ISC MCL – no heaves or thrills; all pulses present); Abdo (Soft, nontender, normal bowel sounds); GU (Normal external make genitalia. The penis is uncircumcised. Smooth walnut-shaped enlarged prostate; urinalysis – unremarkable); MS (ROM WNL, crepitus in both knees); Neuro (WNL).

Differential Diagnosis

Obesity, angina, diabetes, erectile disfunction, and benign prostatic hyperplasia.

Assessment Including Labs/Other

ECG/EKG in clinic. Labs: PSA screen, CMP, Lipids, HbA1C, Thyroid Panel; FBC/CBC with Diff; B12; Folate; Ferritin; Vit D. Urinalysis. Routine CX-R A&P in clinic.

Diagnosis

Await referral reports, labs, and X-rays.

Treatment Plan

Obtain medical records from previous healthcare providers. Refer to orthopaedics for evaluation of both knees. Refer to Cardiology for cardiac evaluation. Refer to Urology for ED and enlarged prostate. Refer to nutritionist for dietary advice. Refer to diabetic nurse specialist (subsequent to lab results). Note that in the obese, weight loss and exercise are associated with improvement of ED.

Counsel the patient: Viagra is contraindicated with Monoket. Consider other options.

References

Ball, J., Dains, J., Flynn, J. et al. (2014a). *Seidel's Guide to Physical Examination*, 8e. St. Louis: Mosby.

Ball, J., Dains, J., Flynn, J. et al. (2014b). *Student Laboratory Manual to Accompany Seidel's Guide to Physical Examination*, 8e. St. Louis: Mosby.

Bickley, L. and Szilagyi, P. (2013). *Bates' Guide to Physical Examination and History Taking*, 11e. New York: Wolters Kluwer/Lippincott Williams & Wilkins.

Collins-Bride, G. and Saxe, J. (2013). *Clinical Guidelines for Advanced Practice Nursing - an Interdisciplinary Approach*, 2e. Burlington, MA: Jones and Bartlett Learning.

Cox, C. (2010). *Physical Assessment for Nurses*, 2e. Oxford: Wiley Blackwell.

Dains, J., Baumann, L., and Scheibel, P. (2012). *Advanced Health Assessment and Clinical Diagnosis in Primary Care*, 4e. St. Louis: Elsevier.

Dains, J., Baumann, L., and Scheibel, P. (2015). *Advanced Health Assessment and Clinical Diagnosis in Primary Care*, 5e. St. Louis: Mosby.

Japp, A. and Robertson, C. (2013). *Macleod's Clinical Diagnosis*. Edinburgh: Churchill Livingstone, Elsevier.

Jarvis, C. (2015). *Physical Examination and Health Assessment*, 7e. Edinburgh: Elsevier.

Rhoads, J. and Paterson, S. (2013). *Advanced Health Assessment and Diagnostic Reasoning*, 2e. Burlington: Jones and Bartlett.

Rundio, A. (2017). Men's health. In: *Lippincott Certification Review: Family Nurse Practitioner & Adult-Gerontology Nurse Practitioner* (ed. A. Rundio and W. Lorman), 224–238. New York: Wolters Kluwer.

Seidel, H., Ball, J., Dains, J., and Benedict, G. (2010). *Mosby's Physical Examination Handbook*, 7e. St. Louis: Mosby-Year Book.

Swartz, M. (2014). *Physical Diagnosis: History and Examination*, With Student Consult Online Access, 7e. London: Elsevier.

Talley, N. and O'Connor, S. (2014). *Clinical Examination: A Systematic Guide to Physical Diagnosis*, 7e. London: Churchill Livingstone, Elsevier.

Tallia, A. and Scherger, J. (2013). *Swanson's Family Practice Review*, 6e. St. Louis: Mosby.

Chapter 8

Examination of the Female Breast

Victoria Lack

General Examination
Introduction

Examination of the female breast needs to be approached with similar care to examination of the remainder of the female reproductive system. Breasts are associated with many things in different cultures such as womanhood, motherhood, and sexuality. In western cultures, the breast is often a focus of sexual attractiveness and stimulation (Burnet 2001). Always explain fully why you need to perform the examination and what you are going to do and always offer a chaperone. Male clinicians should always have a chaperone. Examination is often accompanied by anxiety for the woman, as many of the symptoms women present with could be a sign of breast cancer.

Ask the woman to undress to the waist behind a closed curtain and reassure her there will be no interruptions during the examination. Ask the woman to sit on the edge of the couch and let you know when she is ready. Ensure that your hands are clean and warm.

Review of Anatomy

The breasts are present in both sexes although usually enlarged only in women. Each breast lies over the pectoralis major. For most people the breasts extend from the 2nd to the 6th rib in the midclavicular line. Each breast contains a mammary gland within the subcutaneous tissue of the pectoral fat pad beneath the skin. Each gland is formed of 15–20 lobes which are supported by fibrous tissue and fat. The ducts of each lobe, called the lactiferous ducts, open up onto the nipple. The darker skin surrounding the nipple is called the areola, beneath which are large sebaceous glands which make the area slightly lumpy. The interlobular connective tissue forms suspensory ligaments which attach the breast to underlying muscle fascia and overlying dermis. Breast tissue extends up into each axilla, an area called the 'tail of Spence', where the anterior axillary lymph nodes drain most of the breast and anterior chest wall (Figure 8.1).

Physical Assessment for Nurses and Healthcare Professionals, Third Edition. Edited by Carol Lynn Cox.
© 2019 John Wiley & Sons Ltd. Published 2019 by John Wiley & Sons Ltd.

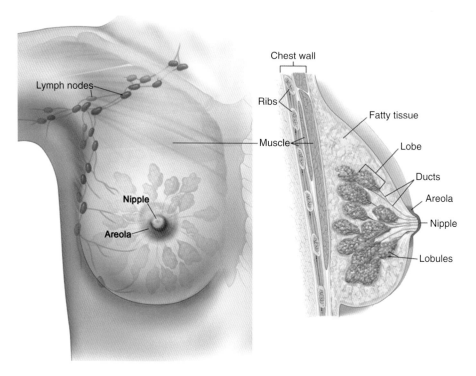

Figure 8.1   Anatomy of the female breast. *Source*: http://www.cancer.gov/types/breast/patient/breast-prevention-pdq.

Inspection

First stand in front of the patient, with the patient in a sitting position with arms resting on her thighs to relax the pectoral muscles. Explain what you are looking for. Note:

- size
- symmetry
- colour
- any scars or stretch marks
- any visible veins
- any dimpling or puckering of the skin (especially look out for an orange peel type appearance 'peau d'orange' due to oedema from breast cancer or radiotherapy).
- any visible lumps
- any lesions, rash, or ulceration (adapted from Thomas and Monaghan 2014).

Inspect the nipples and areolae. Note whether the nipples are:

- symmetrical
- everted, flat, or inverted
- any crusting, eczema type rash, or lesions
- any discharge – from single or multiple ducts.

Ask the patient to put her hands on her hips and press inwards to contract the pectoral muscles. Inspect the breasts again as above. The breasts can also be further inspected with the patient leaning forwards. Ask the patient to put her hands on top of her head near the crown. Inspect the axillae for any lumps or colour change.

These different positions may highlight any changes in the skin and in the contour of the breast (Douglas et al. 2009).

Palpation

Ask the patient to lie back on the couch with the back of the couch raised to approximately 30°. Ask the patient to put one hand behind her head. Explain you are now going to palpate the breast. Starting in the upper outer quadrant, use one hand to palpate the breast tissue firmly but gently. Move in a circular motion around the breast, moving inwards towards the nipple. Ensure that the entire breast is palpated. Note the texture of the breast and ask the patient to tell you if any areas are tender. If any lumps are felt, then assess:

- Size
- Tenderness on palpation
- Consistency
- Does it move with the skin? (lump in the dermis or epidermis)
- Does the skin move over the lump? (lump in the subcutaneous tissue)
- Does it move with muscular contraction? (musculoskeletal)
- Is the border smooth or irregular?

Next palpate from the upper outer quadrant upwards towards the axilla, the tail of Spence. Palpate the axilla. Note any lumps and tenderness. If a change in consistency of the breast or a lump is found in one breast, then check the other breast in same area.

Palpate the nipple by holding it gently between finger and thumb. Try to express any discharge. Massage the breast towards the nipple to further check for discharge. Note the colour, consistency, position, and number of the affected ducts. Axillary nipples and associated breast tissue can occur along the ectodermal ridge (milk line) which extends bilaterally from the axilla to the groin. These are normal developmental variations.

Palpate the axillary lymph nodes; ask the patient to sit up again facing you. Support the full weight of her arm at the wrist and move the flat of the other hand high up into the axilla; then try to compress the contents of the axilla against the chest wall. This examination is often uncomfortable for patients, so warn them in advance. Assess any lumps as above.

Examine for supraclavicular lymph nodes and also all cervical chains.

Key Findings

- skin changes
- nipple discharge
- lumps
- breast abscesses
- breast pain

Skin Changes

Skin changes may be due to dermatological conditions or to underlying conditions, including carcinoma. This can present as dimpling of the skin, indrawing of the skin, or lymphoedema of the breast. This resembles the skin of an orange (peau d'orange).

Eczema of the nipple and or areola can look innocent and may be part of a generalised eczematous condition, but it may be due to Paget's disease (invasion of the epidermis by an intraductal carcinoma). Breast cancer can also present as indrawing of the nipple.

Nipple Discharge

A small amount of fluid may be expressed from multiple ducts on massaging the breast; this may be variable in colour. Single duct discharge may be blood stained (micro or macroscopically). Causes of nipple discharge include duct ectasia, where the major ducts become blocked in the subareolar region, causing secretions from the ducts. This is mainly a condition of older, parous women who are smokers. (Patient 2015).

Periductal mastitis is a similar condition, found more often in younger women smokers, which presents with pain, a periareolar mass, and a puslike discharge from the nipple. Intraductal breast cancer can also produce a discharge; therefore, all nipple discharge needs further investigation. The NICE 2015 guidelines recommend an urgent referral (two-week wait) for all patients over 50 years with nipple discharge (NICE 2015).

A milky discharge from multiple ducts in both breasts in a nonpregnant or breastfeeding woman is called galactorrhoea. It is caused by hyperprolactinaemia. There are various causes including antipsychotic drugs, a prolactin secreting tumour, and hypothyroidism. This always needs further investigation.

Lumps

Finding a breast lump is usually distressing for women, as it is almost invariably associated by patients with breast cancer. There are other reasons for breast lumps as below and most lumps are not cancer, but all reported lumps should be treated with a high index of suspicion.

Fibrocystic Changes

This is irregular nodularity of the breast and is common in young women. The breast feels 'lumpy' but discrete lumps are not found. The tissue feels most 'lumpy' premenstrually. The changes are usually bilateral.

Fibroadenomas

These are benign lumps caused by an overgrowth of the terminal duct tubules. They are the second most common cause of a breast mass in women under 35 (Douglas et al. 2009). They are usually smooth, mobile discrete lumps which have a rubbery texture often known as a 'breast mouse'.

Breast Cysts

These are most common in women aged 35–50 years (Douglas et al. 2009.) They may be soft or hard and tender depending on the amount of fluid in the sac. Cysts may occur in clusters. Most are benign, but not all.

Breast Cancer

Breast cancer affects one in nine women, and incidence increases with age. It may present as a fixed, hard, irregular painless lump, nipple retraction, peau d'orange, and local hard or firm fixed nodes in the axilla. (Lewellyn et al. 2014.)

Breast Abscesses

Most commonly they are associated with lactation and occur in breastfeeding women. They are hot and tender to touch.

Nonlactational abscesses are secondary to periductal mastitis. They are usually associated with nipple inversion. They usually occur in young female smokers. Occasionally the abscess may discharge via a fistula.

Breast Pain

Most women experience breast pain at some point and it is often cyclical due to fluctuating hormone levels during the menstrual cycle. Cyclical breast pain is often worst three to five days prior to the menstrual period and settles with menstruation. Noncyclical breast pain may be associated with musculoskeletal problems originating in the chest wall. It is also associated with more advanced breast cancer.

Referral Guidelines for Breast Cancer

In the United Kingdom (UK), the national guidelines for referral are as follows:

Refer people for breast cancer using a suspected cancer referral pathway (with a two-week wait) for breast cancer if they are:

Aged 30 or over and have an unexplained breast lump with or without pain or aged 50 and over with any of the following symptoms in one nipple only:

- discharge
- retraction
- other changes of concern.

Consider a suspected cancer pathway referral (for an appointment within two weeks) for breast cancer in people:

- with skin changes that suggest breast cancer **or**
- aged 30 and over with an unexplained lump in the axilla.

Consider nonurgent referral in people aged under 30 with an unexplained breast lump with or without pain (NICE 2015).

Breast Awareness and Screening

Breast awareness is 'an important activity that women can carry out themselves in order to maintain their wellbeing' (Taylor and Burnet 2001). It is the practice of encouraging women to look at and feel their own breasts in order to recognise what is normal for them. For more information see Breast Cancer Care 2016; NHS Choices 2015; and NICE 2015.

The national breast screening programme in the UK provides free mammograms every three years for all women aged over 50. This is currently being extended to invite all women aged between 47 and 73 years. The screening programme does not stop after this age. Older women are invited to contact their local breast screening unit for mammography every three years (NHS Choices 2015). It is important to note that the screening, like cervical cytology, is not a diagnostic test; women with symptoms should have a clinical examination and referral as appropriate.

The Male Breast

The male breasts are anatomically equivalent to the female breasts.

Breast Lumps

Breast cancer in men is very rare (approx. 350 men are diagnosed each year in the UK). The symptoms are the same as for women with breast cancer (Cancer Research UK 2015). Gynaecomastia is enlargement of the male breast and often occurs during puberty. It can also occur in chronic liver disease where there are high levels of oestrogens which are not metabolised by the liver. Thyrotoxicosis, some adrenal tumours, and certain drugs can also cause breast enlargement, as can decreased androgen production as in Klinefelter's syndrome (Douglas et al. 2009.)

Case Study of a 40-Year-Old Female with a Lump in Her Right Breast

Presenting problem: 40-year-old woman with a lump in her right breast.

Subjective

History

The patient noticed a lump in her right breast a few months ago whilst in the shower. She says she does not generally check her breasts, so it may have been there for a while before that. She checked her other breast at the time but did not note a similar lump. The lump was about the size of a pea, hard, not tender to touch and is located in the upper outer part of her breast. She is not sure if it is 'mobile' or not. She did not feel anything else unusual in her breasts. She has 'kept an eye on it' for the past few months, but it has not appeared to grow in size. She did not want to come to the doctor as she was worried about it and felt she 'would rather not know'. However, she has come today as the worry is now keeping her awake at night. She has had noted no changes in her nipple or areola, no nipple discharge, no pain and feels otherwise well.

She has one son who is 15. She did not breastfeed her son. She has had an intrauterine system (Mirena coil) *in situ* for the last three years. She does not experience periods with this method of contraception. Prior to this she used the combined oral contraceptive pill.

Family History

The patient thinks her father had prostate cancer in later life, otherwise, no history of cancer in her immediate family.

Social History

The patient is an accountant and lives with her partner and son. Nonsmoker, moderate alcohol. BMI 24.

Medication History

Nil

No known drug allergies

Objective

Physical Examination

Looks well. Vital signs in normal range, apyrexial.

Breast examination (with consent, female chaperone present – practice nurse).

Breasts; small breasts: R breast slightly larger than left. Nipple, no lesions seen, no eczema, no discharge. Areola, no lesions. Skin of breasts; no lesions, dimpling, or puckering noted.

On palpation: R breast was nontender. A 1 cm (approx.) firm, mobile lump was felt in the upper outer quadrant at approx. 2 o'clock. The border felt regular. No other lumps felt. Left breast, nontender, no lumps felt. No nipple discharge was expressed.

No lumps or tenderness felt in the axillae.

Differential Diagnosis

Breast cyst, fibroadenoma, breast cancer

Treatment Plan

Referred to the breast clinic using the suspected cancer referral pathway (two-week wait).

The patient was seen within two weeks in the clinic where on ultrasound and fine needle aspiration she was diagnosed with a benign breast cyst.

References

Breast Cancer Care (2016) Checking Your Breasts. https://www.breastcancercare.org.uk/information-support/have-i-got-breast-cancer/checking-your-breasts (accessed 29 August 2018).

Burnet, L. ed. (2001). *Holistic Breast Care*. Edinburgh: Edinburgh Balliere Tindall.

Cancer Research UK (2015) www.cancerresearchuk.org (accessed 28 August 2018).

Douglas, G., Nicol, F., and Robertson, C. ed. (2009). *Macleod's Clinical Examination*, 12e. Edinburgh: Churchill Livingstone.

Lewellyn, H., Ang, H.A., Lewis, K., and Al'Abdullah, A. (2014). *Oxford Handbook of Clinical Diagnosis*, 3e. Oxford: Oxford University Press.

NHS Choices (2015) Breast Cancer Screening. https://www.nhs.uk/conditions/breast-cancer-screening (accessed 23 September 2015).

NICE (2015) Breast Cancer. https://www.nice.org.uk/Guidance/Conditions-and-diseases/Cancer/Breast-cancer (accessed 28 August 2018).

Patient (2015) Mammary Duct Ectasia and Periductal Mastitis. http://patient.info/doctor/Mammary-Duct-Ectasia.htm (accessed 23 August 2015).

Taylor, M. and Burnet, K. (2001). Breast screening. In: *Holistic Breast Care* (ed. L. Burnet). Edinburgh: Bailliere Tindall.

Thomas, J. and Monaghan, T. ed. (2014). *Oxford Handbook of Clinical Examination and Practical Skills*, 2e. Oxford: Oxford University Press.

Chapter 9

Examination of the Female Reproductive System

Victoria Lack

General Examination

This chapter addresses examination of a nonpregnant adult female. Examination of a woman's reproductive system includes an abdominal examination (discussed in Chapter 6), examination of the external genitalia, a speculum examination, and bimanual examination. A rectal examination may also be needed in some circumstances. Examination of the inguinal lymph nodes should also be performed. The following considers the pelvic examination of a nonpregnant woman.

The examination is regarded by women as very intimate. It is a procedure that most women in western cultures will experience at some point in their lives. It is your responsibility to make the examination as bearable as possible. Some, but not all women will prefer a female examiner to carry out the examination. This wish should be respected. In emergency situations, where it is not practicable to delay the examination, if a female examiner is not available, sensible and practicable measures must be taken (RCN 2013). All women should be offered a chaperone, regardless of the gender of the person carrying out the examination. This is not only to protect the patient but also to protect the clinician. Some women may want to have a friend or relative present. It is important for you as the examiner undertaking the procedure to establish a rapport with the woman prior to examination. It is also important that you explain fully the procedure and why it is necessary, prior to the woman getting undressed and exposed. A diagram or model may help here. However, it is equally important to be aware that some women do not want to have a detailed explanation and would rather you 'just got on with it'.

This chapter does not address the physical examination of a female child, which should be carried out only by specialist staff. Equally, you must assess the capacity of adults to decide if they are fully concordant with the examination prior to procedure. If there is an indication that a child or young person has been sexually abused, you should follow local guidelines and refer immediately. You should not proceed with the examination if you think the woman is not able to cope with the procedure; e.g. if the client is unduly stressed or upset, has had previous vasovagal reactions, or has an imperforate hymen (RCN 2013).

Physical Assessment for Nurses and Healthcare Professionals, Third Edition. Edited by Carol Lynn Cox.
© 2019 John Wiley & Sons Ltd. Published 2019 by John Wiley & Sons Ltd.

Review of Anatomy

The female reproductive system can be divided into the internal and external genitalia. The external female genitalia are composed of the vulva (which includes the labia majora and minora), the vaginal opening (the introitus), urethra, and clitoris.

The internal female genitalia is composed of the uterus, fallopian tubes, ovaries, vagina, and cervix. These lie in the pelvis, posterior to the bladder and anterior to the rectum.

The Uterus

The uterus is a pear-shaped muscular organ with a central cavity and rounded top called the fundus. The cervix, which is the neck of the uterus, lies within the upper vagina and the body of the uterus sits above it. The uterus is most commonly 'anteverted', i.e. it is angled forward. In some women the uterus is 'retroverted', i.e. it tips backward from the axis of the vagina. The muscular uterine wall is called the myometrium, lined internally by the endometrium (Figure 9.1).

The Uterine Adnexa

The fallopian tubes, ovaries, and their attachments form the adnexa. The fallopian tubes lead from the upper outer aspects of the uterus and curve round to meet the ovaries. The ovaries rest on the side wall of the pelvis (Figure 9.2).

FEMALE UROGENITAL SYSTEM (MIDSAGITTAL VIEW)

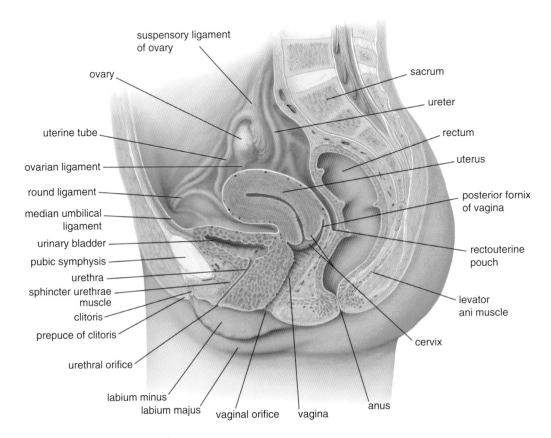

Figure 9.1   Female reproductive system.

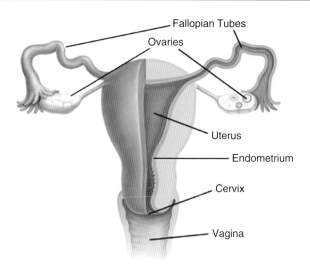

Figure 9.2   The internal female reproductive organs.

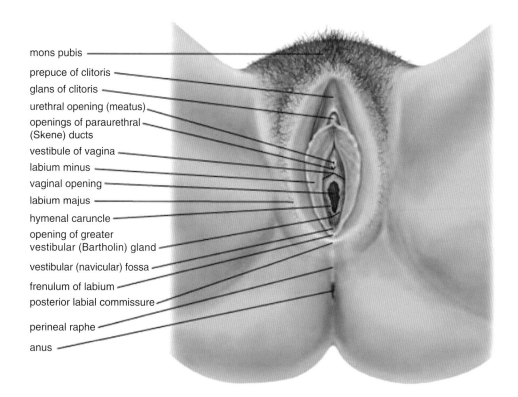

Figure 9.3   External female genitalia.

The Vagina

The vagina is a flattened tube extending backwards from the vulva to the cervix. The cervix is positioned at the superior end of the vagina vault and divides the vault into the anterior/posterior and lateral fornices. The vagina lies parallel and in close proximity to the rectum. The urethra extends along the superior wall of the vagina from the urinary bladder to the external urethral orifice (Figure 9.3).

The Vulva

The area containing the female external genitalia is called the vulva. The vagina opens into the vestibule, which contains the urethral opening, the vaginal orifice, and the clitoris, which is usually covered by the prepuce. The labia minora outline the vaginal vestibule. The hymen is an elastic epithelial fold which partially blocks the entrance to the vagina. It is of variable size and is usually stretched or torn during 1st sexual activity, tampon use, physical activity, or internal examination. The labia vary widely between women, which can give the vulva a very different appearance in different women. The perineum is the area between the vagina and anus.

The muscular base of the pelvis (the pelvic floor) supports the pelvic organs and helps maintain the tone of the urethral and anal sphincters.

Preparation

Ask the woman if she needs to empty her bladder prior to the examination. Make sure everything is ready before asking the woman to get undressed: there is nothing worse than having to leave the bedside to search for a swab that is in another room. Make sure there is a good lighting source, like the Welch Allen speculum light for use with disposable specula, or other source that can be positioned to give the best view of the genitalia. Check the light before the examination to ensure it works. Secure the door to the consultation room and let the woman know that the door is closed and no one else will come in. Explain exactly what you want the woman to do. It may seem evident that you need the woman to remove her underwear, but it may not be evident to the woman. Leave the woman to undress in private, having given her a gown or blanket or paper tissue to put over herself so she is not sitting exposed waiting for you.

In most primary care settings, the woman will be asked to lie on a couch/table in the dorsal position, with her feet either in stirrups or the soles of her feet together and knees apart. In secondary care, the lithotomy position – using leg supports – is more common. The lithotomy position gives a better view of the genitalia. A left lateral position may also be used, which is useful in examining women who have utero-vaginal prolapse or vesicov-aginal fistulae (Arulkamaran et al. 2007). In this case a Sims speculum should be used. This position may also be a more comfortable position for older women, particularly if they have kyphosis or arthritis/bone/joint disease. Once the woman is in the correct position, covered over her abdomen and legs with a gown or sheet, check again that everything is at hand. Always wash your hands and then put on gloves (Table 9.1).

A complete examination of the female genitalia consists of the following components:

- external genitalia – inspection
- external genitalia – palpation
- speculum examination
- bimanual ('per vagina' or 'PV' examination)

(Thomas and Monaghan 2010).

Inspection of the External Genitalia

Tell the woman you are beginning the examination. Look at the perineum. Note hygiene and distribution of pubic hair. Look at the labia majora, which should be generally sym-metrical but may be open or closed, full or thin. Note any lesions. Open the labia majora to inspect the labia minora, which should be darker coloured and soft. Inspect the clitoris, urethral meatus, and vaginal opening. Check for any inflammation, redness or discharge,

Table 9.1   Materials needed for a pelvic examination.

Gloves
Warm water for lubrication
Water-based lubrication jelly
Specula (It may be necessary to use different sizes to ensure comfort and facilitate visualisation of the cervix.) As a
    general rule, short obese women will require a short wide speculum; medium-sized women will require a
    medium-/regular-sized speculum. Tall thin women will require a medium-/regular-sized speculum or a long
    thin speculum. A multipara woman (five vaginal deliveries or more) will require a large speculum to keep the
    vaginal walls from falling in and obscuring your view. Nullipara women will require a small speculum. A female
    child will require a paediatric speculum.
Cervical broom and brush (Note the brush is not normally used.)
Liquid-based cytology container (if cervical cytology is being undertaken.)
Cotton tip applicator (to remove heavy secretions obscuring the cervical os)
Swabs (if samples are being taken for microbiology/virology)
Slides with covers (for microscopy on site)
Culture tube with swabs (for suspected chlamydia or gonorrhoea)
pH paper
Light source
Haemocult test kit (when performing a rectal examination) for occult blood
Disposable gloves in your size
Tissues

ulceration, or atrophy. Ask the patient to 'bear down' and/or to cough to look at the vaginal walls to check for any prolapse.

Palpate the labia majora, which should be pliant and fleshy with the index finger and thumb. Palpate for the Bartholin glands, which are located in the posterolateral labia majora. These will be palpable only if the duct becomes obstructed resulting in a painless lump or acute abscess (Jarvis 2015; Thomas and Monaghan 2010).

Palpate the lateral tissue of the perineum between thumb and forefinger. Check for swelling, tenderness, and masses.

Speculum Examination (Figure 9.4)

Speculum examination is carried out to see further into the vagina, visualise the cervix, take high vaginal and endocervical swabs, and perform cervical cytology. The bivalve Cusco's (disposable) speculum is the most commonly used. Metal bivalve specula, which are reusable following sterilisation, are preferred by some clinicians. Ensure you are familiar with how to open and close the blades. Warm and lubricate the speculum using warm water.

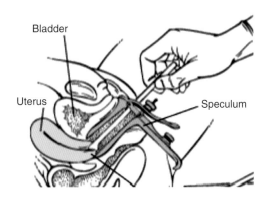

Figure 9.4   Speculum examination.

Lubricating gel can be used as speculum examination is often uncomfortable for women. If a sample for cervical cytology is to be taken use a little water-based lubricant only and avoid putting it over the tips of the blades, so as to not contaminate the sample (NHS Cancer Screening Programme 2006). Tell the woman what you are going to do and then gently part the labia to insert the speculum. In the dorsal position the speculum should be inserted with the handle superior, whereas in the lithotomy position the handle is usually inferior (Arulkamaran et al. 2007). You may choose to insert the speculum sideways and rotate the handle into either the superior or inferior position as using this insertion technique is more comfortable for women. If the handle is superior, make sure that it does not touch the clitoris, which is very sensitive. Insert the speculum in a slightly downwards direction. Check the woman's comfort at this point. Open the speculum when it is fully inserted and flush with the perineum. It may not be necessary to fully open the speculum. Inspect the vaginal walls, which should be pink and moist. The cervix should be visible between the tips of the blades. If you cannot see it try withdrawing the speculum slightly. The cervix may 'drop' into view or you may need to close the speculum, withdraw further, and change direction of the speculum slightly. A digital examination can be used to establish the position of the cervix. Putting a pillow under the woman's buttocks or asking her to put her hands underneath her buttocks may also help to better position the woman in order to visualise the cervix (Jarvis 2015).

Inspect the cervix. It should be symmetrical, pink, and about 3 cm in diameter. The cervix should extend approximately 2 cm into the vagina. More than 3 cm could indicate a vaginal prolapse (Jarvis 2015; RCN 2013). The surface of the cervix should be smooth. The cervix is the point where vaginal squamous epithelium meets the endocervical columnar epithelium at the squamocolumnar junction. The level of the junction varies throughout a woman's life and can give a very different appearance to the cervix. An extension of the endocervical epithelium onto the surface of the cervix is often called an 'ectropion' (sometimes called cervical erosion). This is often present at puberty, during pregnancy, and if a woman is taking oestrogen containing hormonal contraception. The os should be round in a nulliparous woman and slitlike (may look like a smile) in a parous woman. There may be some clear or creamy odourless discharge from the os. Note any secretions, polyps, or other lesions. Note any nabothian cysts or follicles. These are normal findings and have the appearance of small yellow nodules (RCN 2013). In pregnancy the cervix may appear different and have a bluish or purple hue (Chadwick sign). The cervix can also change position and look different according to the time of the menstrual cycle as well as pre- and postmenopausally. Cervicitis causes a red and inflamed cervix which bleeds on contact.

Obtain cervical cytological samples and/or swabs at this point as needed. Note any contact bleeding during taking of the samples. This may not necessarily be abnormal; an enthusiastically taken cervical cytology specimen may cause contact bleeding, especially if the patient has an ectropion. Remove the speculum with as much care as during insertion. Continue to examine the vaginal walls as the speculum is withdrawn, keeping the blades open until they are clear of the cervix to avoid causing pain. Rotate the speculum a quarter turn so the anterior and posterior walls of the speculum can be examined. Close the blades when they are visible near the introitus. Take care not to pinch the labia or hairs.

Taking a Cervical Sample for Cytology

It makes sense to perform cervical cytology, if it is due, during a speculum examination if the woman is not in distress. It is outside the scope of this chapter to discuss fully cervical cytology. You should ensure you are fully trained according to national and local protocols and are competent to carry out the procedure before doing so. In the United Kingdom and United States of America (USA), liquid-based cytology (LBC) is used to perform cervical screening for all women aged 25–64 years every three years (up to age 50) and every five years (aged over 50) (NHS Choices 2015a). It should be remembered that cervical cytology in primary care is a screening test and should not be used for diagnosis. Of note now human papilloma virus (HPV) screening is carried out in conjunction with cervical cytology in the laboratory. There is no difference in how the sample is obtained.

Taking Swabs

Swabs should be taken during a speculum examination if there is concern around infection and/or if there is increased and/or abnormal discharge discussed during history taking and/or found on speculum examination. Swabs should also be taken if the patient is unwell or complaining of abdominal pain. pH paper can also be used to test vaginal discharge; normal pH is < 4.5.

Bimanual Examination

The purpose of a bimanual examination is to bring the pelvic organs closer to the abdominal wall, where they can be felt by the hand on the abdomen (Arulkamaran et al. 2007). Explain again to the woman what you are going to do. Using lubrication on gloved fingers, place the index and middle finger of the right hand into the vagina, palm upwards (Figure 9.5). One finger can be used if the woman is anxious or experiences discomfort. Note vaginal wall tone, any prolapse, tenderness, or protrusions. Locate the cervix. The cervix should feel smooth and firm. Check for 'cervical excitation' or 'cervical motion tenderness' by gently pushing the cervix to one side and then the other. This is the equivalent of rebound tenderness in abdominal examination. Pushing the cervix laterally will stretch the adnexa on the same side of the pelvis. The cervix should move 1–2 cm in either direction without pain. If the procedure elicits pain then this could be because of bleeding from an ectopic pregnancy or inflammation in the adnexa (Cruickshank and Shetty 2009; Jarvis 2015).

Palpate the Uterus

Place the left hand over the lower abdomen. Feel the uterus between the hands. An anteverted uterus should be easy to feel. A retroverted one may not be. However, the body of the uterus may be palpable by the vaginal fingers by moving them to above and below the cervix and exerting pressure inwards. The uterus should be pear shaped, about 5.5–8 cm long in nulliparous women, larger in multiparous women (Seidel et al. 2010). The contour

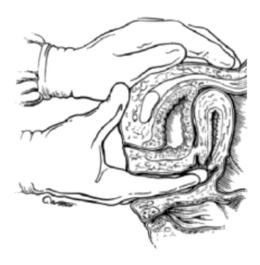

Figure 9.5   Bimanual examination.

should be round, firm, and smooth. The uterus should be slightly mobile in anterior–posterior plane and nontender on movement. Note the presence of any masses.

Next palpate the adnexae by moving the abdominal hand laterally over the lower abdominal quadrant on the same side as the internal fingers, which should be in the lateral fornix of the vagina. Apply firm pressure starting medially to the anterior iliac crest. Note any tenderness or masses. Palpate for the fallopian tubes on either side of the uterus; they should not normally be palpable or the area tender. Try to palpate the ovaries; this can cause discomfort in women. The ovaries are 2–4 cm in length, about the size of an almond. They are sensitive to touch but should not be acutely tender. They should be smooth, firm, and mobile. In postmenopausal women they are smaller and should not be palpable. Finally, place the vaginal fingers in the posterior fornix with the abdominal hand pressing down over the abdomen. The pouch of Douglas and uterosacral ligaments may then be felt. Note any tenderness and nodularity of the ligaments.

Having finished the examination, offer the woman some tissues and sanitary pads if needed and leave her to dress in private. Ensure she is able to wash her hands.

Documentation

See Figure 9.5.

The following points should be included in the records (Jarvis 2015; RCN 2013):

- external genitalia
- vagina
- cervix
- uterus
- adnexae.

They may include reference to:

- size
- position
- consistency
- mobility
- mass
- tenderness.

Provide correct information about the findings and results of the examination. If swabs have been taken or screening performed this should also be included.

Female Genital Mutilation (FGM)

With any discussion concerning examination of the female reproductive system, it is necessary to note the possibility of female genital mutilation. This is defined as procedures which intentionally alter or cause injury to the genital organs for nonmedical reasons. There are four main types of FGM:

- Type 1 – clitoridectomy – removing part of or the entire clitoris.
- Type 2 – excision – removing part or all of the clitoris and the inner labia (lips that surround the vagina), with or without removal of the labia majora (larger outer lips).
- Type 3 – infibulation – narrowing of the vaginal opening by creating a seal, formed by cutting and repositioning the labia.
- Other harmful procedures to the female genitals, which include pricking, piercing, cutting, scraping, and burning the area (NHS Choices 2015a).

FGM is illegal in the United Kingdom and the United States of America (The Guardian 2014; 18 U.S. Code § 116 n.d.) In all cases if you are worried about a child under 18 who is at risk of FGM or has had FGM, you have a legal obligation to share this information with social care and the police. It is then their responsibility to investigate, safeguard, and protect any girls involved. Other professionals should not attempt to investigate cases themselves. However, it is important to note that as with domestic violence and rape, if an adult woman has had FGM and this is identified through the delivery of healthcare, the patient's right to patient confidentiality MUST be respected if they do not wish any action to be taken. No reports to social services or the police should be made in these cases. For detailed guidance for clinicians who encounter FGM please refer to the guidelines available via NHS Choices (2015b).

For women who have undergone FGM, examination may be psychologically difficult and physically painful or impossible. All women who have had FGM should be offered referral to specialist services.

Overview of Common Presentations

examples of common presentations;
abnormal bleeding
vulval symptoms
vaginal discharge
genital prolapse
pelvic pain including dyspareunia
pelvic masses
abnormal bleeding from the vagina

Remember to exclude pregnancy first. Nonpregnancy-related causes of abnormal bleeding patterns can be classified as:

- intermenstrual bleeding (IMB)
- postcoital bleeding (PCB)
- breakthrough bleeding (BTB)
- postmenopausal bleeding (PMB)
- menorrhagia
- amenorrhoea.

Causes of IMB and PMB (many patients will present with a combination of both):

IMB	PMB	BTB
Pregnancy related (including ectopic and molar pregnancy)	Cervical ectropian	Combined oral contraceptive pill
Physiological; around ovulation (spotting) and perimenopausal (diagnosis of exclusion)	Cervical or endometrial polyps	Pre or post
Vaginal cancer	Vaginal cancer	Depot injection
Vaginitis (rare prior to menopause)	Cervical cancer	Intrauterine system
Sexually transmitted diseases (STIs; gonorrhoea, chlamydia, and less commonly trichomoniasis vaginalis)	Trauma	Emergency hormonal contraception
Cervical polyps/warts/ectropion	No specific cause found in approximately 50% of women	
Uterine fibroids		
Uterine cancer		
Oestrogen secreting ovarian tumours		
Iatrogenic (certain drugs, missed pills/following treatment to the cervix)		

Source: Adapted from (Patient 2015a).

The important point is first to rule out pregnancy and second to be aware of the risk of female cancers. In the United Kingdom (UK), refer to the National Institute for Health and Care Excellence (NICE) national guidelines for suspected cancer (NICE 2015). An urgent referral is recommended for women who have postmenopausal bleeding. It needs prompt investigation as it could indicate malignancy. The 2015 UK cancer guidelines state that women should be referred using a suspected cancer pathway referral for an appointment within two weeks for suspected endometrial cancer if they are aged 55 and over with post-menopausal bleeding (unexplained vaginal bleeding more than 12 months after menstruation has stopped because of the menopause). Consider a suspected cancer pathway referral (for an appointment within two weeks) for endometrial cancer in women aged under 55 with postmenopausal bleeding (NICE 2015).

Menorrhagia

Menorraghia is defined as >80 ml of blood loss per period (normal is 20–60 ml) (Thomas and Monaghan 2010). In practice, this is difficult to measure. Some causes of menorrhagia are listed here:

- hypothyroidism
- copper intrauterine device (IUD)
- fibroids
- endometriosis
- polyps of the cervix or uterus
- STIs
- previous sterilisation
- drugs (warfarin/aspirin/nonsteroidal anti-inflammatory drugs)
- clotting disorders (Thomas and Monaghan 2010).

Amenorrhea

Can be primary (failure to menstruate by age 16) or secondary where there is a history of normal menarche, then no menses for six months (Thomas and Monaghan 2010). Of course, it is necessary first to exclude pregnancy, and then further investigations are necessary to determine the cause, which could be endocrine, local ovarian causes, or physical or emotional stress.

Vulval Signs and Symptoms

Conditions affecting the vulva include:

- infection (candida, genital herpes, genital warts)
- vulval dystrophy
- dermatological disorders (lichen planus)
- cancer.

Candida usually presents with itching and burning of vulva and/or the vaginal walls, alongside a 'cottage cheese' looking vaginal discharge. With genital herpes there are usually bilateral crops of vesicles or ulcers on the vulva and sometimes the vagina and cervix. There may also be local oedema of the labia and vaginal discharge. The inguinal lymph nodes will usually be enlarged (Patient 2015b). Genital warts usually present as painless crops of lesions. They may be skin coloured, red, white, grey, or brown and may be broad based or pedunculated. They usually appear fleshy and soft in nonhairy areas but firmer in areas with pubic hair. They may appear on labia, clitoris, urethral meatus, introitus, vagina, and cervix. Visible genital warts are transmitted by the HPV virus but have a low risk of malignancy. They can be associated with increased vaginal discharge, PMB, and IMB. They can also be associated with other STIs and referral to a sexual health clinic is usually indicated (Patient 2015b).

Vulval dystrophy and atrophic vaginitis are caused by a lack of oestrogen, e.g. in postmenopausal women. The labia appear thin, pale, and dry as will the vaginal walls. It can also cause superficial dyspareunia, minor vaginal bleeding, and pain (Thomas and Monaghan 2010).

Almost any skin condition can affect the vulva. Dermatitis can appear as a red rash or area of inflammation of the labia and introitus. It is often secondary to application of products sold for cleansing of the genital area or irritation secondary to urinary incontinence. Lichen planus presents with intense redness and oedema of the vulva and superficial ulceration. It can lead to scarring and narrowing of the introitus over time if not treated, resembling chronic lichen sclerosis. This condition can present with vulval lesions leading to a 'cigarette' paper appearance – thin, white, and crinkly skin. Again, the introitus will shrink and the labia minora may become fused together. Treatment is usually with potent topical steroids (Patient 2015b).

Cancer of the Vulva/Vagina

A lump may be present or ulcer which may be associated with bleeding. Associated symptoms may be itching and pain. The 2015 UK cancer guidelines recommend the following:

Vulval Cancer

- Consider a suspected cancer pathway referral (for an appointment within two weeks) for vulval cancer in women with an unexplained vulval lump, ulceration, or bleeding.

Vaginal Cancer

- Consider a suspected cancer pathway referral (for an appointment within two weeks) for vaginal cancer in women with an unexplained palpable mass in or at the entrance to the vagina (NICE 2015).

Vaginal Discharge

Symptoms suggesting that discharge is abnormal include:

- a discharge that is heavier than usual
- a discharge that is thicker than usual
- puslike discharge
- white and clumpy discharge
- greyish, greenish, yellowish, or blood-tinged discharge
- foul-smelling (fishy or rotting meat) discharge
- a discharge accompanied by bloodiness, itching, burning, rash, or soreness (Patient 2015a).

Discharge can be caused by infection but can also be altered due to noninfective causes such as

- physiological causes; stage in menstrual cycle/pre- postmenopausal
- cervical polyps and ectopy
- foreign bodies – e.g. retained tampon
- vulval dermatitis
- erosive lichen planus
- genital tract malignancy – e.g. cancer of the cervix, uterus, or ovary
- fistulae.

Nonsexually Transmitted

Vulvovaginal candida has been discussed previously and usually produces a thick white discharge which is slightly lumpy and may have a 'cottage cheese' like appearance. There is usually no odour. Bacterial vaginosis usually causes a thin profuse fishy smelling discharge.

Sexually Transmitted

Trichomonas vaginalis may cause a thick, profuse yellowy discharge which may be frothy with an offensive odour. Chlamydia may produce a profuse vaginal discharge, but it is important to remember that the infection is asymptomatic in 80% of women. Gonorrhoea may present with a profuse discharge but again is asymptomatic in up to 50% women (Patient 2015c).

Swabs should be taken, using the correct swab for each procedure according to national and local guidelines. It is acceptable if the woman prefers for her to take her own vaginal swabs.

Normal practice in the UK and USA is to take 'triple swabs'. This will consist of

- High vaginal swab in transport medium (charcoal preferably) to diagnose chlamydia and bacterial vaginosis
- Endocervical swab in transport medium (charcoal preferably) to diagnose gonorrhoea.
- Endocervical swab for a chlamydial nucleic acid amplification test (NAAT) to diagnose chlamydia.

However, current guidelines suggest that high vaginal swabs are needed only if there is treatment failure, in pregnancy, postpartum, posttermination, or postsurgical procedures (RCGP and BASHH 2013).

Genital Prolapse

Genital prolapse is descent of the pelvic organs through the pelvic floor into the vaginal canal. This includes:

- uterocoele: uterus
- urethrocoele: urethra
- cystocoele: bladder
- enterocoele; small bowel
- rectocoele: rectum

The above will present clinically as a bulge in the vaginal wall, either anteriorly (in the case of bladder and or urethral prolapse), apically (uterine prolapse), or posteriorly (rectal prolapse). The degree of uterine descent in a uterine prolapse can be graded by the Baden–Walker or Beecham classification systems:

- 1st degree: cervix visible when the perineum is depressed – prolapse is contained within the vagina.
- 2nd degree: cervix prolapsed through the introitus with the fundus remaining in the pelvis.
- 3rd degree: procidentia (complete prolapse) – entire uterus is outside the introitus (Patient 2015d.)

Treatment can include pelvic floor exercises, vaginal pessaries, or surgical intervention for severe cases.

Pelvic Pain and Dyspareunia

Distinguishing between pain of gynaecological origin and gastrointestinal origin is difficult as the female reproductive organs share the same innervations for the lower ileum, sigmoid colon, and rectum. Careful history taking and abdominal as well as pelvic

Table 9.2 Differential diagnosis of acute pelvic pain.

Category	Diagnosis
Gynaecological	
Pregnancy related	Ectopic Miscarriage Complications in later pregnancy
Ovarian	Mittelschmerz Torsion/rupture/haemorrhage of an ovarian cyst Ovarian hyperstimulation syndrome
Tubal	Pelvic inflammatory disease
Uterine	Dysmenorrhoea Fibroid degeneration
Pelvic	Endometriosis Tumour
Nongynaecological	
Gastrointestinal	Appendicitis Inflammatory bowel disease Diverticulitis Constipation Adhesions Strangulated hernia
Urinary tract	Infection Calculus Retention

Source: Adapted from O'Connor and Kovacs (2003).

examination is needed. As with all pain, it may be acute or chronic in nature. Dyspareunia (pain on sexual intercourse) is often associated with chronic pelvic pain (Table 9.2).

Pelvic Inflammatory Disease (PID)

Pelvic inflammatory disease is a syndrome resulting from the spread of microorganisms to the endometrium and fallopian tubes. It is often caused by a variety of organisms and is not necessarily due to sexually transmitted infections (Patient 2015e). History includes high fever, acute pelvic pain and dyspareunia, abnormal vaginal bleeding, and purulent vaginal discharge. On pelvic examination there is cervical excitation and adnexal tenderness (Sadler et al. 2008).

Endometriosis

Endometriosis is the presence of tissue similar to the endometrium found outside of the uterine cavity, most commonly in the pelvis. History includes pelvic pain, dyspareunia, dysmenorrhoea, menorrhagia, and infertility. On examination, there may be pelvic tenderness, pelvic mass, and fixation of the uterus (Sadler et al. 2008).

Fibroids (Uterine Leiomyoma)

Fibroids are benign tumours of the myometrium. Usually they are asymptomatic, but they may cause menorrhagia, pain, pelvic discomfort, and backache as well as urinary symptoms. On examination, the uterus will feel 'bulky' and there may be a pelvic mass (Sadler et al. 2008).

Ovarian Cancer

Ovarian cancer may present with many symptoms, including abdominal and or pelvic pain as well as abdominal distension or 'bloating', early satiety, and loss of appetite. Late symptoms may include ascites and or pelvic or abdominal mass. The 2015 UK cancer guidelines (NICE 2015) state a two-week referral is indicated if physical examination identifies ascites and/or a pelvic or abdominal mass (which is not obviously a uterine fibroid). For other less well-defined symptoms refer to the guidelines (NICE 2015).

Pelvic Masses

The main differential diagnoses are outlined in the table below:

Pregnancy		
	Example	Nature of mass
Ovarian mass	Benign tumour, functional cysts, ovarian cancer	Painless mass, often one side
Uterine mass	Fibroids	'Bulky' uterus
Tubal mass	Chronic salpingitis	Tender mass

Source: Lewellyn et al. (2014).

As above, all masses should be referred urgently for further investigation unless there is a clear and benign cause.

Case Study of a 24-Year-Old Female Presenting with Acute Pelvic Pain

Presenting Problem

A 24-year-old woman presents to the local general practice out of hours centre at 10 p.m. on a Monday evening with her partner. She is complaining of severe lower abdominal pain and of feeling very unwell.

History

The woman had had some pain in her lower abdomen for the past week. She described it as a dull aching pain in the central lower abdomen. Initially it was mild and she was able to continue to carry out her work (as a carer) and other usual activities. However, over the last two days the pain has become increasingly intense and was waking her from sleep. Today the pain has been getting increasingly severe and she has been in bed most of the day. She has been taking paracetamol at regular intervals without much effect. The pain is now extending round to her back. She is also feeling hot but shivery. She has been able to drink some water today but no food since breakfast. She was feeling nauseous and had vomited one time this evening. She has not passed much urine today but has not had any dysuria; she opened her bowels with a normal movement yesterday. She tried to get a GP appointment this afternoon and has been given one for tomorrow morning but states she can't wait that long because of the acute nature of the pain.

Last Menstrual Period (LMP) three weeks ago, regular cycle approx. 28 days and duration four days. No PCB, no IMB. She has noticed an increase in her vaginal discharge over the last few days, which she says is yellowy and thick and smells bad.

Social History

Lives with partner, works as a carer, originally from Eastern Europe. Nonsmoker, little alcohol.

Past medical history
Usually well
Mild depression
Medhx
Citalopram 20 mg daily
No known drug allergies
Female history
Para 0 + 0. Sexually active. Not using contraception as wishing to conceive. Current partner (male) last 12 months. No history of sexually transmitted infections.

Review of Systems

Feeling generally unwell and feverish. Headache 'all over' today, no visual symptoms, no shortness of breath or chest pain, no rash, no limb pain or paraesthesia, abdominal symptoms as above.

Examination

Looks unwell. Sitting bent over abdomen with hot water bottle. In noticeable pain.
Temperature 38.5; heart rate 120; respiratory rate 20; BP 90/62
Difficulty walking into consulting room. Stooped and using partner for support. Able to talk but tearful at times.
Abdominal examination: Active bowel sounds. Abdomen mainly tympanic (but unable to tolerate percussion well). Light palpation = generalised tenderness over upper quadrants. Tender +++ R and L lower quadrants with guarding bilaterally. Marked rebound tenderness. Rovsing's sign negative, McBurney's point negative for increased tenderness. Psoas stretch test positive. Deep palpation deferred.
Examination of female genitalia (with verbal consent. Chaperone declined, partner present outside curtain.):
Inspection of vulva; Normal appearance of labia majora and minora, no lesions or inflammation seen. Introitus no lesions, but yellowy d/c at entrance. Speculum examination deferred due to condition of the patient.
PV examination: Marked cervical motion tenderness. Tender over adnexae bilaterally. No masses felt. Discharge, white-yellow present on gloved finger.
Urine: pregnancy test negative. Scant specimen. Urine concentrated, blood, and protein present on dipstick.

Diagnosis

Probable PID.

Treatment

Admitted to gynaecology ward as an emergency where she was commenced on IV antibiotics with a provisional diagnosis of PID.
'Triple' swabs taken were positive for chlamydia infection.

Case Study of a 55-Year-Old Woman with Abnormal Vaginal Bleeding

Presenting Problem

A 55-year-old woman presents at her local general practice with bleeding from her vagina three years after cessation of her periods. She says she has been intermittently 'spotting' for a few months and thought nothing of it, but now she needs to use pads on some days as the bleeding has increased. She describes the blood as being pinkish and watery initially but now it is a darker colour, more like menstrual blood. She is currently not sexually active with her partner, mainly because of the bleeding. She has no abdominal pain, has a good appetite, no nausea or vomiting, no urinary symptoms. She is otherwise well.

Social History

Primary school teacher, lives with long-term partner and two teenage children. Nonsmoker, moderate alcohol. Takes regular exercise.

Past medical history
Asthma
No known drug allergies
Medication
Inhalers for asthma
Well woman history
Para 3 + 2 (two children alive and well, one miscarriage.) No hormone replacement therapy.

Physical Examination

Looks well
Temperature 36.5; heart rate 72; BP 130/85.
Abdominal examination; soft nontender, no masses felt.

Per vaginal examination (with consent of patient, chaperone declined). Labia majora and minora no lesions seen. Introitus no lesions. Speculum examination; pink vaginal walls, no lesions, cervix; no lesions seen, small amount of red blood visible around the os. No other discharge seen. Bimanual examination: no cervical excitation, slightly 'bulky' feeling uterus, no masses felt, nontender adnexae. Ovaries and fallopian tubes not palpable.

Differential Diagnosis

Atypical hyperplasia, possible endometrial cancer

Treatment Plan

Referred to gynaecology as per NICE guidelines using suspected cancer pathway referral (two-week wait). Following investigations, the patient was diagnosed with endometrial cancer and underwent a total abdominal hysterectomy.

References

Arulkamaran, S., Symonds, I., and Fowlie, A. (2007). *Oxford Handbook of Obstetrics and Gynaecology*. New York: Oxford University Press.

Cruickshank, M. and Shetty, A. (2009). *Obstetrics and Gynaecology, Clinical Cases Uncovered*. Oxford: Wiley-Blackwell.

Jarvis, C. (2015). *Physical Examination and Health Assessment*, 7e. Edinburgh: Elsevier.

Lewellyn, H., Ang, H., Lewis, K., and Al'Abdullah, A. (2014). *Oxford Handbook of Clinical Diagnosis*, 3e. Oxford: Oxford University Press.

NHS Cancer Screening Programme (2006) *Cervical Screening: Professional Guidance*. https://www.gov.uk/government/collections/cervical-screening-professional-guidance (accessed 28 August 2018).

NHS Choices (2015a) *Cervical Screening*. http://www.nhs.uk/Conditions/Cervical-screening-test/Pages/Introduction.aspx accessed 14 October 2015).

NHS Choices (2015b) *Female Genital Mutilation*. http://www.nhs.uk/conditions/female-genital-mutilation/Pages/Introduction.aspx (accessed 14 October 2015).

NICE (2015) *Suspected Cancer Recognition and Referral Overview*. https://pathways.nice.org.uk/pathways/suspected-cancer-recognition-and-referral (accessed 28 August 2018).

O'Connor, V. and Kovacs, G. (2003). *Obstetrics, Gynaecology and Women's Health*. Cambridge: Cambridge University Press.

Patient (2015a) *Intermenstrual and Postcoital Bleeding*. http://patient.info/doctor/intermenstrual-and-postcoital-bleeding (accessed 22 August 2015).

Patient (2015b) *Vulval Problems*. http://patient.info/doctor/vulval-problems-pro (accessed 22 August 2015).

Patient (2015c) *Vaginal Discharge*. http://patient.info/doctor/vaginal-discharge (accessed 22 August 2015).

Patient (2015d) *Genitourinary Prolapse*. http://patient.info/doctor/genitourinary-prolapse-pro (accessed 21 September 2015).

Patient (2015e) *Pelvic Inflammatory Disease*. http://patient.info/doctor/pelvic-inflammatory-disease-pro (accessed 21 September 2015).

Royal College of General Practitioners & British Association for Sexual Health and HIV) (2013) *Sexually Transmitted Infections in Primary Care (2nd ed.)* http://www.bashh.org/documents/Sexually%20Transmitted%20Infections%20in%20Primary%20Care%202013.pdf (accessed 21 September 2015).

Royal College of Nursing (2013) *Genital Examination in Women*. https://www.rcn.org.uk/professional-development/publications/pub-005480 (accessed 28 August 2018).

Sadler, C., White, J., Everitt, H., and Simon, C. (2008). *Women's Health: Oxford General Practice Library*. Oxford: Oxford University Press.

Seidel, H., Ball, J., Dains, J., and Benedict, G. (2010). *Mosby's Physical Examination Handbook*, 7e. St. Louis: Mosby-Year Book.

The Guardian (2014) FGM is banned but very much alive in the UK. https://www.theguardian.com/society/2014/feb/06/female-genital-mutilation-foreign-crime-common-uk (accessed 21 January 2018).

Thomas, J. and Monaghan, T. (2010). *Oxford Handbook of Clinical Examination and Practical Skills*, 2e. Oxford: Oxford University Press.

18 U.S. Code § 116 –Female genital mutilation. n.d. *LII / Legal Information Institute*. https://www.law.cornell.edu/uscode/text/18/116 (accessed 16 November 2017).

Chapter 10

Examination of the Nervous System

Michael Babcock and Graham M. Boswell

General Examination

Introduction

The nervous system assessment constitutes an essential aspect in evaluating the patient's health. Functions of the nervous system involve the exchange of oxygen and carbon dioxide in the lungs and tissues and regulation of the acid–base balance. Changes in the nervous system affect other systems.

Anatomy and Physiology

Functional Overview of the Brain (Figure 10.1; Table 10.1)

Spinal Nerves

There are 31 pairs of spinal nerves with one pair leaving the spinal cord at each vertebral level (Table 10.2). The cervical region has one extra pair because the 1st pair leave above C1 but all other pairs leave at the bottom of the vertebral level. All pairs of spinal nerves contain both motor and sensory fibres (Crossman and Neary 2014; Martini et al. 2014; Tortora and Derrickson 2012).

Physical Assessment for Nurses and Healthcare Professionals, Third Edition. Edited by Carol Lynn Cox.
© 2019 John Wiley & Sons Ltd. Published 2019 by John Wiley & Sons Ltd.

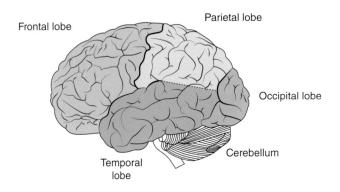

Figure 10.1   The brain.

Table 10.1   The brain.

Lobe	Functions the lobe is involved in
Frontal lobe	Motor function, mood, behaviour, decision making, memory, personality
Parietal lobe	Sensation, touch, pain, temperature, left/right determination
Temporal lobe	Hearing, language, memory, emotion, vision
Occipital lobe	Vision
Cerebellum	Modifies motor commands, balance, equilibrium, muscle tone

Cerebral Blood Supply

The cerebral blood supply comes from two vertebral and two carotid arteries. The right common carotid artery and the right vertebral artery branch from the brachiocephalic artery (1st branch from the aorta). The left common carotid artery branches directly from

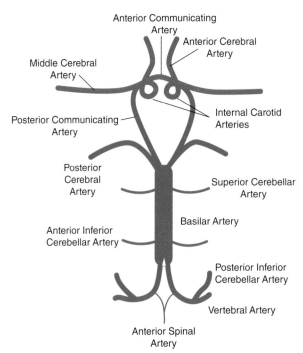

Figure 10.2   Cerebral blood supply.

the aorta (2nd branch from the aorta). The left vertebral artery branches from the left sub-clavian artery (3rd branch from the aorta). The common carotid arteries divide at the upper level of the larynx to form the internal and external carotid arteries. The external carotid arteries supply the face, neck, larynx, thyroid, and scalp.

The left and right internal carotid arteries provide ophthalmic, posterior communi-cating, and anterior choroidal arteries before dividing into the anterior and middle cerebral arteries. The left and right anterior cerebral arteries are then linked by the anterior communicating artery.

The left and right vertebral arteries provide anterior spinal and posterior inferior cerebellar arteries before joining to form the basilar artery in front of the medulla oblon-gata. This provides anterior inferior cerebellar and superior cerebellar arteries as well as pontine branches. The basilar artery divides at the upper border of the pons to form the right and left posterior cerebral arteries. The posterior communicating arteries join with the posterior cerebral arteries to complete the circle of Willis (Figure 10.2) (Crossman and Neary 2014; Martini et al. 2014; Tortora and Derrickson 2012).

The Nerve and Action Potential

The resting membrane potential is when the inside of the nerve (cytoplasmic side) is negatively charged compared to the outside (Figure 10.3). This varies from −40 to −90 mV in different types of neurons and the membrane is polarised (ready to fire) in this state. The resting mem-brane potential is created by differences in the ionic solution inside and outside of the cell. The cell cytosol contains less sodium (Na^+) and more potassium (K^+) than extracellular fluid.

Table 10.2 Spinal nerves.

Region	Number
Cervical	8
Thoracic	12
Lumbar	5
Sacral	5
Coccygeal	1

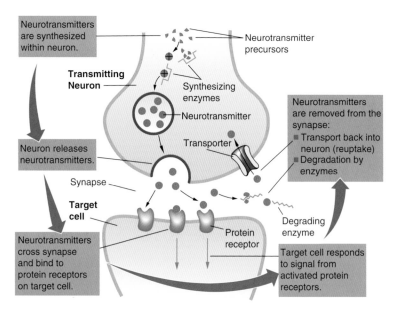

Figure 10.3 Nerve and action potential.

A nerve impulse begins when the dendrite is stimulated (for example, the receptor sites being activated by a neurotransmitter such as acetylcholine). This causes some local sodium channels to open and as Na$^+$ enters the cell it becomes a bit less negatively charged. If the change reaches a critical threshold (usually about −55 mV) many more local voltage gated sodium channels (VGSC) open which allows a large influx of sodium into the local cell region raising the charge to +40 mV (depolarisation). This process creates a self-generating stimulus to the next part of the cell membrane affecting nearby VGSCs and allows the action potential (+ve charge) to move wave-like (propagate) along the nerve until it reaches the synaptic end bulb. Here the action potential causes the release of a neurotransmitter and the stimulus passes to another nerve, a muscle, gland, or organ. After transmission any unused neurotransmitter is either reused by the transmitting neuron or degraded by enzymes (such as cholinesterase).

After the depolarisation the VGSCs close and the local voltage gated potassium channels open, which allows K$^+$ out making the outside of the cell positively charged and the inside negative (repolarisation). Because the K$^+$ gates do not begin to shut until the cell membrane resting state (−80 mV) is reached and they are a little slow closing the charge inside the cell becomes lower than the resting state (hyperpolarisation). The refractory period is when the sodium-potassium pump corrects the hyperpolarisation by active transport against the concentration gradient of Na$^+$ and K$^+$. Powered by adenosine triphosphate (ATP) the voltage gated channel changes shape to attract three Na$^+$ ions to bind, when open to the inside of the cell. It then closes to the inside and opens to the outside and changes shape to release the Na$^+$ ions but it then attracts two K$^+$ ions to bind and the process reverses. This transfer of three Na$^+$ ions out to 2 K$^+$ ions in is then supported by passive diffusion channels, which allow small amounts of K$^+$ to leak out and much smaller amounts of Na$^+$ to diffuse in. The entire process of activation, polarisation, depolarisation, and refraction takes approximately 4 thousandths of a second and then another wav can pass along the nerve (Crossman and Neary 2014; Martini et al. 2014; Tortora and Derrickson 2012).

Action Potential

The action potential travels at different speeds in different nerves depending upon the size and type of nerve Figure 10.4. Myelinated nerves travel at up to 20 times the speed of unmyelinated fibres (up to approximately 120 m per second). Myelin is an insulating

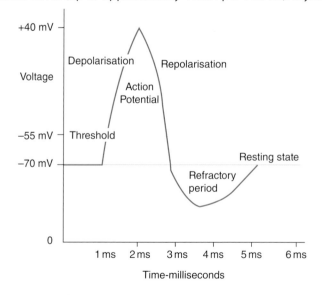

Figure 10.4   Action potential.

membrane approximately 1–1.5 mm long with very small gaps (nodes of Ranvier; Figure 10.5) in between. It is formed from oligodendrocytes in the central nervous system and from Schwann cells in the peripheral nervous system. The insulating quality of myelin means that Na⁺ and K⁺ can change places at only the nodes of Ranvier, which means that the action potential travels down a nerve in blocks (saltatory conduction) and so is quicker (Crossman and Neary 2014).

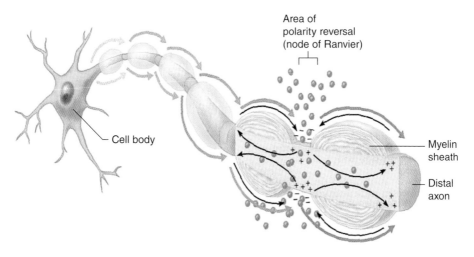

Figure 10.5 Node of Ranvier.

General Examination

Assessment of a patient's problem(s) is essential in planning effective care. An accurate history facilitates assessment of the pathology and helps guide the examination and identify appropriate tests. The examination reveals the location and extent of the lesion. The examination should address three questions: (i) Does the patient have a neurological illness? (ii) Where in the nervous system is the pathology located? (iii) What is the pathology? (Jarvis 2015; Swartz 2014).

The mnemonic SOCRATES is widely used to help explore symptoms especially pain (Table 10.3).

Table 10.3 SOCRATES.

S – Site	Where are the symptoms?
O – Onset	When did the symptoms begin?
C – Characteristics	If there is pain, is it dull, sharp, stabbing, burning, etc.?
R – Radiation	Is it localised, or does it spread and if so in what direction?
A – Associated factors	Any signs or symptoms associated with the pain?
T – Timing	Since it began, has it progressed?
E – Exacerbating or alleviating factors	Things that make the symptoms better or worse?
S – Severity	Grading symptoms such as pain scales, breathlessness, etc.

The following features in the history can be informative:

- speed of onset
- rapid, abrupt – *vascular*, *oedema*, or *infective*
- seconds – *seizure*
- minutes – *migraine*
- hours – *infective, inflammatory*
- slow, progressive – *neoplasm* or *degenerative disorder*
- duration
- brief episodes with recovery, e.g. *transischaemic attack (TIA), epilepsy, migraine, syncope*
- longer episodes with recovery – *mechanical, obstruction,* or *pressure*
- demyelination, e.g. *multiple sclerosis*
- frequency
- witness description – particularly if the patient has episodic loss of consciousness or is confused (Ball et al. 2014; Bickley and Szilagyi 2013; Japp and Robertson 2013; Jarvis 2015; Sirven and Malamut 2008; Swartz 2014; Talley and O'Connor 2013).

The minute examination of the nervous system can be elaborated almost indefinitely. Of far greater importance is to acquire the ability to conduct a thorough but comparatively rapid examination with confidence in the findings. As with other examinations, it is best to develop your own basic system and perform it consistently because this will help avoid omissions.

- Adapt your examination to the situation. The order in which functions are examined may be varied according to the symptoms, but the routine examination must be mastered.

From the history, usually it will be obvious whether it is necessary to examine the mental functions in detail. A patient with sciatica would rightly be dismayed by an examination that began by asking him to name the parts of a watch.

The examination of the nervous system is approached under the following headings:

- Motor and sensory function
- Mental function
  - appearance and behaviour
  - mood
  - orientation
  - geographical orientation
  - memory
  - intelligence
  - speech and comprehension
- Cranial nerves (Ball et al. 2014; Bickley and Szilagyi 2013; Japp and Robertson 2013; Jarvis 2015; Sirven and Malamut 2008; Swartz 2014; Talley and O'Connor 2013).

Motor and Sensory Function

The motor examination should be carried out in a systematic way. You should begin by assessing the upper limbs to the neck and trunk and finally to the lower extremities of the patient. When examining the limbs and the trunk you will need to observe the patient's posture, muscle tone, presence or absence of involuntary movements, and muscular wasting and/or fasciculation. Your limb evaluation and examination should proceed from proximal to distal. Assess the major muscle groups first and if you note problems in any particular area then carry out a more detailed examination.

The assessment will examine the patient's proprioception, balance, gait, sensory stimuli, cortical sensory function, and reflex activity.

The nervous system cannot effectively be examined in isolation.

Other points of relevance may include:

- configuration of the skull and spine
- neck stiffness
- ear drums for otitis media
  - blood pressure
  - heart, e.g. arrhythmia, mitral stenosis
  - carotid arteries – palpation and bruit
  - neoplasms – breast, lung, abdominal
  - jaundice.

191

Mental Function

General Observation

- appearance, e.g. unkempt
- behaviour, e.g. bewildered, restless, agitated
- emotional state, e.g. depressed, euphoric, hostile.

Observe, and ask for comments from nurses, other healthcare practitioners, and relatives.

Consciousness Level

If the patient is not fully conscious shake him gently and/or speak to him loudly but clearly. Record:

- drowsy but able to rouse to normal level
- drowsy but not able to rouse.

Glasgow Coma Scale (GCS) (Appendix F)

The GCS provides a rapid, widely used assessment of a patient's level of consciousness (Table 10.4). The GCS is an indirect measure of consciousness because it measures behaviours that are associated with conscious activity. Patterns of change in these behaviours when linked with alterations with pupil size, temperature, pulse, respirations, and blood pressure provide an effective guide to the extent of damage within the central nervous system. These observations can be even more effective when computer tomography (CT) and magnetic resonance imaging (MRI) scan evidence is also utilised.

Monitor responses to verbal command and if there is no response then a painful stimulus should be utilised. The painful stimuli should elicit a localising response which requires a central application. The trapezius pinch is the preferred option and is produced by squeezing the trapezius muscle between the thumb and index finger. Supraorbital pressure is usually the secondary choice for painful stimuli. Locate the supraorbital notch by feeling along the supraorbital arch at the nasal end and apply pressure with the thumb. If there is a risk of facial fractures this is contraindicated. The sternal rub (with knuckles over sternum) will damage the patient's skin and should be used only in extremis. Nail bed pressure (with smooth round object such as a torch) is sometimes used if there is no localising response to indicate that the limb is able to move but because this may be due to a spinal arc reflex it is an unreliable measure of cerebral function.

The GCS is the total score for the patient's response, but when communicating the GCS also provide the breakdown of scores as this ensures greater clarity for other healthcare professionals.

Table 10.4   Glasgow Coma Scale.

Scoring the GCS
There are three subscales: Eye opening (4), Verbal response (5), and Motor response (6). Each subscale must score a minimum of 1 to a maximum of 4–6 depending upon the subscale. This provides a score range of 3–15. A score between 3 and 8 necessitates airway management and a rapidly deteriorating score such as 2 points between observations requires urgent intervention.

A Eye opening	4 – Spontaneous with normal blinking 3 – Eyes open to command 2 – Eyes open to pain 1 – Eyes remain closed
B Verbal response	5 – Normal speech – able to hold a reasonable and relevant conversation 4 – Confused speech – language is in a reasonable structure for the conversation but the meaning is inappropriate 3 – Inappropriate words – single words spoken (expressing cerebral irritation) but no conversational structure 2 – Incomprehensible sounds – moaning sounds only 1 – No response
C Motor response	6 – Voluntary – responds normally to commands 5 – Localising – attempts to protect site of pain 4 – Flexion response – normal withdrawal of limb to pain 3 – Abnormal flexion – exaggerated withdrawal of limb to pain with shoulder and elbow moving to the midline 2 – Extension response to pain – adduction and internal rotation at shoulder, extension at elbows, pronation of forearms 1 – No response

Confusion

If a patient appears confused, move on to assess cognitive state, including disorientation.

Language/Speech

Assess from conversation:

- Is there difficulty in articulation?
  If necessary, ask patient to say for example 'British Constitution', 'West Register Street'.
  - Dysarthria – difficulty moving and controlling the muscles of the lips, face, tongue, and the upper respiratory system that control speech.
  - Cerebellar or ataxic dysarthria – The cerebellum processes proprioceptive information that refines muscle activity in speech. Damage may result in scanning (slow, deliberate speech with each syllable equally stressed) or the voice may have a drunken quality, i.e. slurred because of the distorted vowels.
  - Lower motor neuron or flaccid dysarthria – Either bulbar or peripheral nerve lesions affect the muscles of articulation which may result in a rasping or monotonous voice, tongue wasting, and reduced lip control.
  - Upper motor neuron or spastic dysarthria – Damage to the pyramidal and extrapyramidal tracts affects muscle tone and strength especially of the lips and tongue. This results in slow speech, which requires more effort to produce and has a 'harsh' vocal quality.
- Is there altered voice tone?
  - extrapyramidal (monotonous and slow)
  - lower motor neuron (slurred)

- upper motor neuron (slurred)
- acute alcohol poisoning (slurred)
- dysphonia – disorder of voice
- cord lesion – hoarse
- hysterical dysphonia is a stress related difficulty
- Is there difficulty in finding the right word?
  - dysphasia or aphasia – disorder of use of words as symbols in speech, writing, and understanding; nearly always the result of left hemisphere lesion
  - N.B. The centres for language are in people's dominant hemisphere. In right-handed and 75% of left-handed people, the dominant hemisphere is the left.
  - expressive dysphasia or slight dysphasia – difficult to detect; look for mispronounced words and circumlocutions in spontaneous speech; test for nominal aphasia by asking patient to name objects you point to, e.g. wristwatch, pen, chair, etc.; understanding should be intact
  - receptive dysphasia – speech fluent, but comprehension poor; patient may seem 'confused'; test for by asking patient to follow commands – a three-step command is a good screening test (e.g. 'please pick up the glass, but first point to the curtain and then the door'); caused by a lesion in Wernicke's area
  - gross dysphasia or missed dysphasia – most common; usually obvious; the patient's spontaneous speech will be scanty, small vocabulary, often with the wrong words used; there are also other dysphasias produced by interruption of the connecting pathways between the speech centres
  - aphasia or mutism – no speech at all, just grunts; this may be due to aphasia, anarthria, psychiatric disease, or occasionally diffuse cerebral pathology (Ball et al. 2014; Bickley and Szilagyi 2013; Japp and Robertson 2013; Jarvis 2015; Sirven et al. 2008; Swartz 2014; Talley and O'Connor 2013).

193

Other Defects Occurring in Absence Motor or Sensory Dysfunction
First Establish the Normal Reading and Writing Skills of the Person

- dyslexia – inappropriate difficulty with reading; read few lines from newspaper (having established that comprehension and expressive speech are intact)
- dysgraphia – inappropriate difficulty writing
- agraphia – loss of ability to write
- acalculia – loss of ability to do mental and written sums
- apraxia – inability to perform a learned purposeful task when there is no paralysis, e.g. opening matchbox, waving goodbye; apraxia for dressing is common in *diffuse brain disease*
- visual agnosia – inability to visually recognise familiar objects
- auditory agnosia – inability to recognise familiar sounds
- astereognosis – tactile agnosia – With their eyes closed, it is the inability to recognise common objects (e.g. a key or coin when placed in the hand)
- parietal lobe lesions – can cause a neglect of the opposite side of the body, there are no perceived sensations and so the half of the body is not recognised by the conscious brain; right parietal lobe lesions cause particular problems with spatial awareness: getting lost in familiar places, inability to lay table, to draw or make patterns, and neglect of left side of space (Ball et al. 2014; Bickley and Szilagyi 2013; Japp and Robertson 2013; Jarvis 2015; Sirven et al. 2008; Swartz 2014; Talley and O'Connor 2013).

Cognitive Function

Take account of any evidence you have about the patient's intelligence, education, and interests.

'Cognitive' is a term that covers orientation, thought processes, and logic.

Orientation

In the process of normal conversation, you can check the patient's awareness of time, place, and person. The ability to respond and contribute appropriately to a conversation with the consequent changes of parameters inherent to a 'normal' conversation would indicate that understanding (Wernicke's area) and speech (Broca's area) are able to function. Issues of time, place, and person provide some details that you may find easier to check but which require less use of the patient's language centres. The patient's sentence construction demonstrates how well the speech process is working; therefore, questions that require one-word answers should be avoided.

Disorientation indicates disruption of the pathways between language understanding and expression. *Depressed patients* may be unwilling to reply although they know the answers.

Attention, Concentration and Calculation

- Test the concentration of a patient by asking them to take away 7 from 100, 7 from 93, etc. or by asking them to say the months of the year backwards.

Concentration may be impaired with many cerebral abnormalities, depression, and anxiety.

Memory (Appendix E: Mini-Mental State Examination)
Immediate Recall – Digit Span

- Ask the patient to repeat a random series of numbers. Speak slowly and start with an easy short sequence and then increase the numbers. Most people manage seven digits' forwards, five backwards.

Short-Term Memory

- Ask patient to tell you:
  - what they had for breakfast
  - what they did the night before
  - what they read in today's paper.

Demented patients will be unable to do this. They may confabulate (make up impressive stories) to cover their ignorance.

New Memory

- Ask patient in early part of your assessment to remember four or five common objects such as orange, apple, pen, book, and teddy bear, make sure the patient has learnt it. After 10 minutes or so ask the patient to recall your objects. It is a good idea to note the objects and order.

Longer-Term Memory

- Ask patient and if necessary check with relatives, etc.
  - events before illness, e.g. last year, or during last week
  - 'What is your address?'

General Knowledge
- Assess in relation to anticipated performance from history.
  - What is the name of the President/Prime Minister or other political leader.
  - Name six capital cities.
  - What were the dates of a major event relevant to the patient's societal grouping that happened approximately two to five years ago. You may need to ask about several events because depending upon the questions, a person's inability to answer may just reflect a lack of interest rather than an inability to recall.

In *acute organic states* and *dementia*, new learning, recent memory, and reasoning are usually more impaired than remote memory. Vocabulary is usually well preserved in *dementia*. In *depression*, patients may be unwilling to reply, and appear demented.

- A history from a relative or employer is very important in early dementia (Ball et al. 2014; Bickley and Szilagyi 2013; Japp and Robertson 2013; Jarvis 2015; Sirven et al. 2008; Swartz 2014; Talley and O'Connor 2013).

Reasoning (Abstract Thought)
- What does this proverb mean: 'Let sleeping dogs lie?'.

Skull and Spine
- Inspect and palpate skull if there is any possibility of a head injury.
- Check neck stiffness – meningeal irritation.
- Inspect spine – usually when examining back of chest.
- If there is any possibility of pathology, stand patient and check all movements of spine; if there is possible trauma then X-ray first.

Cranial Nerves (I – XII)
- Examine cranial nerves and upper limbs with patient sitting up, preferably on side of bed or on a chair (Table 10.5).

I Olfactory Nerve
Not normally tested unless there are other neurological deficits, including papilloedema, undiagnosed headache (especially frontal), or head injury. Ask the patient to close eyes, then close one nostril by palpation. Then present a smell such as oil of cloves, peppermint, coffee, etc. to the open nostril. Test each nostril in turn. It is normal not to be able to name all smells, but one smell should be distinguished from another. Pungent or noxious smells such as ammonia should not be used, as they are perceived by the 5th cranial nerve and confuse results. A loss of the sensation of smell indicates possible:

–	*base of skull fracture*	especially if loss of smell is one sided
–	*olfactory groove meningioma*	
–	*rhinitis*	more likely if loss of smell is bilateral
–	*smoking*	

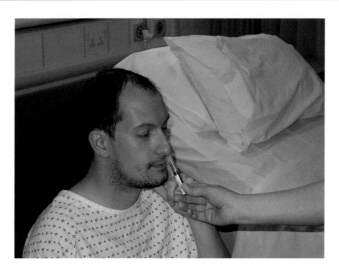

Test Olfactory 1 - smell

Table 10.5   'Examine the cranial nerves'.

I	Olfactory	Smell
II	Optic	Visual acuity Visual field Fundi
III, IV and VI	Occulomotor, trochlear, and abducens	Ptosis Nystagmus Eye movements Pupils
V	Trigeminal	Facial sensation Corneal reflex Jaw muscles/jerk Tongue taste
VII	Facial	Face muscles
VIII	Vestibuloauditory	Hearing Rinne/Weber tests Nystagmus/gait
IX, X	Glossopharyngeal, vagus	Palate Swallowing Taste – posterior third of tongue
XI	Spinal accessory	Trapezius
XII	Hypoglossal	Tongue wasting

II Optic Nerve
Visual Acuity (Appendixes A and B Acuity Charts)

- Test each eye separately.
- Check patient can read a language you understand and then ask them to read small text such as newspaper print with each eye separately, with reading glasses if used.

196

- If sight poor, test formally:
  - ○ near vision – newsprint or Jaeger type (each eye in turn) (see Appendix A)
  - ○ distant vision – Snellen type (more precise method) (see Appendix B)

Stand patient at 6 m from Snellen's card (each eye in turn). Results expressed as a ratio:

- 6 – distance of person from card
- x – distance at which patient should be able to read type

i.e. 6/6 is good vision, 6/60 means the smallest type the patient can read is large enough to be normally read at 60 m.

If the patient cannot read 6/6, try after correction with glasses or pinhole. Looking through a pinhole in a card obviates refractive errors, analogous to a pinhole camera. If vision remains poor, suspect a neurological or ophthalmic cause.

A 3 m Snellen chart is shown in Appendix B.

A pinhole is not effective for correcting near vision for reading.

Visual Fields

- Quick method for temporal peripheral patient fields by confrontation of patient and examiner with both eyes open Figure 10.6. Always test fields. Patients are often unaware of visual loss, the most dramatic of which is Anton's syndrome (blindness with lack of awareness of the blindness).
  - ○ Sit opposite the patient and ask them to look at your nose with both eyes open.
  - ○ Examine each eye in turn.
  - ○ Bring waggling finger forwards from behind patient's ear in upper and lower lateral quadrants and ask when it can be seen.
  - ○ Normal vision is approximately 100° from axis of eye.

The patient must fully understand the test. The extreme of peripheral vision can be tested with both eyes open, because the nose obstructs vision from the other eye. If peripheral field seems restricted, retest with the other eye covered to ensure each eye is being tested separately.

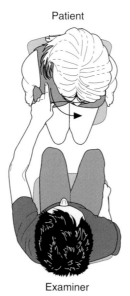

Patient

Examiner

Figure 10.6   Testing temporal peripheral patient fields of vision.

Patient

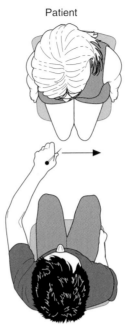

Examiner

Figure 10.7 Visual field assessment.

- A peripheral defect in the visual field of one eye would indicate a nasal defect in the other eye. To test this, the patient covers the eye with the peripheral defect and then the examiner moves the waggling finger from the expected defect towards the area of better vision.
- Normal vision is approximately 50° from each axis of eye.
- Standard method: (Figure 10.7)

Hold a small red pinhead in the plane midway between the patient and examiner. With the other eye covered, compare the visual fields of the patient with that of the examiner, with a pin brought in from temporal or nasal fields.

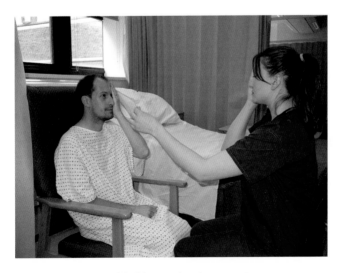

Visual field examination - optic

Defects in the central field can be assessed by the standard method with a small red pin held in the plane midway between the patient and examiner:

- scotoma – defects in the central field (*retinal or optic nerve lesion*)
- enlarged blind spot (*papilloedema*)

Map by moving the pin from inside scotoma or blind spot outwards until red pinhead reappears.

This is a crude test and small areas of loss of vision may need to be formally tested with a perimetry.

- Test for sensory inattention when fields are full with both eyes open.
  - Hold your hands between you and the patient, one opposite each ear and waggle forefingers simultaneously. Ask which moves. With a parietal defect, the patient may not recognise movement on one side, although fields are full to formal testing.

The patterns of visual field deficit will indicate where the lesion is on the optic pathway from the optic disc to the occipital cortex. The changes in the visual field deficit occur because at the optic chiasma half of the optic nerve crosses over to enable stereoptic vision (Figure 10.8). A review of visual pathways is that all light from the right reaches the left-hand side of both optic discs and then travels to the left occipital cortex (blue) and vice versa. Deficits before the optic chiasma (1) cause problems in one eye only. Deficits at the optic chiasma are usually central (2 – bitemporal hemianopia) and caused by an enlarged pituitary (such as pituitary adenoma). At the optic chiasma the problems are mirrored in both visual fields whereas after the optic chiasma the deficits affect one side of the visual field in both eyes (3, 4, and 5). Partial damage to the optic radiation will produce a partial deficit (4), with a top-quadrant defect being caused by temporal damage or an occipital lesion and a lower-quadrant defect being caused by parietal damage or an occipital lesion.

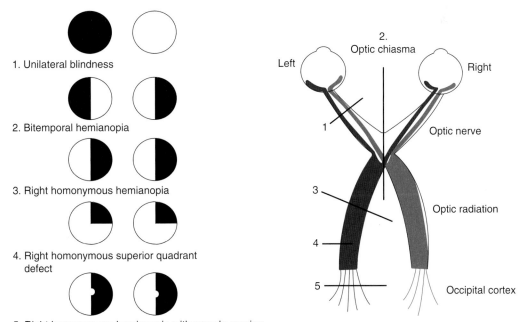

1. Unilateral blindness

2. Bitemporal hemianopia

3. Right homonymous hemianopia

4. Right homonymous superior quadrant defect

5. Right homonymous hemianopia with macula sparing

Figure 10.8   Visual field defects.

Examine the Fundi

- Lesions particularly relevant to the neurological system:
  - *optic atrophy* – pale disc and demyelination, e.g. *multiple sclerosis: pressure on nerve*
  - *papilloedema* – caused by a raised intracranial pressure (RICP); RICP pushes cerebral tissue through the superior orbital fissure, which squashes the back of the eye; this is more likely with conditions that cause acute changes in intracranial pressure such as *tumours, trauma*, and *obstructive hydrocephalus*
- Nystagmus – a sensitive test for nystagmus is to ask the patient to cover the other eye during fundoscopy. This removes fixation and can help to elicit nystagmus.

II Optic Nerve and III Oculomotor Nerve

Assessment of the cranial nerves related to the eye and eye function will have a degree of overlap: a constriction of a pupil to light involves the optic nerve transmitting the light stimuli and the occulomotor nerve stimulating the pupils to constrict.

- Look at pupils. Are they round and equal? (Normal pupils for adults are between 2 and 5 mm in diameter.)
  - Symmetric small pupils: (< 2 mm)
    old age
    opiates
    Argyll Robertson pupils (syphilis) are small, irregular, eccentric pupils, reacting to convergence but not light
    pilocarpine eye drops for *narrow-angle glaucoma*
  - Symmetric large pupils: (> 6 mm)
    youth
    alcohol
    sympathomimetics, anxiety
    atropine-like substances
  - Asymmetric pupils (anisocoria):
    - *3rd-nerve palsy* – affected pupil dilated, often with ptosis and diplopia
    - *Horner's syndrome* (sympathetic defect) – affected pupil constricted (miosis – smaller pupil), often with partial ptosis (drooping eye lid), enophthalmos (backward displacement of the eyeball into the orbit) and anhydrosis (abnormal deficiency of sweat)
    - *iris trauma*
    - *drugs* (see above) – e.g. tropicamide 1.0% or cyclopentolate 1.0% will be used in the treatment of anterior uveitis
- Light reflex: Shine bright light from torch into each pupil in turn in a dimly lit room. Do pupils contract equally?
  - *Holmes–Adie pupil*: large, slowly reacting to light
  - *afferent defect, ocular or optic nerve blindness*: neither pupil responds to light in blind eye; both conditions respond to light in normal eye (consensual response in blind eye)
  - *relative afferent defect* – direct response appears normal but when light moves from normal to deficient eye, paradoxical dilation of pupil occurs
  - *efferent defect–3rd-nerve lesion*, pupil does not respond to light in either eye
- Accommodation reflex (Figure 10.9): Ask patient to look at distant object, and then at your finger 10–15 cm from nose – do pupils contract?
  - Response to accommodation but not light:
    Argyll Robertson
    Holmes–Adie
    occular blindness
    midbrain lesion
    some recovering *3rd-nerve lesions*

Looking ahead

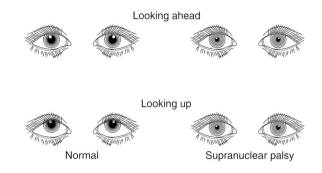

Looking up

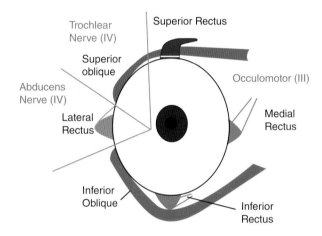

Normal   Supranuclear palsy

Figure 10.9   Accommodation reflex.

Figure 10.10   Muscles of the eye and relevant cranial nerves.

III Oculomotor Nerve
IV Trochlear Nerve
VI Abducens Nerve

Smooth movement of the eye is achieved through the opposing muscles equally contracting and relaxing, a process controlled by three cranial nerves. The oculomotor (III) controls the superior, medial, and inferior rectus; the inferior oblique; pupil; and the levator palpebrae (raises upper eyelid). Moving the eye up, down, and inwards to the nose. The trochlear (IV) controls the superior oblique and moves the eye up and out. The abducens (VI) controls the lateral rectus and moves the eye out (Figure 10.10).

External Ocular Movements

- Test the eye movements in the four cardinal directions (left, right, up, and down as though you were printing a large H in the air) and convergence using your finger at 1 m distance.

    Look for abnormal eye movements (Figure 10.11 Testing external ocular movements [EOM]).

- Ask: 'Tell me if you see double'.

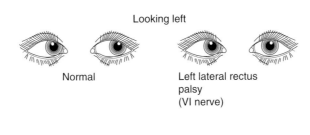

Looking left

Normal   Left lateral rectus
palsy
(VI nerve)

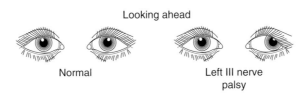

Looking ahead

Normal   Left III nerve
palsy

Figure 10.11   Testing external ocular movements (EOM)

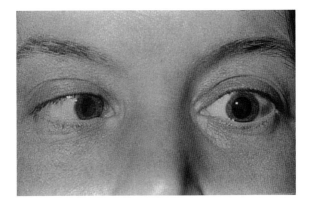

Figure 10.12   Left 6th nerve lesion.

Upward gaze and convergence are often reduced in uncooperative patients.

- To detect minor lesions (Figure 10.12):
  - Find direction of gaze with maximum separation of images.
  - Cover one eye and ask which image has gone.

Peripheral image is seen by the eye that is not moving fully.

Peripheral image is displaced in direction of action of weak muscle, e.g. maximum diplopia on gaze to left. Left eye sees peripheral image, which is displaced laterally. Therefore left lateral rectus is weak.

- Diplopia may be due to a single muscle or nerve lesion (N.B. monocular diplopia usually implies ocular pathology):
  - paralytic strabismus (squint)
  - III palsy: diploplia, ptosis (drooping eye lid), large fixed pupil, eye can be abducted only; eye is often looking 'down and outwards'
  - IV palsy: diplopia when eye looks down or inwards
  - VI palsy: abduction paralysed, diplopia when looking to side of lesion

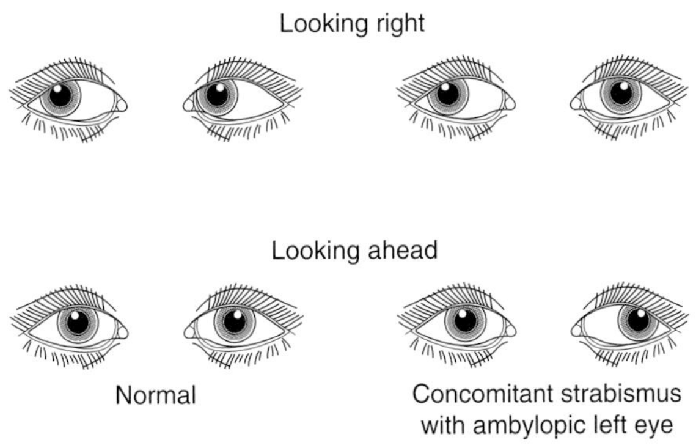

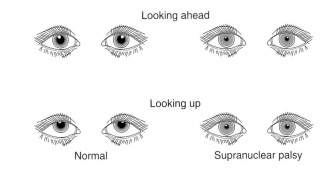

Looking right

Looking ahead

Normal

Concomitant strabismus
with ambylopic left eye

Figure 10.13 Concomitant nonparalytic strabismus.

Looking ahead

Looking up

Normal

Supranuclear palsy

Figure 10.14 Supranuclear palsies.

- ○ concomitant nonparalytic strabismus, e.g. *childhood ocular lesion* – constant angle between eyes. Usually no double vision as one eye ignored (amblyopic) (Figure 10.13).
- ○ conjugate ocular palsy
- ○ *supranuclear palsies* affecting coordination rather than muscle weakness; inability to look in particular direction, usually upwards
- ○ *intranuclear lesion*: convergence normal but cannot adduct eyes on lateral gaze
- ○ if patient sees double in all directions
  - — may be *3rd-nerve palsy*
  - — *thyroid muscle disease* – worse in morning
  - — *myasthenia gravis* – worse in evening
  - — manifest strabismus (Figure 10.14).

Ptosis

Drooping of upper eyelid can be:

- complete – *3rd-nerve palsy*
- incomplete
- *partial 3rd-nerve palsy*
- muscular weakness, e.g. *myasthenia gravis* (from anti-acetylcholine receptor antibodies)
- sympathetic tone decreased – *Horner's syndrome* (also small pupils – miosis and enophthalmos and decreased sweating on face)

- partial Horner's syndrome (small irregular pupils with ptosis) in *autonomic neuropathy* of *diabetes* and *syphilis*
- lid swelling
- *levator dysinsertion syndrome* (from chronic contact lens use)

Nystagmus

This is an involuntary rapid back and forth movement of the eye in a horizontal, vertical, or a combination of directions. Nystagmus is labelled by the direction of the fast movement (the return movement is a little slower). A small amount of end-position (at the extremes of gaze) lateral nystagmus is normal. Horizontal nystagmus is often associated with problems in the labyrinth and vertical nystagmus frequently with brain stem problems. (Swartz 2014)

- Test first in the neutral position and then with the eyes deviated to right, left, and upwards. Keep object within binocular field as nystagmus is often normal in extremes of gaze. Keep your movements smooth.
  - cerebellar nystagmus (Figure 10.15).
    - fast movement to side of gaze (on both sides)
    - increased when looking to lesion
    - *cerebellar* or *brainstem lesion* or *drugs (ethanol, phenytoin)*
  - vestibular nystagmus
    - fast movement only in one direction – away from lesion
    - reduced by fixation if peripheral in origin
    - more marked when looking away from lesion
    - *inner ear, vestibular disease* or *brainstem lesion*

Labyrinthine nystagmus may be positional – particularly in benign positional vertigo and can be induced by hyperextension and rotation of the neck (Hallpike manoeuvre) which after a latency of a few seconds will produce a vertical/torsional type of nystagmus for about 10–15 seconds, along with symptoms of vertigo.

- congenital nystagmus – constant horizontal wobbling
- downbeat nystagmus – foramen magnum lesion or Wernicke's disease
- retraction nystagmus – midbrain lesion
- complex nystagmus – brainstem disease, usually multiple sclerosis

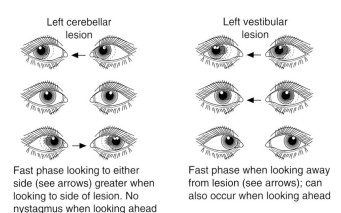

Left cerebellar lesion

Left vestibular lesion

Fast phase looking to either side (see arrows) greater when looking to side of lesion. No nystagmus when looking ahead

Fast phase when looking away from lesion (see arrows); can also occur when looking ahead

Figure 10.15   Cerebellar nystagmus.

Saccades

This is the rapid eye movement used to change eye position. It is tested in the horizontal and vertical planes by asking the patient to switch fixation between two targets (e.g. the examiner's fingers). Slow saccades may be seen in a variety of disorders including degenerative disorders such as progressive supranuclear palsy.

V Trigeminal Nerve

Sensory V

- Test light touch in all three divisions with cotton wool. (Figure 10.16). Ask the patient to close his eyes and to tell you when and where he is being touched. Pinprick usually only if needed to delineate anaesthetic area.

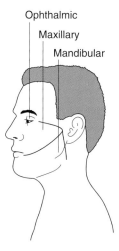

Figure 10.16   Assessment areas for trigeminal nerve sensation.

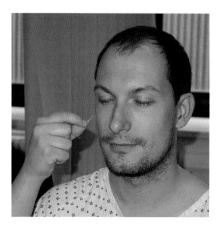

Assess facial sensation - Trigeminal V

Corneal Reflex–Sensory V (Trigeminal) and Motor VII (Facial)

- Ask the patient to look up and away from you and touch the cornea from the opposite side to the gaze, with a wisp of cotton wool. Both eyes should blink. The corneal reflex (Figure 10.17) is easily prompted incorrectly by eliciting the 'eyelash' or 'menace' reflex.

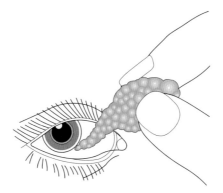

Figure 10.17   The corneal reflex.

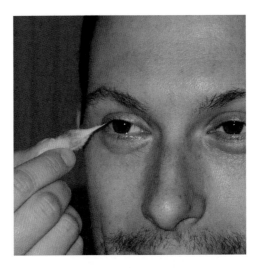

Assess corneal reflex (blink) - trigeminal V & facial

Motor V – Muscles of Jaw

- Ask the patient to open their mouth against resistance and look to see if the jaw descends in midline. Palsy of the nerve causes deviation of the jaw to the side of the lesion. Fifth-nerve palsies are very rare in isolation (Figure 10.18).
- Jaw jerk (Figure 10.19) – only if other neurological findings, e.g. upper motor neuron lesion. Increased jaw jerk is only present if there is a bilateral upper motor neuron 5th-nerve lesion, e.g. *bilateral strokes* or *pseudobulbar palsy*.
  - Put your forefinger gently on the patient's loosely opened jaw. Tap your finger gently with a tendon hammer. Explain the test to the patient or relaxation of the jaw will be impossible. A brisk jerk is a positive finding.

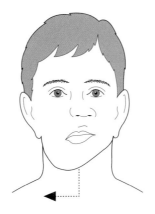

Weak right pterygoid

Figure 10.18 Fifth nerve palsy.

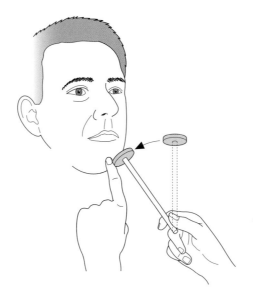

Figure 10.19 Jaw jerk test.

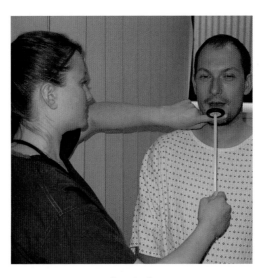

Jaw jerk

VII Facial Nerve

- Ask the patient to:
  - ○ raise eyebrows
  - ○ close eyes tightly
  - ○ smile
  - ○ frown
  - ○ show you their teeth
  - ○ puff out cheeks

Demonstrate these to the patient yourself if necessary.

Lower motor neuron lesion: all muscles on the side of the lesion are affected, e.g. *Bell's palsy*: widened palpebral fissure, weak blink, drooped mouth.

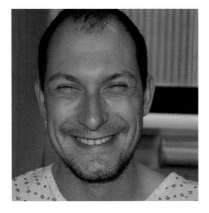

Smile - facial VII

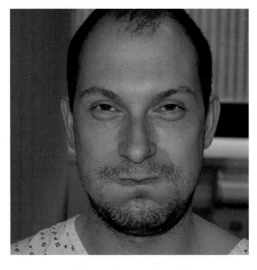

Puff out cheeks - facial VII

Upper motor neuron lesion: only the lower muscles are affected, i.e. mouth drops to one side but eyebrows raise normally. This is because the upper half of the face is bilaterally innervated. This abnormality is very common in a hemiparesis (Figure 10.20).

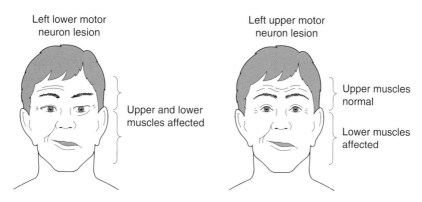

Figure 10.20   Upper and lower motor neuron lesions.

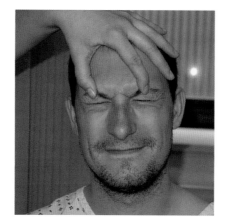

Assess strength of oculomotor nerve for levator palpebrae superioris and sympathetic nerves for superior tarsal muscle

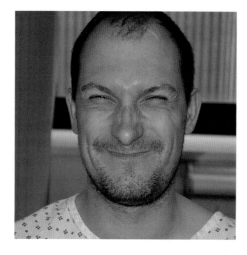

Grimace - facial VII

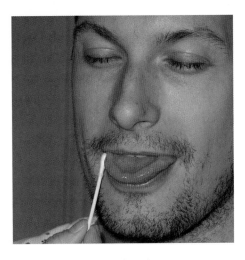

Assess taste - facial nerve VII

- Taste – can be tested easily only on anterior two-thirds of tongue.

Ask patient to close eyes and stick their tongue out, small amounts of glucose (sweet), lemon (sour) or sodium chloride (salt) in solution can be placed on the tongue.

VIII Vestibuloauditory Nerve
Vestibular
No easy bedside test for this nerve except looking for nystagmus.

Acoustic
- Block one ear by pressing the tragus. Whisper numbers increasingly loudly in the other ear until the patient can repeat them.

More accurate tests are as follows:
Rinne's test. Compares a patient's hearing of a tone conducted via the bone and air. Place a high-pitched vibrating tuning fork on the mastoid (1 in figure). When the patient says the sound stops, hold the fork 1 in. from the external auditory meatus (2 in figure). Ask the patient whether the tone is louder at point 1(bone) or point 2 (air) (Figure 10.21).

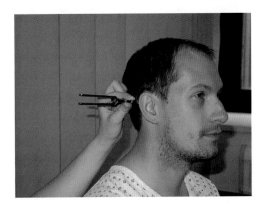

Assess hearing - Rinne 1

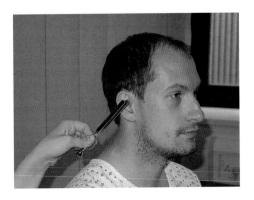

Assess hearing - Rinne 2

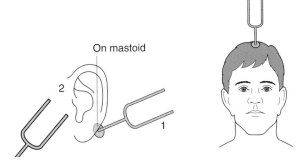

Figure 10.21   Rinne's and Weber's tests.

- If there is nerve deafness then the tone is audible at the external auditory meatus because air and bone conduction will be reduced equally. As such air conduction will be better than bone conduction (as it would be normally). A positive Rinne's test.
- If the tone is not heard at the external auditory meatus then bone conduction is better than air conduction (conductive hearing loss). A negative Rinne's test

Weber's test. Hold a lightly vibrating tuning fork firmly on the top of the patient's head or on the forehead. The sound should be heard equally in both ears. If the sound is heard to one side, either there is a conductive hearing loss on that side or there is a sensorineural hearing loss on the other side (Figure 10.21).

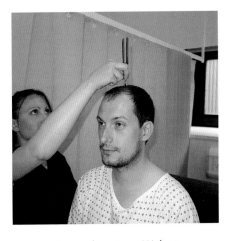

Assess hearing - Weber

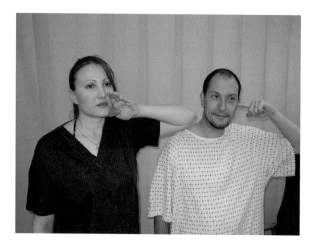

Assess hearing by whispering 'apple' or 'elephant' 18 inches from the patient's ear

IX Glossopharyngeal

- Ask patient to say 'Ahh' and watch for symmetrical upwards movement of uvula – pulled away from weak side.
- Touch the back of the pharynx with an orange stick or spatula gently. If the patient gags the nerve is intact (Figure 10.22).

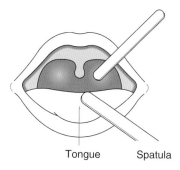

Tongue   Spatula

Figure 10.22   Stimulating the gag reflex.

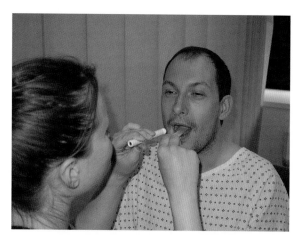

Assess gag reflex - glossopharyngeal IX

This gag reflex depends on the IX and X nerve, the former being the sensory side and the latter the motor aspect. It is frequently absent with ageing and abuse of tobacco.

X Vagus Nerve

- Ask if the patient can swallow normally.

There are so many branches of the vagus nerve that it is impossible to be sure it is all functioning normally. If the vagus nerve is seriously damaged, swallowing is a problem; spillage into the lungs may occur. Swallowing can be assessed by initially ensuring that cranial nerves V, VII, IX, and XII are working correctly (oral stage) and listening and watching a person talk will give a good indication of the function of these cranial nerves. Then asking the patient to swallow (without food or fluid), the pharyngeal stage lasts one second. Observe that the throat muscles (pharyngeal constrictor muscles) move evenly, effectively, and at normal speed. If the dry swallow is effective, then ask the patient to take a small drink of water. Coughing on attempted swallow indicates a high risk of aspiration. Check speech afterwards. A change of voice quality ('wet' speech) indicates pooling of fluids on the vocal cords and indicates a high risk of aspiration. Check for a voluntary cough as this can become quiet and ineffective. Check speech for dysarthria. Whenever patients have been intubated and had an endotracheal tube *in situ*, a swallowing assessment should be undertaken before fluids or food is given by mouth to ensure aspiration is prevented.

XI Spinal Accessory Nerve

- Ask the patient to flex neck, pressing the chin against your resisting hand. Observe if both sternomastoids contract normally (Figure 10.23).
- Ask the patient to raise both shoulders. If they cannot, the trapezius muscle is not functioning.

Failure of the trapezius muscle on one side is often associated with a *hemiplegia* (particularly anterior cerebral artery infarctions).

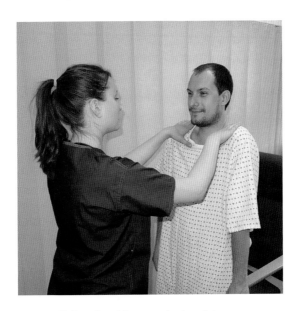

Raise shoulders against resistance

- Ask the patient to turn their head against your resisting hand. This tests the contralateral sternomastoid and can help to demonstrate normal motor functioning in a *hysterical hemiplegia*.

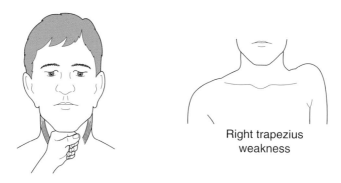

Right trapezius
weakness

Figure 10.23   Flexing the neck and raising both shoulders.

214

XII Hypoglossal Nerve

- Ask the patient to put out their tongue. If it protrudes to one side, this is the side of the weakness, e.g. deviating to left on protrusion from left hypoglossal lesion (Figure 10.24)
- Look for fasciculation or wasting with mouth open.

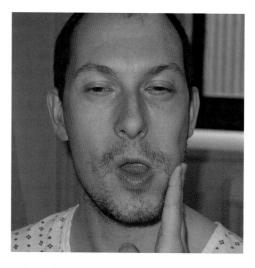

Assess strength of the tongue against your fingers - hypoglossal XII

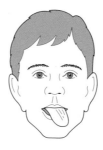

Figure 10.24   Left hypoglossal lesion.

Limbs and Trunk
General Inspection
- Look at the patient's resting and standing posture:
  - flexed upper limb, extended lower limb – *hemiplegia*
  - wrist drop – *radial nerve palsy*
- Look for abnormal movements:
  - tremor
  - *Parkinson's* – coarse rhythmical tremor at rest, lessens on movement
  - *essential tremor* (*thyrotoxicosis*) – tremor present on action; look at outstretched hands
  - *chorea* – abrupt, involuntary repetitive semipurposeful movement
  - *athetosis* – slow, continuous writhing movement of limb
  - *spasm* – exaggerated, involuntary muscular contraction
- Look for muscle wasting. Check distribution:
  - symmetrical, e.g. *Duchenne muscular dystrophy*
  - asymmetrical, e.g. *poliomyelitis*
  - proximal, e.g. *limb-girdle muscular dystrophy*
  - distal, e.g. *peripheral neuropathy*
  - generalised, e.g. *motor neuron disease*
  - localised, e.g. with *joint disease*
- Look for fasciculation. This is irregular involuntary contractions of small bundles of muscle fibres, not perceived by the patient.

This is typical of denervation, e.g. *motor neuron disease* when it is widespread. It is caused by the death of anterior horn cells.

215

Arms
Inspection
In addition to the general inspection it is important to make an initial assessment.

- Ask the patient to hold both arms straight out in front them with palms up and eyes shut. Observe gross weakness and posture and whether the arms remain stationary:
  - hypotonic posture – wrist flexed and fingers extended
  - drift – gradually upwards with sensory loss, may be *cerebellar damage*
  - gradually downwards may be *pyramidal weakness*
  - downwards without pronation can be seen in *hysteria* or in profound *proximal muscle weakness*
  - athetoid tremors – *sensory loss* (peripheral nerve) or *cerebellar disease*
- Tap both arms downwards. They should by reflex return to their former position.
     If the arm overswings in its return to its position, weakness or *cerebellar dysfunction* may be present (Figure 10.25).
- Ask the patient to do fast finger movements. Quickly touch each fingertip on one hand to the thumb and repeat several times, or ask them to pretend they are playing a fast tune on the piano. You may have to demonstrate this yourself. Clumsy movements can be a sensitive index of a slight *pyramidal lesion*. The dominant side should always be quicker than the nondominant side.

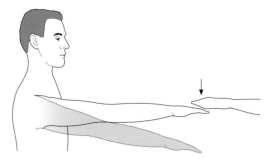

Figure 10.25   Tapping both arms downwards.

Coordination

- Ask the patient to touch their nose with index finger (Figure 10.26).
- With the patient's eyes open, ask them to touch their nose, then your finger, which is held up in front of the patient. This can be repeated rapidly with your finger moving from place to place in front of the patient, but your finger must be in position before the patient's finger leaves their nose (Figure 10.27).

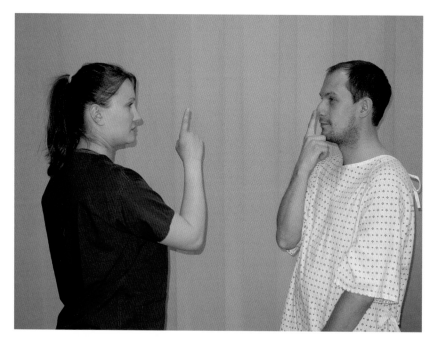

Assess cerebellar function (index finger to nose to examiner's moving finger.)

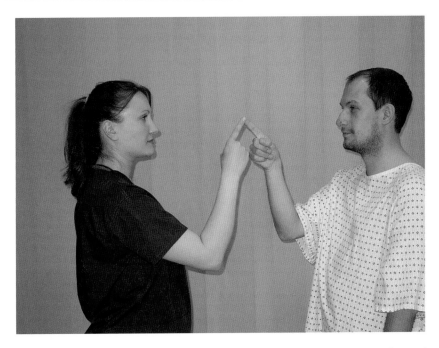

Assess cerebellar function (index finger to nose to examiner's moving finger.)

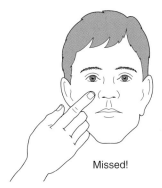

Missed!

Figure 10.26 Testing coordination – index finger to nose.

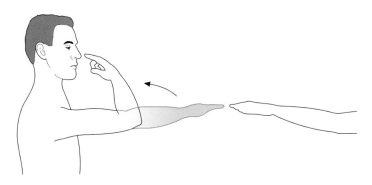

Figure 10.27 Cerebellar function – index finger to nose to examiner's moving finger.

Past pointing and marked intention tremor in the absence of muscular weakness suggests *cerebellar dysfunction*. If you suspect a cerebellar abnormality check rapid alternating movements (*dysdiadochokinesia*):

- fast rotation of the hands on the patient's lap (supination and pronation)
- tapping back of other hand as quickly as possible

Damage to the cerebellum results in a loss of proprioception, the brain's unconsciousness awareness of the position of the joints, muscles, and limbs. Proprioception enables normal movement to be a smoothly coordinated process. Any disruption creates clumsiness, especially at night when vision is less able to compensate (Swartz 2014).

Tone

(Refer to the Musculoskeletal Examination for examples of assessment.)

Always check tone before you assess strength. This is a difficult test to perform as patients often do not relax. Try to distract the patient with conversation.

- **Ask the patient to relax the arm and then you flex and extend the wrist or elbow.** Move through a wide arc moderately slowly, at irregular intervals to prevent patient cooperation.
- **Ask the patient to let the leg go loose, lift it up, and move at the knee joint** (hip and ankle if required). It can be difficult to assess this in the legs because patients often cannot relax. Ankle clonus can be assessed at the same time (refer to examination technique below).

Hypertonia (increased tone):

- pyramidal: more obvious in flexion of upper limbs and extension of lower limbs; occasionally 'clasp knife', i.e. diminution of tone during movement
- extrapyramidal: uniform 'lead pipe' rigidity. If associated with tremor the movement feels like a 'cog wheel'
- hysterical: increases with increased movement

Hypotonia (decreased tone):

lower motor neuron lesion
recent upper motor neuron lesion
cerebellar lesion
unconsciousness

Muscle Power

For screening purposes, examine two distal muscles, one flexor and one extensor (e.g. finger flexion and extension), and two proximal muscles in each limb. Compare each side. Confirm the weakness suspected by palpation of the muscle.

Strength/power is usually graded:

- No active contraction.
- Visible as palpable contraction with *no* active movement.
- Movement with gravity eliminated, i.e. in horizontal direction.
- Movement against gravity.
- Movement against gravity plus resistance.
- Normal power.
  - Look for patterns of weakness:
    - *hemiplegia* – muscles weak all down one side
    - *monoplegia* – weakness of one limb
    - *paraplegia* – weakness of both lower limbs

— *tetraplegia* – weakness of all four limbs
— *myasthenia* – weakness developing after repeated contractions – most obvious in smaller muscles, e.g. repeated blinking
— proximal muscles, e.g. *myopathy*
— nerve root distribution, e.g. *disc prolapse*
— nerve distribution, e.g. wrist drop from *radial nerve palsy*

Upper Limbs

- As indicated previously, compare each side and confirm the weakness suspected by palpation of the muscle. For example (Figure 10.28):
  o 'Squeeze my fingers'. Present the two forefingers of each hand. The patient may hurt you if they squeeze your whole hand.
  o Ask the patient to extend arms (demonstrate) and then say, 'Stop me pressing them down'.
  o Ask the patient to bend the arm and as you hold the wrist ask him to force the arm down against resistance to check extension (Figure 10.29).

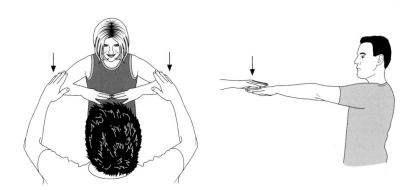

Figure 10.28 Testing muscle power.

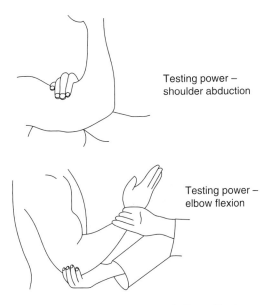

Testing power – shoulder abduction

Testing power – elbow flexion

Figure 10.29 Testing power: shoulder abduction and elbow flexion.

- Resistance to extension:
  - Ask patient to bend the arm and as you hold the wrist ask them to pull the arm up against resistance to check flexion.

Gross power loss will have been noted on inspection of extended arm position or on walking.

- If the patient is in bed, start the examination by asking them to:
  - raise both arms
  - raise one leg off the bed
- Test power at joints against your own strength – shoulder, elbow, wrist.
  - power at main joints cannot normally be overcome by permissible force.
- If there is weakness or other neurological signs in a limb, test the individual muscle groups:
  - shoulder – abduction, extension, flexion
  - elbow – flexion, extension
  - wrist – flexion, extension: 'Hold wrists up, don't let me push them down'.
  - finger – flexion, grasp, extension, adduction (put a piece of paper between straight fingers held in extension and ask the patient to hold it; *as you* remove it), abduction (with fingers in extension, ask patient to spread them apart against your force)

Tendon Reflexes
Arms

- Place arms comfortably by side with elbows flexed and hands on upper abdomen. Tell the patient to relax because reflexes are easier to see; continuing to talk with the patient during this part of the examination may provide distraction and help accuracy. Compare sides.
  - supinator reflex: tap the distal end of the radius with a tendon hammer
  - biceps reflex: tap your forefinger or thumb over biceps tendon
  - triceps reflex: hold arm across chest to tap your thumb over the triceps tendon (Figure 10.30)

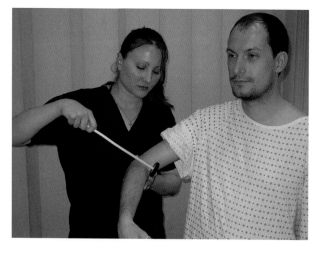

Assess biceps reflex

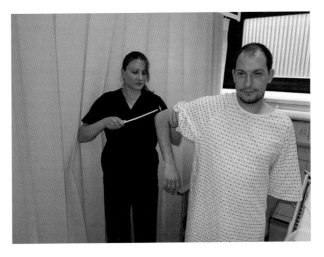

Assess deltoid reflex

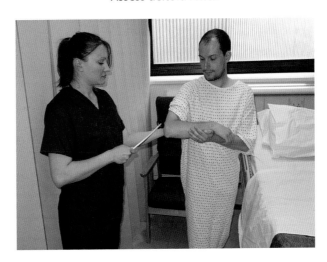

Assess triceps reflex

Increased jerks – *upper motor neuron lesion* (e.g. hemiparesis).

Decreased jerks – *lower motor neuron lesion* or acute *upper motor neuron lesion*.

Clonus – pressure stretching a muscle group causes rhythmical involuntary contraction. If a brisk reflex is obtained, test for clonus. Found in *marked hypertonia* from stretching tendon. No need to strike tendon with tendon hammer. Clonus confirms an increased tendon jerk and suggests an upper motor neuron lesion. A few symmetrical beats may be normal.

Trunk

- The superficial abdominal reflexes rarely need to be tested.
  - Lightly stroke each quadrant with an orange stick or the back of your fingernail. Note the contractions of the muscles and movement of the umbilicus towards the stimulus. These reflexes are absent or decreased in an upper or lower motor neuron lesion (Figure 10.31).
- Cremasteric reflex T12–L1
  - Stroke inside of leg – induces testis to rise from cremaster muscle contraction.

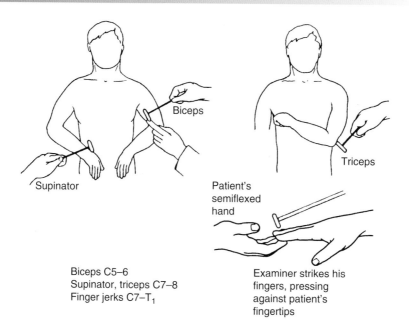

Biceps C5–6
Supinator, triceps C7–8
Finger jerks C7–T$_1$

Examiner strikes his
fingers, pressing
against patient's
fingertips

Figure 10.30 Tendon reflexes.

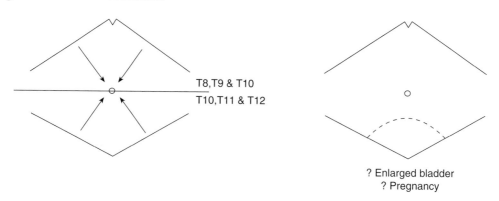

T8,T9 & T10
T10,T11 & T12

? Enlarged bladder
? Pregnancy

Figure 10.31 Trunk reflexes.

- Palpate the bladder.
  The patient with a distended bladder will feel very uncomfortable as *you* palpate it.
  Many neurological lesions, sensory or motor, will lead to a distended bladder, giving
  the patient *retention with overflow incontinence*.
- Examine the strength of the abdominal muscles by asking the patient to attempt to sit
  up without using hands.

Lower Limbs
Inspection
As for arms.

Coordination
- Ask the patient to run the heel of one leg up and down the shin of the other leg. Lack of
  coordination will be apparent (Figure 10.32).
  Gait may become broad based, and the patient may be unable to perform a tandem gait
  (heel–toe walking).

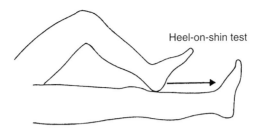

Heel-on-shin test

Figure 10.32   Lower limb coordination.

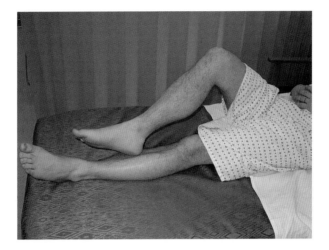

Assess lower limb coordination heel on shin test

Tone

- Ask the patient to let limb go loose, lift it up, and move at knee joint (hip and ankle if required)

It may be difficult to assess in the legs because patients may have difficulty relaxing. Ankle clonus can be assessed at the same time (see below).

Muscle Power

Bending and straightening the knee as well as dorsiflexion and plantarflexion of the ankle against resistance will demonstrate the muscle power in the legs. Lifting the straight leg off the bed against resistance will demonstrate hip flexion (Figure 10.33).

- hip flexion: ask the patient to lift leg, and say, 'Don't let me push it down'.
- hip extension: ask the patient to keep leg straight on the couch or bed surface and try to lift at the ankle; you can test for abduction and adduction against resistance as well; refer to Chapter 13 for further information on performing these tests (Figure 10.34).
- knee – flexion and extension
- ankle – plantarflexion, dorsiflexion, eversion, and inversion

Only severe weakness will be detected because the legs are stronger than the arms. If no weakness is detected and the patient is complaining of weakness, then more sensitive tests can be helpful, e.g. walking on tiptoes, heels, arising from a squat position, hopping on either leg.

Hip weakness is easily overlooked. If a weakness is suspected, test the patient's ability to lift their own weight, i.e. rising from a chair or climbing stairs.

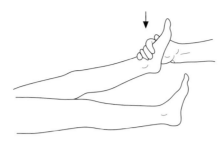

Figure 10.33   Muscle power in the legs. Hip flexion.

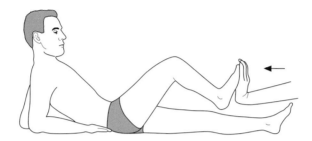

Figure 10.34   Knee flexion.

Occasionally patients will have hysterical weakness. A useful test is Hoover's sign. This is tested by placing your hand under the ankle of the patient's paralysed leg. The patient is first asked to extend the paralysed leg (which should produce no effort), and then by asking for hip flexion of the nonparalysed leg, resulting in contraction of the 'paralysed' hip extensor (a reflex fixation that we all do). Unlike other tests for nonorganic illness, this test demonstrates normalcy in the paralysed limb (Jarvis 2015; Swartz 2014).

Tendon Reflexes

Deep tendon reflexes are tested to demonstrate how well the central nervous system is operating. In testing the patella reflex when the leg is relaxed and dangling the tendon is tapped – this suddenly stretches the tendon (as if the knee was further bent), the muscle spindles (stretch receptors) are stimulated and a spinal arc reflex is generated to effectively return the tendon (and therefore the lower leg) to the resting position but because the leg is still dangling the effect is to kick the lower leg forwards normally just a few inches. Reflexes are exaggerated in upper motor neuron damage because the spinal arc reflex operates without the cerebral controls. Reflexes are absent in lower motor neuron damage because the spinal arc reflex is interrupted.

Although muscle tone can increase in the older adult (reducing flexibility) the muscle power is mostly well preserved. Deep tendon reflexes do not normally diminish in the elderly, but ankle jerks may be compromised by inelasticity of the achilles tendon. As such alteration of reflexes are indicative of disease (Sirven and Malamut 2008).

- Test knee reflexes by passing left forearm behind both knees, supporting them partly flexed. Ask the patient to let leg go loose and tap the tendons below patella (Figure 10.35).
  - Compare both sides.

Reflexes can be normal, brisk (can occur in normal subjects or *upper motor* neuron lesion), decreased, absent (always abnormal).

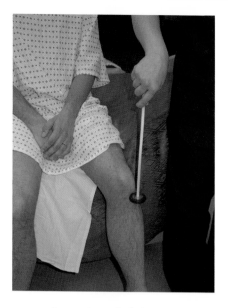

Assess knee jerk 1

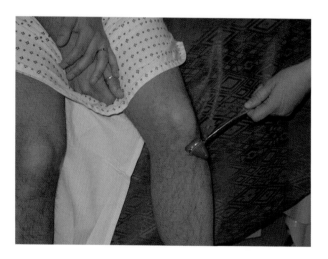

Assess knee jerk 2

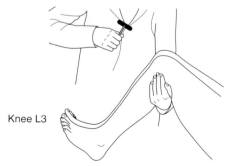

Knee L3

Testing the knee reflexes

Figure 10.35 Testing knee reflexes.

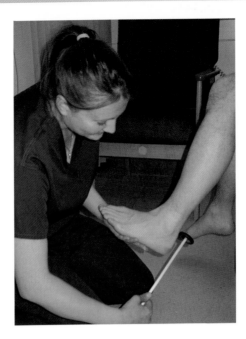

Assess ankle jerk

- Test ankle reflex by flexing the knee and abducting the leg. Apply gentle pressure to the ball of the foot, with it at a right angle and tap the tendon.
  Ankle jerks are often absent in the elderly.
- Compare sides – right versus left and arms versus legs. It is essential that the patient is relaxed when reflexes are tested. This is not always easy for the patient, particularly the elderly. You can elicit reinforcement (an apparently absent reflex may become present) by asking the patient to clasp his hands together and pull one hand against the other just as you strike with the hammer (Figure 10.36).

Increased jerks – *upper motor neuron lesion* (e.g. hemiparesis).
Decreased jerks – *lower motor neuron lesion* or *acute upper motor neuron lesion*.
Clonus – if a brisk reflex is obtained, test for clonus. A sharp, then sustained dorsiflexion of the foot by pressure on ball of the foot, may result in the foot 'beating' for many seconds. Clonus confirms an increased tendon jerk and suggests an *upper motor neuron lesion*. A few symmetrical beats may be normal.

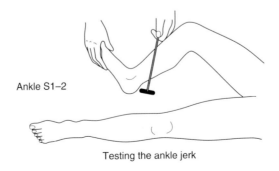

Ankle S1–2

Testing the ankle jerk

Figure 10.36   Testing ankle jerk.

Plantar Reflexes

- Tell patient what you are doing and scratch the side of the sole with a firm but not painful implement (orange stick or rounded spike on tendon hammer). Watch for flexion or extension of the toes (Figure 10.37).

Normal plantar responses = flexion of all toes.

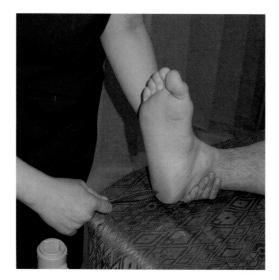

Assess for Babinski

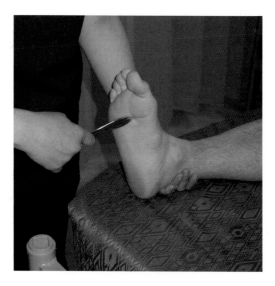

Plantar response

Extensor (Babinski) response = slow extension of the big toe with spreading of the other toes. Withdrawal from pain or tickle is rapid and not abnormal. In individuals with sensitive feet, the reflex can be elicited by noxious stimuli elsewhere in the leg; stroking the lateral aspect of the foot can be very useful or testing for sharp sensation on the dorsum of the great toe. (Do not use needles or pins to test for 'pinprick' sensation. Use a disposable 'neurostick', 'neuropin', or paper clip and ask the patient to tell you whether the sensation is sharp or dull.)

An extensor reflex is normal up to six months of age.

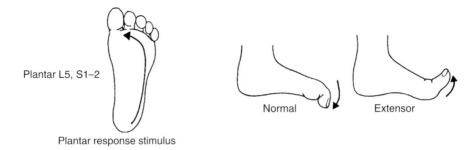

Plantar L5, S1–2

Normal   Extensor

Plantar response stimulus

Figure 10.37   Plantar response stimulus.

228

Sensation

If there are no grounds to expect sensory loss, sensation can be rapidly examined.

Briefly examine each extremity. Success depends on making the patient understand what you are doing and cooperating effectively with you. This examination is very subjective. As in the motor examination you are looking for patterns of loss, e.g. nerve root (dermatome), nerve, sensory level (spinal cord), glove/stocking (peripheral neuropathy), dissociation (i.e. pain and temperature versus vibration and proprioception – e.g. syringomyelia).

Vibration Sense

- Test vibration sense using a 128 Hz tuning fork. Place the fork on the sternum first, so that the patient appreciates what vibration is. Ask the patient to close eyes, then place the vibrating fork on the lateral malleoli and wrists. Ask the patient to tell you when it stops vibrating. You stop the vibrating fork and if vibration sense is normal, the patient will tell you the vibration has stopped. If the periphery is normal, proximal sensation need not be examined. Occasionally a patient will claim to feel vibration when it is absent. If this is suspected, try a nonvibrating fork or surreptitiously stop the fork vibrating and see if the patient notices. If the patient says they can feel it vibrate, testing is not valid. Vibration sense often diminishes with age and may be absent in the legs of the elderly patient.

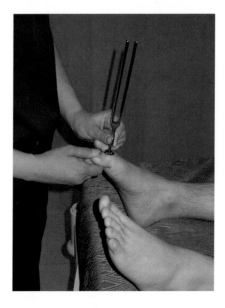

Assess vibratory sense 1

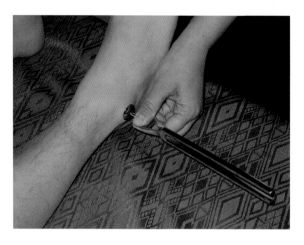

Assess vibratory sense 2

Position Sense – Proprioception

- Show the patient what you are doing. 'I am going to move your finger/toe up or down' [doing so]. 'I want you to tell me up or down each time I move it. Now close your eyes'.
- Hold distal to joint and either side with your forefinger and thumb so that pressure does not also indicate the direction of movement. Make small movements in an irregular, not alternate, sequence. e.g. up, up, down, up, down, down, down (Figure 10.38).

Normal threshold is very low – the smallest, slowest passive movement you can produce in the terminal phalanges should always be correctly detected.

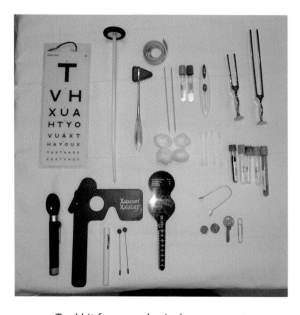

Tool kit for neurological assessment

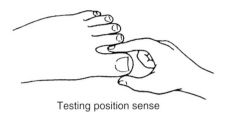

Testing position sense

Figure 10.38   Testing position sense.

Pain, Touch, and Temperature

Pain and Touch

- Take a new clean neurostick/neuropin (do not reuse same neurostick/neuropin on another patient). Also take a tongue depressor.
- With the patient's eyes open touch the sharp end of the neurostick/neuropin on the skin. Do not draw blood. Ask, 'Does this feel sharp?'
- Also touch the skin with the tongue depressor. 'Does this feel blunt?'

Ask the patient to close eyes and to tell you where you touch the skin and whether it is sharp or blunt. Then randomly assess the patient's sensory function. If you find sensory loss, map out that area by proceeding from the abnormal to normal area of skin.

Temperature

- This process can be repeated with test tubes of 'hot' (but not burning) and cold water to test perception of temperature. Ask the patient to close eyes and then tell you if they feels 'hot' or cold as you touch the skin with the test tube.

Light Touch

- Close patient's eyes.
- Ask the patient to tell you when and where you touch them with a wisp of cotton wool. Touch at irregular intervals.
- Compare both sides of body.

Two-point discrimination. Normal threshold on fingertip is 2 mm. If sensory impairment is peripheral or in cord, a raised threshold is found, e.g. 5 mm. If cortical, no threshold is found.

Stereognosis tested by placing coins, keys, pen top, etc. in the patient's hand and, with eyes closed, the patient attempts to identify by feeling.

Sensory exclusion is assessed by bilateral simultaneous, e.g. touch; sensations are felt only on the normal side, whilst each is felt if applied separately. Indicates a parietal lobe lesion as brain is unable to process all stimuli.

Dermatomes

Most are easily detected with a neurostick/neuropin (Figure 10.39). Map out from area of impaired sensation.

Note in arms: middle finger – C7 and dermatomes either side symmetrical up to mid upper arm.

Note in legs: lateral border of foot and heel (S1), back of legs and anal region have sacral supply.

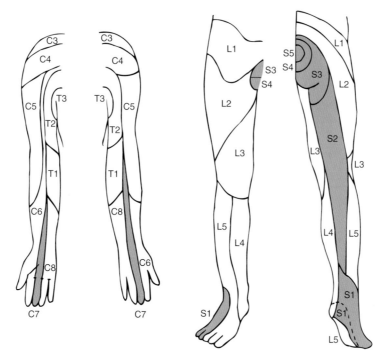

Figure 10.39 Dermatomes.

Gait

- Observe the patient walking. If ataxia is suspected but not seen on ordinary walking, ask the patient to do heel-to-toe walking. (Demonstrate it yourself.)

There are many examples of abnormal gait.

- Parkinson's disease. Patient has stooped posture with most joints flexed and walks with small shuffling steps without swinging arms; tremor of hands (Figure 10.40).
- Spastic gait. Patient scrapes toe on one or both sides while walking; to prevent this the patient moves foot in a lateral arc (Figure 10.41).
- Sensory ataxia. Patient has a high stepping gait, with a slapping-down of feet. Seen with peripheral neuropathy (Figure 10.42).
- Cerebellar gait. Patient has feet wide apart while walking (Figure 10.43).
- Foot drop. Patient's toe scrapes on ground in spite of excessive lifting-up of leg on affected side.
- Shuffling gait. Patient takes multiple little steps – typical of diffuse cerebrovascular disease.
- Hysterical gait. Patient usually lurches wildly but without falling over, with the pattern marked by inconsistency.

Romberg's test is often performed at this time but is mainly a test of position sense. Ask the patient to stand upright with feet together and eyes closed. If there is any falling noted, the test is positive. Be sure you stand to the side of the patient with one arm held out in front and one arm held out to the patient's back in case the patient begins to fall so that you can steady them (Figures 10.44 and 10.45).

Elderly patients may fail this test and may begin to fall sideways but stop just before they topple over because of reduced proprioceptive awareness. Test positive with posterior

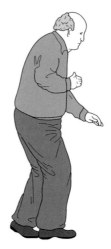

Figure 10.40   Parkinson's disease gait.

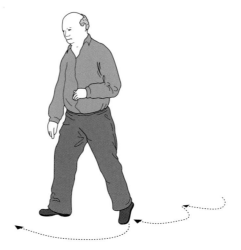

Figure 10.41   Spastic gait.

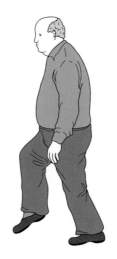

Figure 10.42   Sensory ataxia gait.

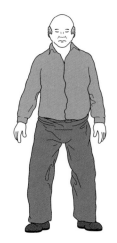

Figure 10.43   Cerebellar gait.

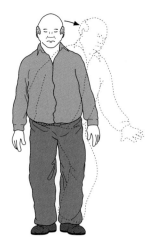

Figure 10.44   Romberg's test.

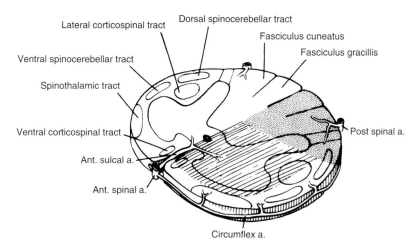

Figure 10.45   Anatomy and vascular supply of the spinal cord. Note: Anterior spinal artery occlusion spares posterior column function. *Source*: Reproduced from Talley and O'Connor (2006).

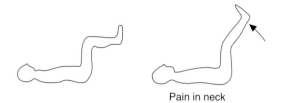

Pain in neck

Figure 10.46   Signs of meningeal irritation.

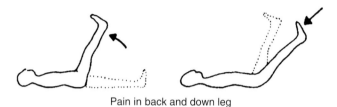

Pain in back and down leg

Figure 10.47   Straight-leg raising for sciatica.

column loss of tabes dorsalis of syphilis. Anxious patients may sway excessively; try distracting them by testing stereognosis at the same time – the excess swaying may disappear (Jarvis 2015; Swartz 2014).

Dorsal Column Loss of Sensation
- decreased position, vibration, and deep pain sensation (squeeze achilles tendon)
- touch often not lost, as half carried in anterior column

Cortical Loss of Sensation
Defect shown by deficient function:

- position sense
- tactile discrimination
- sensory inattention

Signs of Meningeal Irritation

- neck rigidity – try to flex neck, is there resistance or pain?
- Kernig's sign – not as sensitive as neck rigidity (Figure 10.46).

Straight-Leg-Raising for Sciatica
- Lift straight leg until there is pain in back. Then slightly lower leg until there is no pain and then dorsiflex the foot to 'stretch' the sciatic nerve until the patient says there is pain present down the back of the leg (Figure 10.47).

Summary of Common Illnesses
Lower Motor Neuron Lesion

- wasting
- fasciculation
- hypotonia

- power diminished
- absent reflexes
- + or − sensory loss
- T1 palsy
- weakness of the intrinsic muscles of the hand: finger adduction and abduction, thumb abduction (cf. median nerve palsy and ulnar nerve palsy)
- sensory loss: medial forearm
- median nerve palsy
- abductor pollicis brevis weakness (other thenar muscles may be weak) wrist drop
- sensory loss: thumb, 1st two fingers, and palmar surface
- ulnar nerve palsy
- interversion, hypothenar muscles wasted (Figure 10.48), weakness of finger abduction and adduction; clawhand, cannot extend fingers
- sensory loss: half 4th, all 5th fingers, palmar surface.
- radial nerve palsy
- wrist drop
- sensory loss: small area/dorsal web of thumb (Figure 10.49)

235

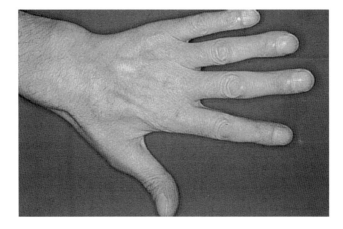

Figure 10.48   Wasted interossei and hypothenar eminence from an ulnar nerve orT_1 lesion.

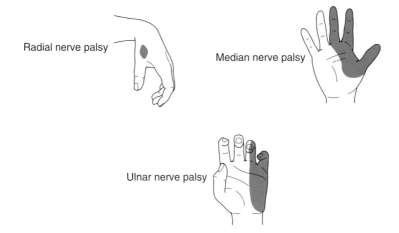

Figure 10.49   Radial, median, and ulnar nerve palsies.

- L5 palsy – foot drop and weak inversion; sensory loss on medial aspect of foot
- peroneal nerve palsy – foot drop and weak eversion; minor sensory loss of dorsum of foot
- S1 palsy – cannot stand on toes, sensory loss of lateral aspect of foot, absent ankle reflex

Upper Motor Neuron Lesion

- no wasting
- extended arms – hand drifts down
- overswing when hands are tapped
- hypertonia
- spastic flexion of upper limbs, extension of lower limbs
- clasp knife
- power diminished
- increased tendon reflexes (+ or – clonus)
- extensor plantar response
- + or – sphincter disturbance
- spastic gait
- extended stiff leg with foot drop
- arm does not swing, held flexed

N.B. Check 'level' first, then pathology.

Cerebellar Dysfunction

- no wasting
- hypotonia with overswing; irregularity of movements
- intention tremor
- inability to execute rapid alternating movement smoothly (dysdiadochokinesia)
- ataxic gait
- nystagmus
- scanning or staccato speech
- incoordination not improved by sight (whereas it is with a defect of proprioception)

Extrapyramidal Dysfunction – Parkinson's Disease

- flexed posture of body, neck, arms and legs
- expressionless, impassive face, staring eyes
- 'pill-rolling' tremor of hands at rest
- delay in initiating movements
- tone – 'lead pipe' rigidity, possibly with 'cog-wheeling'
- normal power and sensation
- speech quiet and monotonal
- gait – shuffling small steps, possibly with difficulty starting or stopping
- postural instability: test by having the patient standing comfortably; stand behind the patient and give a sharp tug backwards; normal patients should show a slight sway; taking steps backwards, particularly multiple steps, is abnormal

Multiple Sclerosis

- evidence of 'different lesions in space and time' from history and examination; usually affects cerebral white matter; common sites:
  - optic atrophy – optic neuritis
  - nystagmus – vestibular or cerebellar tracts
  - brisk jaw jerk – pyramidal lesion above 5th nerve

- cerebellar signs in arms or gait – cerebellar tracts
- upper motor neuron signs in arms or legs – pyramidal, right or left (absent superficial abdominal reflexes)
- transverse myelitis with sensory level – indicates level of lesion
- urine retention – usually sensory tract
- sensory perception loss – sensory tract

System-Oriented Examination
'Examine the Higher Cerebral Functions'
- general appearance
- consciousness level
- mood
- speech
- cognitive
- confusion
- orientation
- attention/calculation
- memory – short term, long term
- reasoning – understanding of proverb

'Examine the Arms Neurologically'
- Inspect:
  - abnormal position
  - wasting
  - fasciculation
  - tremor/athetosis
- Ask patient to extend arms in front, keep them there with eyes closed, then check:
  - posture/drift
  - tap back of wrists to assess whether position is stable
  - fast finger movements (pyramidal)
  - touch nose (coordination) – finger – nose test
  - 'Hold my fingers'; push and pull against resistance
- Tone
- Muscle power – each group if indicated
- Reflexes
- Sensation
  - light touch
  - pinprick
  - vibration
  - proprioception

'Examine the Legs Neurologically'
- **Inspect**:
  - abnormal positions
  - wasting
  - fasciculation
- 'Lift one leg off the bed'
- 'Lift other leg off the bed'
- Coordination – heel–toe

- Tone
- Power – 'Pull up toes. Push down toes'. against resistance
- Reflexes
- Plantar reflexes
- Sensation (as hands)
- Romberg test
- Gait and tandem gait

'Examine the Arms or Legs'
- Inspect:
  - colour
  - skin/nail changes
  - ulcers
  - wasting (are both arms and legs involved?)
  - joints
- Palpate:
  - temperature, pulses
  - lumps (see above)
  - joints
  - active movements
  - feel for crepitus, e.g. hand over knee during flexion
  - passive movements (do not hurt patient)
  - reflexes
  - sensation

Case Study of a 63-Year-Old Female Presenting with Recurrent Episodes of Right Sided Weakness and Difficulty Speaking

Presenting Problem
63-year-old female presents with recurrent episodes of right sided weakness and difficulty speaking

Subjective
The patient was in her usual state of health when she began to experience weakness in her right hand which progressed to her entire right arm, advancing to complete paralysis of her right arm within 30 minutes. Her right leg then became involved in an identical fashion. At this time, she began to have slurred speech and considerable difficulty speaking. Whilst on the way to the emergency department, she also began to have some drooping of the right side of her face. She did report a mild headache at the onset of symptoms. She denies any sensory loss, visual changes, auditory changes, dizziness or vertigo, chest pain, palpitations, shortness of breath, nausea, or vomiting. Past medical history is significant for four previous episodes in the past three years that were identical to her current symptoms, each with full recovery within three days. Previous workups were negative for transient ischemic attack or stroke, and the patient was started on levetiracetam after her last episode two months prior for the presumptive diagnosis of seizures with postictal (Todd) paralysis. Patient denies familial history of stroke, epilepsy, or similar episodes. She denies alcohol, tobacco, or drug use.

Objective
Vitals: Temp. 98.2 °F, Pulse 94, Respiratory rate 22, blood pressure 143/68, O_2 sat. 100% on room air

Patient is alert, oriented, and in no acute distress. Exam is significant for R lower facial drooping, complete flaccid paralysis of right upper and lower extremities, and R-sided hyperreflexia (3+ right-sided biceps, triceps, patellar, and achilles tendon reflexes) with an upgoing Babinski on the right side. Language is intact despite some dysarthria. Sensation is completely intact bilaterally, including light touch, pain, temperature, vibration sense, and joint-proprioception. Cranial nerves II, III, IV, V, VI, VIII, IX, X, XI, and XII are intact. The cardiovascular exam is benign with a normal heart rhythm, no murmurs, rubs, or gallops, and no carotid bruits.

Differential Diagnosis
Transient ischemic attack, stroke, seizure with postictal hemiparesis (Todd paralysis), hemiplegic migraine

Test Results
CT-angiography (CTA) of head: no evidence of large vessel occlusion or haemorrhage
MRI of head: no evidence of ischemia, haemorrhage, or intracranial mass or abnormality
Carotid ultrasound: negative for carotid artery stenosis
Echocardiogram: normal ejection fraction, no valvular stenosis or regurgitation
Electrocardiogram (ECG/EKG): sinus rhythm with no abnormalities
Electroencephalogram (EEG): no evidence of seizure activity or any other abnormalities

Assessment
The most likely diagnosis is hemiplegic migraine, a subtype of migraine with aura. The negative CTA, MRI, and carotid ultrasound rule out TIA and stroke, particularly given the lack of abnormalities on ECG and echocardiogram and the benign cardiovascular exam findings. Although a normal EEG alone cannot completely rule out seizures with postictal paralysis (Todd paralysis), such episodes are usually characterised by sudden onset rhythmic jerking movements, often with loss of consciousness and postictal confusion. Furthermore, this patient's presentations fulfils the diagnostic criteria as described by the International Classification of Headache Disorders (ICHD-3):

A. At least two attacks fulfilling criteria B and C
B. Aura consisting of both of the following:
   - fully reversible motor weakness
   - fully reversible visual, sensory, and/or speech/language symptoms
C. At least two of the following four characteristics:
   - At least one aura symptom spreads gradually over ≥ five minutes, and/or two or more symptoms occur in succession
   - Each individual nonmotor aura symptom lasts 5–60 minutes, and motor symptoms last < 72 hours
   - At least one aura symptom is unilateral
   - The aura is accompanied, or followed within 60 minutes, by headache
D. Not better accounted for by another ICHD-3 diagnosis, and transient ischemic attack and stroke have been excluded

Plan
Discontinue levetiracetam and start topiramate for migraine prophylaxis.

References

Ball, J., Dains, J., Flynn, J. et al. (2014). *Seidel's Guide to Physical Examination*, 8e. St. Louis: Elsevier Mosby.

Bickley, L. and Szilagyi, P. (2013). *Bates' Guide to Physical Examination and History Taking*, 11e. Philadelphia: Wolters Kluwer Health Lippincott Williams & Wilkins.

Crossman, A.R. and Neary, D. (2014). *Neuroanatomy: An Illustrated Colour Text*, 5e. London: Churchill Livingstone Elsevier.

Japp, A. and Robertson, C. (2013). *Macleod's Clinical Diagnosis*. Edinburgh: Churchill Livingstone, Elsevier.

Jarvis, C. (2015). *Physical Examination & Health Assessment*, 7e. St. Louis: Elsevier Saunders.

Martini, F., Ober, W., Nath, J. et al. (2014). *Visual Anatomy and Physiology*, 2e. San Francisco: Benjamin Cummings.

Sirven, J. and Malamut, B. (2008). *Clinical Neurology of the Older Adult*, 2e. Wolters Kluwer Health Lippincott Williams & Wilkins.

Swartz, M. (2014). *Physical Diagnosis, History and Examination*, 7e. Philadelphia: Elsevier Saunders.

Talley, N. and O'Connor, S. (2006). *Clinical Examination: A Systematic Guide to Physical Diagnosis*, 5e. Edinburgh: Churchill Livingstone.

Talley, N. and O'Connor, S. (2013). *Clinical Examination: A Systematic Guide to Physical Diagnosis*, 7e. London: Churchill Livingstone Elsevier.

Tortora, G. and Derrickson, B. (2012). *Principles of Anatomy and Physiology*, 13e. Oxford: Wiley.

Chapter 11

Examination of the Eye

Helen Gibbons

General Examination

Introduction

The purpose of examining the eye is to assess the function of the eye and its anatomy and to discern pathology that affects vision. Until recently patients with ophthalmic conditions were seen in specialist eye centres. Today more and more clinicians are assessing ophthalmic conditions in outreach centres, accident and emergency, walk-in-centres, and general practice settings. Your assessment of the eye is important because, according to the Royal National Institute of the Blind one in five people over the age of 75 live with sight loss, the main cause being age-related macular degeneration (RNIB 2015).

Many patients that you will see will be unaware that they have any pathological conditions of the eye; therefore, your assessment and intervention are essential and recommended if for example, your patient has had a recent fall. This chapter begins by reviewing the anatomy and physiology of the eye and then presents examination techniques.

Anatomy and Physiology of the Eye

The eyeball is approximately 25 mm in diameter.

Orbit

- The eye sits within the orbit; the optic nerve leaves the eye at the optic disc and transports the entire visual image to the brain. The ophthalmic artery also leaves here running underneath the optic nerve.

Eyelids

- Provide protection to the eye itself (blinking action).
- Secrete oily part of the tear film.

Physical Assessment for Nurses and Healthcare Professionals, Third Edition. Edited by Carol Lynn Cox.
© 2019 John Wiley & Sons Ltd. Published 2019 by John Wiley & Sons Ltd.

- Help the tear film to spread over the eye.
- Prevent the eye drying out.
- Contain the puncta whereby tears drain into the lacrimal system.
- Eyelid opening performed by the levator muscle.
- Eyelid closed by orbicularis muscle.

Cornea

- A transparent structure, convex shaped (like a watch glass cover). It is 0.5 mm thick. This allows light rays to pass through and the shape allows light rays to bend.
- It is highly sensitive and protects the front of the eyeball.
- It has five layers with the epithelium being the only layer to regenerate. The layers are:
  - epithelium
  - Bowman's membrane
  - stroma
  - Descemet's membrane
  - endothelium (damage to these cells results in a hazy cornea).
- The cornea is avascular.

Anterior chamber

- The area between the posterior surface of the cornea and the anterior surface of the iris.
- When the eye has inflammation, cells may be visible here.

Posterior chamber

- The area between the posterior surface of the iris and the anterior surface of the lens and suspensory ligaments.

Both the anterior and posterior chambers are filled with aqueous; this nourishes the lens and maintains intraocular eye pressure. Aqueous is made up of 99% water and 1% nutrients.

Ciliary body

A triangular structure lying between the choroid and iris. It consists of the ciliary processes and the ciliary muscle.

Iris

The coloured circular diaphragm which lies behind the cornea and in front of the lens. It forms the pupil at its centre. It is attached at the periphery to the ciliary body.

- The sphincter muscle constricts the iris restricting the amount of light allowed in the eye.
- The dilator muscle dilates the pupil.
- The sphincter muscle is more powerful than the dilator muscle so if inflammation in the eye affects both muscles the sphincter muscle will be dominant and constrict the pupil.

Posterior chamber

- The area where the lens is suspended.
- Aqueous is present.

242

Lens

- The focussing mechanism of the eye.
- It is held in place by zonules (suspensory ligaments).

Vitreous

- The vitreous is transparent and fills the posterior segment of the eye (between the lens and the retina).
- It consists of 98–99% water, 1–2% hyaluronic acid, and collagen fibres.
- It maintains the shape of the eye; if taken out and not replaced with artificial replacement substance the eye would collapse.
- It helps with refraction of light.

Sclera

- The sclera extends from the cornea (limbal area) to the optic nerve.
- It is often described as the hard protective coating of the eye.
- It composed of dense, white, nonuniform collagen fibres.

Choroid

- The choroid lies between the sclera and the retina.
- Its function is to provide nourishment to the underlying retina.
- It contains blood vessels to supply the underlying retina.

Retina

- The retina has 10 layers:
  - Layer 1 pigmented epithelium
  - Layers 2–10 neural layers.
- The retina is transparent; it gets its colour from the choroid's blood supply.
- The retina is responsible for converting light into electrical signals.
- Contains rods and cones:
  - Rods are important for night vision, they are sensitive to light and do not signal colour information.
  - Cones are responsible for daytime vision. Some of the cones are responsible for red, green, and blue colour vision.
  - Cones are concentrated at the fovea, which is responsible for reading vision and fine print.

Optic disc

- The area where the retinal fibres leave the eyeball as the optic nerve.

Macula

- The region of the retina where precise central vision occurs.
- Not fully developed in the child until six months of age.

Fovea centralis

- Found in the centre of the macula and is responsible for detailed vision, e.g. fine print.

(Figure 11.1)

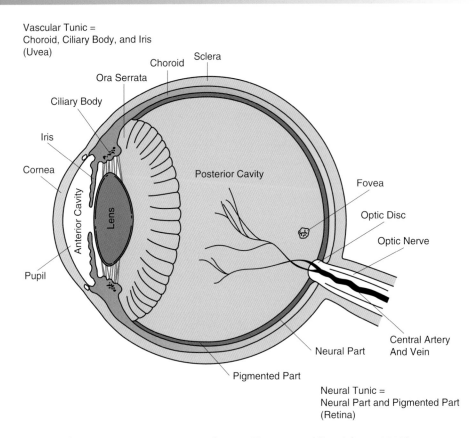

Vascular Tunic =
Choroid, Ciliary Body, and Iris
(Uvea)

Choroid   Sclera

Ora Serrata

Ciliary Body

Iris

Cornea

Anterior Cavity

Lens

Pupil

Posterior Cavity

Fovea

Optic Disc

Optic Nerve

Central Artery
And Vein

Neural Part

Pigmented Part

Neural Tunic =
Neural Part and Pigmented Part
(Retina)

Figure 11.1   The Eye. (*Source*: Martini et al. 2012; Tortora and Derrickson 2012).

History Taking in the Ophthalmic Assessment

It is fundamentally important when examining a patient with an ophthalmic condition to have a logical and systematic approach to history taking, visual assessment, examination, and diagnosis. If this approach is not adopted, then vital signs and symptoms may be missed during the examination.

Patients with ocular symptoms often have high levels of anxiety and therefore need tact and understanding during their examination (Walsh 2006). It is therefore important to appear calm and confident in your approach Goldblum (2004) suggests that if patients are not treated in a friendly and professional manner then often they will not express all their concerns to the examiner.

In the 1st two years of life the eyeball grows rapidly. Between 10 and 13 years of age the eyeball will have reached its adult size. The scleral thickness and rigidity also increase from around 0.5 mm in childhood to 1 mm by adulthood (Wright 2003).

Children need to be treated with special care when being examined as they will often remember negative experiences which then make reexamination more traumatic, especially if they need regular follow-up. There are local anaesthetics on the market which don't smart and can be instilled before other drops that do smart to make the child's experience more comfortable.

As noted previously, it is essential to use a systematic approach in your examination and treatment of ophthalmic patients. It is good practice to:

- Take a history.
- Perform visual assessment using a Snellen Visual Acuity Chart, near vision chart, and colour vision, or Amsler Grid as required.
- Carry out a detailed examination using a good quality torch, magnifying light, and preferably a slit lamp.

The following features in the history are a requirement:

Presenting Complaint
- Why has the patient attended?
- Which eye is the problem (If both, did it start in one eye and transfer to the other?)

Duration of Symptoms
Identify:

- How long the symptoms have been present.
- Whether the symptoms are there all the time or whether they come and go.
- Whether the pain occurred suddenly or gradually.
- What the patient was doing at the time *(Be very suspicious of penetrating injury if the patient has been drilling, chiselling, hammering, or carrying out a task that could have caused a high-speed injury.)*.
- If it was a chemical injury, what it was *(These patients need immediate irrigation with at least 1 l of normal saline, ensuring the eyelids are everted.)*. Establish whether the pH of the chemical is alkaline or acid and contact the local ophthalmology unit for advice.
- If the eye has a foreign body sensation, was the patient wearing eye protection and whether the protection chosen was a good fit.
- If the patient has a discharge, it is relevant to ask whether the patient has had a recent cough or cold, as a high proportion of conjunctivitis comes from viral aetiology. Establish colour and consistency of discharge.
- Whether the patient has tried any over the counter treatments themselves at home; if yes, whether the treatments had any effect.
- If the eye has a photophobic red eye with a foreign body sensation that came on gradually, do they suffer with cold sores on their face or lip? *(It could be a Herpes simplex keratitis.)*
- If the complaint is of a headache in what region of their head is the headache positioned? Does the patient suffer with migraine? If the headache is temporal is the patient well; have they suffered weight loss, pain on touching the temporal area, or jaw claudication? *(If yes to these questions and the patient has visual symptoms this could be temporal arteritis. Thus, the patient needs urgent bloods drawn and tested for C-reactive protein [CRP] and erythrocyte sedimentation rate [ESR] and an urgent referral to an ophthalmologist. Listen for bruits over the temporal artery as on occasion this may be heard over the temporal artery.)* If temporal pain and no visual symptoms refer to a general practitioner urgently.
- Whether the patient has any nausea and or headache. If yes, is the eye red, has a hazy cornea, and a fixed dilated pupil? *This could indicate an attack of acute glaucoma. The patient needs urgent referral to an ophthalmologist for urgent treatment.*
- Whether the patient is complaining of vision loss. Ask whether the vision is blurred. Did it worsen rapidly or over a course of weeks or months? Was it like a camera shutter closing over their eye with complete loss of vision or can they make out blurred images? Is their vision distorted when they are reading? *In sudden onset of loss of vision check blood pressure and blood sugar to exclude underlying medical conditions.*
- Whether the patient is experiencing flashing lights±floaters; are they experiencing a cobweb or net curtain like appearance in their vision. Are they high myopes? *These patients are at higher risk of retinal detachment* (James and Bron 2011) *and require prompt referral to an ophthalmologist.*

Past Ocular History
Identify:

- Whether the patient has had anything similar before. If yes does the patient know what eye condition the patient had and what treatment was required?

- Whether the patient had a history of:
  - *iritis/uveitis*
  - *episcleritis/scleritis*
  - *previous eye trauma*
  - *diabetic eye disease*
  - *previous corneal abrasion/recurrent erosion syndrome*
  - Whether they wear glasses for distance or reading
  - *If the patient wears contact lenses, what type are they? How does the patient clean them? What is the average length of time that lenses are worn? (Overwear of contact lenses is a common cause of the red eye in contact lens wearers.).*

Family Ocular History

Does the patient have a history of familiar eye problems?

- *glaucoma*
- *diabetic eye disease*
- *retinal detachment*
- *diabetic eye disease*
- *squints/glasses/lazy eye.*

General Medical Health

Do they have?

- *hypertension*
- *diabetes (how is it controlled, type and duration of symptoms)*
- *heart disease*
- *thyroid disorders*
- *joint complaints, e.g. rheumatoid arthritis*
- *bowel problems such as Crohn's disease*
- *chest problems such as asthma or sarcoidosis*
- *any other relevant problems*

Questions Relevant to Child's History Taking

Who is accompanying child?

- *parent*
- *carer*
- *sibling*
- *other relative*

What source has the referral come from?

- *school*
- *Accident and Emergency*
- *parent*

Child's Birth and Developmental Information

- *Was the child full term or premature?*
- *Was it a normal delivery, C–section or assisted, e.g. forceps?*
- *Does the parent have any concerns over development?*
- *Did the mother experience any problems during pregnancy, e.g. infections, amniocentesis?*

Other Questions Relevant to Child's History

In the young child ask the parent. In a child who is able to verbalise, direct the question to the child.

- *When do you notice the problem?*
  - *All the time*
  - *When tired*
  - *When unwell*
- *Is the problem getting worse?*
- *Does your child complain of headaches?*
- *Does your child bump into things?*
- *Have you noticed your child sitting close to the television?*
- *Do you sit near the board where your teacher writes?*
- *Can you see what your teacher is writing on the board?*
- *When your teacher uses different colours on the board are some colours missing?*
- *Are they frightened of the dark?*
- *Are they scared when you cover one eye?*

Allergies

What allergies does the child have? What reaction occurs when the child uses/takes this medicine, food, or product (e.g. swelling/rash)?

Occupation

- Consider what the patient's occupation is.
- Consider whether a child is at school or nursery as this may have implications for them. For example, a patient with acute bacterial or viral conjunctivitis working in a school environment or attending a nursery school needs to be advised that their condition is highly contagious, and they should refrain from work until symptoms resolve (can be anything from 24 hours to 1 week) as this can be spread to the child and staff.

Examination
Visual Acuity Assessment

It is an essential requirement to check and fully document a formal visual acuity. The standard assessment tool for measuring distance visual acuity is a Snellen Chart, with acuity measured at a distance of 6 m from the chart (United Kingdom Standard). *(Some charts are designed for use at shorter distances; for example, if using a reverse Snellen Chart in a mirror the vision can be measured at 3 m but still be recorded as 6 m. North American standard, 21 or 9 ft.)* The main advantage of Snellen Charts is that they are relatively straightforward to use.

Snellen Chart

A Snellen Chart (refer to Appendix B) is a commonly used method of measuring visual acuity. It consists of nine rows of letters that get progressively smaller (Chen et al. 2016). The letters are heavy block letters, numbers, or symbols printed in black on a white background. The top letter can be read by a normal eye at a distance of 60 m and the smallest line at a distance of 4 m. The vision recorded is expressed as a fraction; for example, if the patient is sitting at a distance of 6 m away from the chart and they can read the top line only then their vision in the eye being tested is 6/60. It is essential that when you record the vision you record whether the patient had their glasses or contact lenses in situ. It is not acceptable practice to record 'vision normal' or 'not affected'. If the patient is reassessed at a later date, there will not be any recordings to compare the results with, and if the patient requires referral to an eye clinic, visual acuity will be one of the 1st questions that will be asked.

Procedure

- Ensure the patient is seated comfortably with their feet firmly on the floor or footrest of the chair.
- Ask the patient to use distance glasses if needed. Test each eye individually starting with the right eye and then the left. Cover the untested eye with an occluder or a fresh tissue. (The occluder needs to be cleaned in between patients according to local policy.)
- Ask the patient to read down the chart from left to right as far as they can read. Encourage them to try another couple of letters and reassure them that it doesn't matter if they get a letter wrong.
- If the patient's visual acuity is anything less than 6/9 with or without glasses, it is advisable to use a pinhole to establish whether the decreased vision is correctable or not, as in some cases reduced vision is due to a refractive error and nothing more serious.
- If the patient cannot read any letters on the chart move the patient forwards 1 m closer to the chart and try the test again. If they are still unable to read the top letter, continue to move the patient forwards 1 m at a time. If at 1 m from the chart they are still unable to read the top letter, stand about 1 m away and ask the patient to count the number of fingers held up and record as counting fingers (CF). If they cannot recognise the number of fingers held up, wave your hand 30 cm in front of patient's eye and ask them if they can see your hand moving. If they can, record this as hand movements (HM). If the patient is unable to visualise hand movements, using your bright torch shine the light from different directions whilst asking the patient if they can see the light and which direction it is coming from. If they can see the light it can be recorded as perception to light (PL). If unable to see the light in any direction record as no perception to light (NPL).

The Sheridan–Gardiner Method

This test can be used in illiterate patients or in young children to obtain a Snellen Vision determination. The examiner holds a card at 6 m from the patient and asks the patient to match the letter on the corresponding card which they are holding. This gives a Snellen recording.

LogMAR Vision Testing

Although more complex, LogMAR vision testing is well documented as being more accurate in its measurement of visual acuity (Rosser et al. 2001). The main advantage of a LogMAR chart is that there are five letters on each line each of which is scored and therefore gives the patient a fairer chance of being able to read the letters. The main disadvantage to the tester is that it takes longer in the early stages and clinicians are put off at having to work out the scores for each individual patient. However, most departments have a conversion chart which can be used to easily record the patients score (Elliott 2007). The LogMAR vision chart is primarily used in low vision, glaucoma, and macular degeneration clinics.

Near Vision Testing

Near vision is assessed using a specifically designed reading card using different sizes of ordinary printer's type; each size is numbered. As in testing distance vision the patient's eyes are tested individually and using the patient's reading glasses if applicable. The chart should be used in good light, preferably with a reading light positioned over the patient's shoulder. The chart should be positioned at approximately 25 cm from the patient. Record the number of the lowest line read (e.g. N8).

248

Colour Vision Assessment

Colour vision assessment should be carried out in any patient who presents with painful loss of vision and who you suspect may have an optic nerve condition or the patient who requests a colour vision assessment for work purposes. The standard method for colour vision assessment is performed by pseudoischromatic plates such as Ishihara colour plates. These are a series of plates that test for red/green colour blindness. The plates appear as a circle of dots and within the circle a number will be placed. The patient covers one eye and reads the number. If a number on a plate cannot be distinguished a number is taken away from the total score (e.g. 16/17 read).

Contrast Sensitivity Testing

This test is designed to assess subtle levels of vision changes not accounted for in the normal visual acuity testing, for example, in patients with cataracts. It measures real life vision compared to black on white (Yannoff and Duker 2014). It is not routinely assessed in ophthalmology clinics but more often in research clinics. The standard chart used is a Pelli-Robson, which has six letters on each line all the same size on all eight lines. The letters fade in blackness until on the 8th row they are barely visible. Like the LogMAR test each letter is given a score. A printed conversion sheet is provided with the Pelli-Robson chart to ensure correct interpretation of results is recorded.

Testing Amsler Grid

This test is used for assessing the patient's central vision. It is an A5 sheet of paper with a grid of black lines. In the centre of the grid is a black spot.

- Each eye is tested individually. The patient needs to wear their reading glasses and holds the test at a distance of approximately 25 cm and looks at the centre spot. They inform the examiner of any distortion, blurring, wavy or missing parts on the grid and this is then recorded on the chart. This test is of great importance in patients with suspected macular degeneration. In these cases, the patient would note wavy or distorted lines.

Testing Eye Movements

This test must be done in all patients who complain of double vision.

- The examiner sits in front of the patient at the same height. Explain to the patient that they must follow the pen torch with their eyes.
- Using a light from a pen torch. Ask the patient to cover their left eye and then move the light slowly up and down left and right asking the patient to report any double vision or any pain on eye movement.
- Observe for full eye movement in all directions in both eyes. Repeat the process for the other eye.

Recording Visual Fields

Confrontational Field Testing

- Make sure your patient is seated comfortably with their feet on the floor or footrest. You should adjust the patient's chair to ensure the patient is seated at arms-length distance from you and at eye level. You face the patient.
- Holding a large red hat pin, ask the patient to close or cover their left eye (you do the same to your opposite eye – right eye). Bring the red coloured pin into vision and ask the patient to verbalise when they can see the pin in their visual field upper right, middle and lower right.

- Once the right eye is examined repeat on the left eye.
- The examiner uses their observation of the pin as a guide to when the pin should come into view. Note you must have good visual fields to perform this assessment.

Perimetry Visual Field Testing

These tests are carried out in optometry practices and ophthalmic clinics. They measure the degree of peripheral and central visual field loss.

- They are used most frequently in glaucoma clinics to detect progression of the disease.
- The most common machine is a Humphrey field analyser. This provides an electronic record of the patient's visual field. Each eye is tested individually with the patient's refractive error corrected.
- The patient is given a buzzer to press when they see a light being shone. These lights are shone in all 360°. Recordings will show any changes to that of a normal visual field.
- The test records not only the spots correctly identified but can tell when the patient has pressed the buzzer incorrectly and whether there was any loss of fixation.

Testing the Child's Vision

There are several methods for checking a child's visual acuity. How it is performed greatly depends on the child's age and ability. Testing of a young child's visual acuity is best performed by an orthoptist in an ophthalmic unit as they are best equipped and experienced to obtain the best vision assessment from a young child. Vision in the child varies. At birth visual acuity is very poor and newborn babies are unable to fix on an object. By the age of two to four months' babies are able to fix and their vision starts to develop and will continue to do so until its peak of development at around age seven to nine years (Wright 2003).

Nonverbal Children

Young babies should be able to fix on a bright toy or object even if only for a few moments. By the ages of six months and over the infant will try and reach out for the toy or object or pick up small sweets (small cake decorations are a useful tool for this test).

Verbal Children

From the age of one year there are tests specifically designed to test children's vision and are outlined below.

The Cardiff Acuity Test

- This is a preferential test based on the perspective that children like to look at complex rather than plain targets.
- It is aimed at young children from about 12 months of age to three years of age.
- The test works by the examiner observing eye movements and response from the child to establish whether or not the child can see the target or not on a card.
- The cards are of a grey background with a white picture. If the picture is too small for the child to see the picture card will appear grey and the child will lose interest.
- The test is carried out at a distance of 1 m and covers vision down to 6/3.75.

Kay Pictures

This test is aimed at children as young as two years of age and requires the examiner to hold a series of pictures at 3 or 6 m distance.

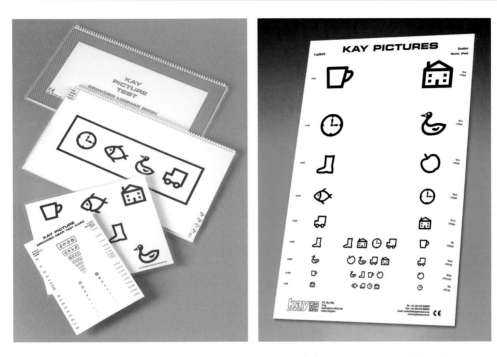

Figure 11.2 Kay Picture Charts. *Source*: Reproduced with kind permission of Hazel Kay.

Each card has a picture, or if using a LogMAR equivalent will have five pictures on each card getting smaller as each new card is presented. The child is asked to say what picture is on each card. If child is shy or not communicating they can be asked to match the pictures on a corresponding card that they are holding. Once the child reaches school age they can try matching the letters on a Snellen or LogMAR chart until they are able to read the letters for themselves (Figure 11.2).

Visual Electrophysiology Testing

In some children it is impossible to obtain a visual acuity or colour vision measurement and therefore electrophysiology in the form of an electroretinogram (ERG), visual evoked potential (VEP) and electro-oculogram (EOG) tests may be performed. These are noninvasive tests and serve as integrated parts of the ophthalmology examination. They determine how the retina and the visual cortex are functioning. These tests provide important and objective information for eye disease diagnosis, prognosis, and treatment. These tests are carried out in specialist units.

Ocular Examination of the Adult

The eye should always be examined from the outside in. When examining the patient's eye, first look at the patient's face as a whole to ensure facial symmetry and note any obvious palsy, ptosis, proptosis, or allergic reaction. Always consider the patient's age and psychological state. Patients with Parkinson's disease may, for example, find it very difficult to position themselves when a slit lamp is used to carry out the examination (Stollery 2010).

At the beginning of the examination, ask the patient to open both eyes as this is easier to do than open one alone. Use of good pen torch or magnifying light is essential (if a slit lamp is unavailable) to examine the eye and to check pupil reactions. If the patient is in pain, local anaesthetic drops may be required prior to the examination. In the case of a glass foreign body, or the history indicates a possible penetrating injury or perforation

251

from drilling or using high-speed equipment, local anaesthetic should **not** be instilled. These patients need referral immediately to an eye unit or ophthalmic A&E (emergency) department day or night. **Do not pad the eye or put any pressure on it.** (A cartella eye shield should be used to cover the entire eye to prevent further accidental injury. A cartella eye shield is a transparent plastic shield used to protect the eye after operations.)

It is essential to look under the patient's top eyelid by everting it, if they are complaining of a foreign body sensation and a corneal foreign body can't be seen. Use fluorescein eye drops to highlight any scratches or abrasions to the eye.

Ocular Examination of the Child

When a child attends with an eye problem requiring examination, it is essential that the child feel at ease as much as possible. Encourage young children to bring in their favourite comforter and to sit on their parent's lap if they wish. Offer the child lots of patience and reassurance. If, however, you are unsure of a diagnosis or you find a corneal foreign body for example, contact your local eye unit for advice.

The following chart gives clear guidance on what to look for when examining eyes in both adults and children.

Face	Evaluate	• Facial symmetry, look for drooping mouth and eyelids (Common in Bell's palsy.)
Eye movements	Can they Is there	• Look upwards, downwards, left, and right comfortably • Any obvious squint present
Eyelids	Look for	• Swelling of the lids *(Is the swelling hard or soft? Is it hot to touch?)* • Ptosis *(Droopy eyelid)* • Entropion *(Inturning lid)* • Ectropion *(Outturning lid)* • Trichiasis *(Ingrowing eyelashes)* • Any lacerations to lids • Chalazions • Blepharitis *(Inflammation to the eyelid margins)*
Conjunctiva	Assess	• Redness *(Position and degree of redness. Is it all over? Is it localised or limbal?)* • Is there any haemorrhage • Any swelling • Can a foreign body be visualised • Is there a laceration • Any conjunctival cysts *(Look like a balloon filled with water.)* • Pterygium *(Wing-shaped growth that can encroach onto cornea causing irritation.)*
Cornea	Is it Is there Are there	• Clear/hazy • Any scarring • Staining when fluorescein dye instilled • Any ulcers • Any foreign bodies • Any lacerations
Anterior chamber	Is it Is there	• Shallow/deep *(Compare both eyes together.)* • A hyphaema *(Blood in the anterior chamber.)* • A hypopyon *(Pus in the anterior chamber.)* • Cells *(Seen when carrying out a slit lamp examination.)*
Iris	Are they Are there Is there	• The same colour *(Some patients have different colour irises; some medications change the iris colour.)* • Any nevus present • Any trauma *(Has the patient had any previous surgery?)*

Pupil	Is it Are they	• Round *(A peaked pupil could indicate posterior synechiae in uveitis; an oval pupil with a hazy cornea indicates acute glaucoma.)* • Equal and reactive • Black in colour *(In an adult a white or grey pupil often indicates a cataract; in an infant a cataract or more seriously retinoblastoma.)*

Use of a Slit Lamp

It is almost impossible to give a definite diagnosis of an eye condition without using a slit lamp (Figures 11.3 and 11.4).

- The slit lamp consists of a microscope and a light source.
- Slit lamp examination is indicated in any condition of the eyelids or eyeball. Ocular conditions can be better diagnosed and treated by having a highly illuminated, magnified view.
- **Technique**
- Explain to patient that the light may be a little bright but that it will give a highly magnified view of the eye; thus, aiding diagnosis.
- Patient and examiner are seated (both must be comfortable) with the patient chin height adjusted, to ensure the eye is aligned with the slit lamp guide.
- Patient places chin and forehead on bars; examiner looks through the eyepieces (The examiner has adjusted the eyepieces to their own glasses prescription.)

253

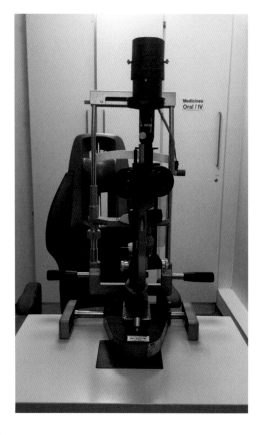

Figure 11.3   Slit lamp.

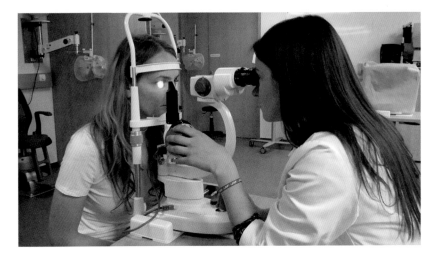

Figure 11.4   Examination of the retina with the slit lamp.

- The lids, cornea, anterior chamber, and iris can be easily viewed by moving the focus from the joystick, forwards and backwards as required.
- Use fluorescein and the blue cobalt light to look for corneal staining and corneal abrasions.
- Use slit beam, approximately 1 mm wide and 3 mm long with high magnification to look for anterior chamber cells and flare.

The Use of a 90 Dioptre Lens with a Slit Lamp to View the Retina

This examination is usually carried out in optometry practices and hospital clinics. Extra training should be undertaken prior to carrying out this procedure. It gives a much better view of the retina than direct ophthalmoscopy and is therefore used more in the hospital setting than a direct ophthalmoscope.

- This procedure can be carried out with an undilated pupil; however, a better image will be seen through a dilated pupil.
- Ensure the 90 D lens is clean and smear free. (Clean only with a lens cloth to prevent scratching on the lens coating.)
- Ensure that the patient is comfortably and correctly positioned at the slit lamp with their chin on the chin rest, forehead firmly pressed against the plastic strap, head pointing straight ahead, and patient's eye in line with the mark on the metal frame of the slit lamp.
- Adjust the power of the light so that it is not too bright for the patient. Adjust the width of the slit so that it is 2–3 mm wide and the height of the beam to about 8 mm.
- Pull the slit lamp joystick towards you
- To examine the patient's right eye, hold the 90 D lens in your left hand.
- Ask the patient to look at your right ear or use the fixation light.
- Hold the 90 D lens just in front of the patient's right eye without touching the eye with the lens. Hold the lens with the thumb and index finger.
- Using your right hand, slowly advance the slit lamp towards the eye. At first the lens will be seen with an inverted image of the eye in its centre. (The image is vertically and laterally inverted and virtual.)

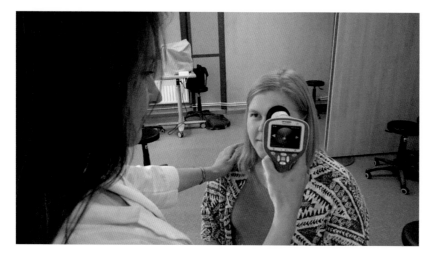

Figure 11.5   Alternative method for examination of the fundus.

Fundus Examination

- As the slit lamp is moved closer to the patient the vitreous and then the retina should come into view. With the patient looking in the direction you tell them to, the disc should come into view. From the nasal side to the disc the macula can be seen. Examine the retinal vessels for any signs of haemorrhages or occlusion.
- To examine the temporal retina, ask the patient to look to their right.
- To examine the nasal retina, ask the patient to look to their left.
- Get the patient to look up for the superior retina, then down for the inferior retina. The patient's upper lid will need to keep open by gently lifting it with a finger when the patient looks down.
- The image seen in all directions of gaze is vertically and laterally inverted, for example. On up gaze, the superior most part of the retina is in the inferior field. This must be remembered when drawing the image, but a useful tip is to turn the page upside down; thus you can draw what you are seeing and on turning the page round the image will be presented correctly.
- Repeat the entire process to examine the patient's left fundus; this time using your right hand to hold the lens, with the patient looking at your left ear, to see the disc (Figure 11.5).

Measurement of Intraocular Pressure (IOP)

This test is carried out on most patients who attend an ophthalmology clinic and on all patients who are over the age of 40 in optometry practices. The usual intraocular eye pressure is between 10 and 21 mmHg (Coakes and Holmes 1995)

Goldmann Tonometry

- The gold standard method is by Goldmann tonometry. This provides the most accurate measurement, but it is difficult to master and should be carried out only after specialist training.
- Fluorescein dye and anaesthetic dye is instilled in the eye.
- A clear plastic prism is advanced until it touches the cornea. Two semicircles are seen, and the two inner circles meet. The measurement can then be read on the dial at the side of the instrument which gives you the measurement (Figure 11.6).

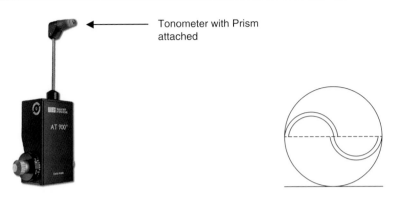

Figure 11.6 Tonometer with diagram to illustrate correct alignment of the semicircles (mires) in Goldmann tonometry.

Perkins Applanation Tonometry
- This is a handheld device useful to patients unable to be seen on a slit lamp.
- Same principles as Goldmann tonometry
- Difficult to master
- In order to obtain this measurement, the examiner needs to get very close to patient.

Tonopen
- This is easy to use and is good for emergency departments and patients who are unable to reach a slit lamp.
- It is a penlike device which when gently tapped on an anaesthetised cornea will give you an IOP reading.

Air Puff
- Most commonly used in optometry practices.
- Can give abnormally high readings as it makes the patient jump or hold their breath.
- The time taken to flatten the cornea is converted into a figure to give an IOP.

Palpation of the Globe
- Palpation of the eye using two fingers on a closed eyelid with the patient looking downwards.
- Is of no value other than to detect the hardness in an acute glaucoma (Coakes and Holmes 1995).

Use of an Ophthalmoscope
- Make sure that the ophthalmoscope is fully charged and has a bright light and the bulb is in working order before the examination commences.
- The patient should be sitting. Remove spectacles from yourself and the patient.
- Begin by setting the lens dioptre dial at 0 if you do not use spectacles. If you are myopic, you should start with the 'minus' lenses. Set the lens dioptre at −4 to begin, which is indicated as a red number. If you are hyperopic you should use the 'plus' lenses, which are indicated by black numbers. Keep your index finger on the dial to permit easy focusing. Hold the ophthalmoscope about 30 cm from the patient. Shine the light into the patient's pupil, identify the red reflex (from the retina), and approach the patient at an angle of 15°. Approach on the same horizontal plane as the equator of the patient's eye. This will bring

you straight to the patient's optic disc. After observing the disc examine the peripheral retina fully by following the blood vessels to and back from the four main quadrants.

- Hold the ophthalmoscope in your right hand in front of your right eye to examine the patient's right eye, and in your left hand in front of your left eye to examine the patient's left eye. Try to hold your breath when using the ophthalmoscope. Do not breathe into the patient's face.
- If the patient's pupils are small, dilate with 1% tropicamide, one drop per eye. Tropicamide works in 15–20 minutes and lasts 2–4 hours. Warn the patient that their vision will be blurred for approximately 4 hours. Do **not** dilate if neurological observation of pupils is needed.
- The patient should be told they cannot drive, if their pupils have been dilated, for at least four to six hours.

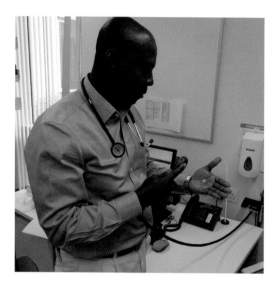

Check the light on the ophthalmoscope

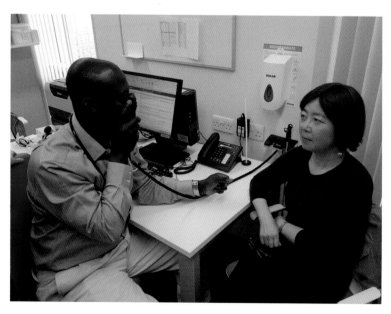

Look for the red reflex

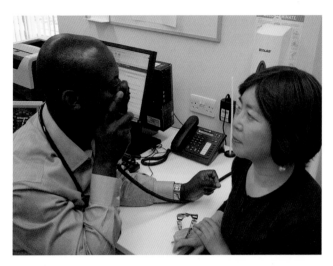

Prepare to 'zoom in' to inspect the anterior and posterior portions of the eye

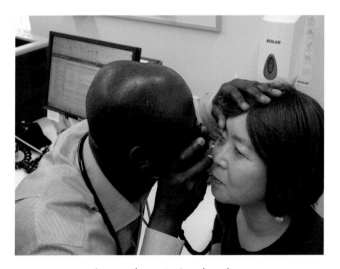

Assess the anterior chamber

Look at Optic Disc

- normally pink rim with white 'cup' below surface of disc
- *optic atrophy*
- disc pale: rim no longer pink
  multiple sclerosis
  after optic neuritis
  optic nerve compression, e.g. tumour
- papilloedema
  - *disc pink, indistinct margin*
  - *cup disappears*
  - *dilated retinal veins*
    increased cerebral pressure, e.g. tumour
    accelerated hypertension
    optic neuritis, acute stage

- glaucoma – enlarged cup, diminished rim
- new vessels – new fronds of vessels coming forwards from disc
- ischaemic *diabetic retinopathy*

Look at Arteries

- arteries narrowed in hypertension, with increased light reflex along top of vessel
  Hypertension grading:

  1. narrow arteries
  2. 'nipping' (narrowing of veins by arteries)
  3. flame-shaped haemorrhages and cotton-wool spots
  4. papilloedema

- occlusion artery – pale retina
- occlusion vein – haemorrhages

259

Look at Retina Figure 11.7

- hard exudates (shiny, yellow circumscribed patches of lipid)
  - *diabetes*
- cotton-wool spots (soft, fluffy white patches)
  - microinfarcts causing local swelling of nerve fibres
    diabetes
    hypertension
    vasculitis
    human immunodeficiency virus (HIV)
- small, red dots
  - microaneurysms – retinal capillary expansion adjacent to capillary closure
    diabetes
- haemorrhages
  - round 'blots': haemorrhages deep in retina larger than microaneurysms
    diabetes

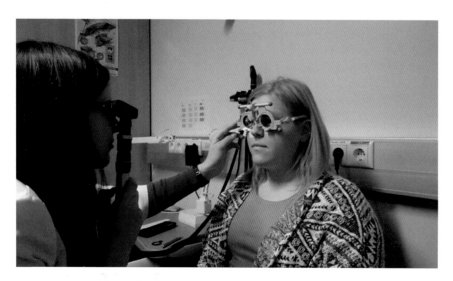

Figure 11.7   Retinoscopy

- ○ flame shaped: superficial haemorrhages along nerve fibres
    hypertension
    gross anaemia
    hyperviscosity
    bleeding tendency
  - ○ Roth's spots (white-centred haemorrhages)
    microembolic disorder
    subacute bacterial endocarditis
- • pigmentation
  widespread
    retinitis pigmentosa
  localised
    choroiditis (clumping of pigment into patches)
    drug toxicity, e.g. chloroquine
  tigroid or tabby fundus: normal variant in choroid beneath retina
- • peripheral new vessels
  ischaemic diabetic retinopathy
  retinal vein occlusion
  - ○ medullated nerve fibres – normal variant, areas of white nerves radiating from optic disc

Pupil Assessment for Relative Afferent Pupillary Defect (RAPD)

This is an essential test to perform prior to dilating drops being instilled, especially in patients who you suspect have optic nerve conditions.

- • Assess size and shape of pupils
- • Sit the patient in a dimly lit room
- • Ask the patient to gaze into the distance
- • Shine the bright torch from one eye to the other (hold light on pupil for two to three seconds on each eye); if there is a pupil defect the pupil will dilate instead of constricting when the eye is illuminated. The normal response would be for the pupil to constrict when the light is shone on pupil.

Documentation

When documenting your findings, it is essential to document in a systematic format. An example is outlined below.

Right eye		Left eye
	Visual acuity	
	Lids	
	Conjunctiva	
	Cornea	
	Anterior chamber	
	Iris	
	Pupil	
	Intraocular pressure	

Right eye		Left eye
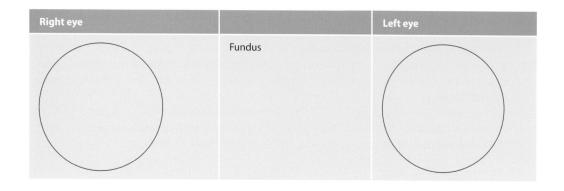	Fundus	

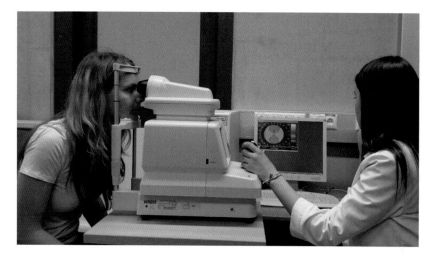

Figure 11.8 Corneal topography.

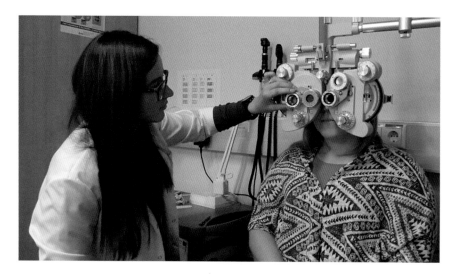

Figure 11.9 Phoropter.

Corneal topography is also known as photokeratoscopy or videokeratography. It is a noninvasive medical imaging technique for mapping the surface curvature of the cornea, which is the outer structure of the eye (refer to Figure 11.1). Its topography is of critical importance in determining the quality of vision and corneal health because the cornea is responsible for approximately 70% of the eye's refractive power (Figure 11.8).

Phoropter is an ophthalmic testing device that is also called a refractor. It contains different lenses used for refraction of the eye during sight testing. It measures a person's refractive error and determines the spectacle prescription (Figure 11.9).

Case Study of a Patient with Episcleritis

History
A 24-year-old woman attends your clinic complaining of a red aching left eye for three days

Presenting Ocular History
- A red aching left eye for three days, (she describes it as a bruised feeling)
- No discharge/watering
- No change in vision
- No swelling
- No change in sleep pattern
- No history of injury
- No other ocular complaints
- Doesn't wear any glasses/contact lenses or had any previous refractive laser surgery

General History
- Fit and well

Medication
- Ocular cicatricial pemphigoid

Allergies
- Latex allergy

Social History
- Lives with boyfriend and six month old baby
- Works as a teacher (currently on maternity leave)
- Doesn't drink any alcohol or smoke

Pain Score
4 out of 10

Differential Diagnosis
Scleritis (but this would be deep red and pain intense), viral conjunctivitis (but the patient has no discharge), blepharititis, no other symptoms

Examination

Visual acuity
6/4 u/a 6/4

Nasal redness

No crusting or blocked glands seen **Lids** No crusting or blocked glands seen
White **Conj** Redness noted nasally
Clear **Cornea** Clear
Quiet and deep **AC** Quiet and deep

NAD **iris** NAD
Round **Pupil** Round

11 T 11

Diagnosis
Left episcleritis

Treatment
Ibruprofen 400 mg TDS (no stomach problems)
Over the counter lubricant QDS left eye

Patient Education
Explanation that symptoms will resolve, but patient should return if pain worsens or any deterioration in visual acuity.

Case Study of a Patient with Viral Conjunctivitis

A 16-year-old girl attends your clinic with a two-day history of bilateral red eyes with a watery discharge. Her eyes feel gritty and sore.

Presenting Ocular History
- Two-day history of red sticky eyes, reported that started in left eye and then in right eye next day.
- Discharge is clear, but eyes stuck on waking
- No history of injury
- No other ocular complaints
- Doesn't wear any glasses/contact lenses or had any previous refractive laser surgery

General History
- Had tonsillitis and an earache last week needing a week off school

Medication
- None

Allergies
- No known allergies

Social History
- Lives with mother, her partner, and stepbrother
- At school, taking examinations next month
- Smokes socially
- Drinks at parties (Given advice on alcohol and smoking.)

Pain Score
4 out of 10

Differential Diagnosis
Bacterial conjunctivitis but the patient has no coloured discharge; blepharitis, unlikely as no symptoms before this episode; corneal ulcer/abrasion, no history of trauma or exposure to chemicals; scleritis, unlikely as not painful, just gritty

Examination

Visual acuity

6/9 u/a 6/6

Periacular nodes palperable submandibular area

Follicles visible and injected on eversion **Lids** Follicles visible and very injected on eversion

Mild swelling top lid

 Injected +   **Conjunctiva**   Injected ++

Clear, No staining with Fluorescein **Cornea** Clear, No staining with Fluorescein
Quiet and deep **AC** Quiet and deep
NAD **iris** NAD
Round **Pupil** Round

11 T 11

Diagnosis
Bilateral viral conjunctivitis

Treatment
Warm compresses. Use disposable kitchen towels then dispose and wash hands.
  Over the counter lubricants if required; separate bottle for each eye

Explanation to Patient
Highly contagious
   Antibiotics are not prescribed unless a secondary bacterial infection is evident as it is a viral infection similar to the common cold virus

Patient Education
Explain that symptoms will resolve, but patient should return immediately if pain worsens, or any deterioration in visual acuity or if discharge changes colour to a green purulent discharge.

- No towel sharing
- Change pillowcases on a daily basis
- No sharing of make-up (Throw away mascara and wash all make-up brushes with baby shampoo and hot water, air dry.)
- Not to touch eye but dab with a paper tissue then throw away; wash hands immediately
- Symptoms can take between a week and six weeks to resolve.

References

Coakes, R. and Holmes, S. (1995). *Outline of Ophthalmology*, 2e. Oxford: Butterworth Heineman.

Chen XM, Cui LG, He P, Shen WW, Qian YJ, Wang JR. et al. (2016). Diagnostic and Interventional Imaging, 97: 71–79.

Elliott, D. (2007). *Clinical Procedures in Primary Eye Care*, 3e. Edinburgh: Butterworth Heineman.

Goldblum, K. (2004). Obtaining a complete and pertinent patient history. *The Journal of the American Society of Ophthalmic Registered Nurses* XXIX (2): 17–20. April–June.

James, B. and Bron, A. (2011). *Lecture Notes on Ophthalmology*, 11e. Oxford: Wiley-Blackwell Publishing.

Martini, F., Nath, J., and Bartholomew, E. (2012). *The Eye, in Fundamentals of Anatomy & Physiology*, 9e. San Francisco, CA: Pearson Benjamin Cummings.

RNIB (2015) www.RNIB.co.uk (accessed 30 December 2015).

Rosser, D., Laidlaw, D., and Murdoch, I. (2001). The development of a "reduced LogMAR" visual acuity chart for use in routine clinical practice. *British Journal of Ophthalmology* 85: 432–436.

Stollery, R. (2010). *Ophthalmic Nursing*, 4e. Oxford: Wiley-Blackwell Publishing.

Tortora, G. and Derrickson, B. (2012). *Principles of Anatomy and Physiology*, 13e. Oxford: Wiley.

Walsh, M. (2006). *Nurse Practitioners: Clinical Skills and Professional Issues*, 2e. Edinburgh: Elsevier.

Wright, K. (2003). *Paediatric Ophthalmology for Primary Care*, 2e. Edinburgh: Elsevier.

Yannoff, M. and Duker, J. (2014). *Ophthalmology*, 4e. London: Mosby.

Chapter 12

Mental Health Assessment

Patrick Callaghan

Introduction

A mental health assessment can be carried out to identify a person's needs, to assist in developing and using appropriate interventions, to contribute to diagnostic accuracy, and to define problems that need solving. Assessing the mental state of people involves judging their psychological health and this requires experience, a degree of intelligence, self-insight, social skills, objectivity, and the ability to deal with cognitive complexities. A mental health assessment is usually done during an assessment interview. This chapter examines the role of motivational interviewing (MI) in the mental health assessment process, describes different approaches to assessment, and demonstrates how these may be used in practice. It also analyses contested issues in risk assessments and suggests ways to address the pitfalls inherent in the risk approach, summarises the clinical features of common mental disorders, and presents a case study showcasing assessment in practice.

Motivational Interviewing (MI)

Mental healthcare often involves helping people change from being overwhelmed by mental distress to a position where they recover to lead lives that are meaningful and satisfying to them (Andrews and Jenkins 1999; Attenborough 2006). People seeking mental healthcare are often looking to change aspects of their lives. However, people seeking change are often ambivalent and may lack the will, ability, or readiness to change (Hettema et al. 2005). MI is a person-centred, but directive, therapeutic intervention designed to help people improve their readiness to change (Miller and Rollnick 2002). MI has its practical origins in humanistic approaches to therapy based upon the work of Carl Rogers (1961).

MI may lead to a more accurate assessment and involves exploring the pros and cons of the person's current state, their general life satisfaction, and what help they need in making decisions about care.

Physical Assessment for Nurses and Healthcare Professionals, Third Edition. Edited by Carol Lynn Cox.
© 2019 John Wiley & Sons Ltd. Published 2019 by John Wiley & Sons Ltd.

MI has a robust evidence base. Studies testing the effect of MI show:

- A 56% reduction in problem drinking and a 51% reduction in substance misuse (Burke et al. 2003)
- A 59% improvement on general health and mental health outcomes (Hettema et al. 2005)
- Improvements in psychotic symptoms and satisfaction with medication (Maneesakorn et al. 2007)
- Improvements in participants' self-esteem, quality of life, depression, and social support (Callaghan et al. 2010).

Key characteristics of MI that are relevant to assessment are:

Working with ambivalence: ambivalence is not seen as unwillingness to seek help; instead it may reflect the conflict the person feels between wanting help and wanting to remain the same.

Empathic listening: not making value judgements, but displaying an attitude of acceptance, for example, by reflecting comments back to the person to allow them to explore the possibility of help.

Self-motivational statements: eliciting comments from the person that indicates a willingness to accept help.

Counselling skills: for example, the use of open-ended questions, reflective listening, affirmations, and summarising.

Resistance: roll with the resistance by using nonconfrontational methods. For example, the person may indicate they do not want to accept treatment; you may reply that they cannot see a reason to accept treatment.

There are three phases in MI:

1. The eliciting phase
2. The information phase
3. The negotiation phase.

The *eliciting phase* is characterised by assessing readiness to change. For example, the use of a Readiness to Change questionnaire or ruler will help establish how ready the person is to change any harmful behaviour that has led them to need professional help. For example, when using the Readiness Ruler, you ask the person to rate on a score of 1–10 how ready they are to change. For people seeking your help to change, three specific questions are of interest:

1. How important is it to change the unhelpful behaviour?
2. How confident are they that they can change their behaviour?
3. How realistic is it that they will avoid the harmful behaviour in the long term?

In the *information phase*, you seek the person's views as to their goals for changing harmful behaviour. For example, in relation to the behaviour, you pose the question: 'What is your goal for your harmful behaviour?' You may want to anchor the responses as:

- 'eliminating it completely'
- 'reducing it'
- 'continuing with it or undecided'.

In the *negotiation phase*, you work with the person to agree a plan for how change may occur. For example, you may ask the person to consider:

What actions they have taken in the past to change their harmful behaviour?
'What worked well, less well or what did not work at all'?

For those actions that had some success previously, ask the person to consider, 'What made them successful and what they can learn from these to change current behaviour'?

Assessment of Mental Health Status

An increasing number of people with mental health problems will be seen in general health settings. Assessment of mental health status may be necessary in all people, not just those seen in mental health settings. An assessment of mental health status is not something you do to a person, but activity undertaken in partnership with them and during which you elicit their views of their needs. Barker (2004) suggests different levels of assessment of people's lives:

the physiological self – assessment of basic physiological needs
the biological self – needs in relation to any symptoms a person may be experiencing, e.g. pain
the behavioural self – the effects of our thoughts, feelings, attitudes, and values on behaviour
the social self – how people relate to others
the spiritual self – The person's values, hopes, and experiences of the world.

When considering mental health status, in addition to the aforementioned, general health determinants should be remembered that can affect a person's mental health and overall health outcome. These include:

individual behaviour
health services
policy making
social functions
biology and genetics (Figure 12.1)

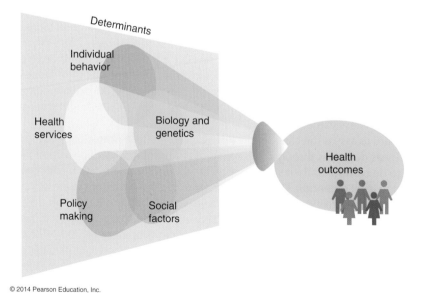

© 2014 Pearson Education, Inc.

Figure 12.1   Healthy people 2020 – health determinants. *Source*: https://www.bing.com/images/search?q=healthy+people+2020+health+determinants+pearson+drawing&qpvt=healthy+people+2020+health+determinants+pearson+drawing&FORM=IGRE (accessed 25 January 2018).

Gamble and Brennan (2006) suggest several elements of a comprehensive mental health assessment. Risk – an assessment of the likelihood of risk to self or others – is recommended by the authors and is common in many mental health assessments. However, risk has come to be a highly contested issue in mental health assessment. Prior to unpacking Gamble and Brennan's components of a comprehensive assessment, the possibilities and pitfalls of risk assessment are examined.

Possibilities and Pitfalls in Risk Assessment

Possibilities

A useful starting point for an examination of the possibilities of risk assessment is to consider its purpose. The purpose of risk assessment is to identify the likelihood of harm to self or others with a view to preventing or minimising such harm (Large and Nielson 2011). According to the latest data from the National Confidential Inquiry into Suicide and Homicide by People with Mental Illness in England (University of Manchester 2015) between 2009 and 2013 30% of all suicides in the United Kingdom (UK) were patient suicides, an increase of 3%. In the same period, the homicide rates remained fairly static. Only 7% of all stranger homicides were committed by people living with a mental illness. Thus, more than three times as many people with a mental health problem will take their own life than will take the life of others. Preventing or minimising this harm is an important public health issue and risk assessment offers this possibility.

Actuarial measures of risk are based on probabilistic reasoning that allows data to be coded in a predetermined manner using risk algorithms such as the Area under the Curve (AUC). An AUC of 0.50 or below suggests that the efficacy of the prediction is due to chance, not the risk assessment measure (Buchanan 2008). Evidence shows that the predictive accuracy of most actuarial measures exceeds chance (Singh et al. 2011; Yang et al. 2010). Therefore, using actuarial measures of risk offers the possibility of being able to predict risk accurately.

Notwithstanding the limitations of using AUC scores, they allow for a calculation of clinical utility similar to numbers needed to treat (NNT). NNT is an important measure of clinical utility. For example, before using a particular intervention to reduce harm – harm to others – it would be useful to know how many people would need to be treated using the intervention in order to reduce harm by at least one incident; the lower the NNT, the more clinical utility of the intervention. An NNT of 10 would mean that 10 people would need to be treated to reduce harm by at least one incident. Thus the intervention might be seen to have value. An NNT of 100 would mean that 100 people would need to be treated to reduce harm by at least one incident. In this case the intervention might be seen to have less value.

It is hard to assess the clinical utility of AUC scores; Buchanan (2008), using the principles of NNT, has done this through calculation of the numbers needed to detain (NND). People likely to be harmful to their selves or others as a result of a mental health problem may be subject to legal detention. One of the purposes of risk assessment using actuarial measures is to predict the likelihood of harm with a view to preventing it through detention. NND is an attempt to calculate how many people would need to be detained to prevent at least one harmful act. Generally there is an inverse relationship between the NND and the prevalence of harm; the NND rises as the harm prevalence falls. Therefore, calculation of the NND using the AUC score would lend more clinical utility to risk assessment measures.

Another possibility to using risk assessment measures is developing interventions from significant factors in the measure. These factors may be static, such as history of harm, and would not be amenable to change. Other factors, such as social support, are dynamic and would be amenable to change (Yang et al. 2010). Therefore, interventions may be suggested to improve an individual's social support level, e.g. increasing social networks have been shown to reduce harm (Budde and Schene 2004).

A final possibility of using risk assessment measures concerns the use of legal detention. Requirements for legal detention using mental health law in most jurisdictions are that a person who is judged to have a mental disorder of a nature or severity that threatens the safety of the person or others may be detained involuntarily (Katona et al. 2008). The issue of risk is pertinent here. As long as risk is linked to decisions around legal detention, mental health practitioners with the powers to detain people involuntarily may benefit from access to the best available risk assessment measures.

Notwithstanding the possibilities of risk assessment measures, there are several pitfalls that need consideration.

Pitfalls

A starting point for a discussion of the pitfalls in risk assessment of harm concerns the issue of risk assessment in decisions as to the detention of people under mental health law. In his Gresham College lecture, 'How mental health legislation discriminates unfairly against people with mental illness,' George Szmukler, Professor of Psychiatry at the Institute of Psychiatry, Psychology and Neuroscience in London (Szmukler 2010) illustrated how the issue of risk, crucial to detention decisions, discriminates against people thought to be mentally ill. A person deemed to be mentally ill who is thought to be at risk of harm to self or others can be detained even if they have never committed a violent act, have insight into their risk, and have plans to manage it, i.e. they have mental capacity. Conversely, a person with a life-threatening physical illness who refuses treatment that can save their life and who is deemed to have mental capacity can refuse treatment without fear of involuntary detention.

There is evidence of an association between having a mental disorder and being a risk to others (University of Manchester 2015); but this risk is small (10%). The number of people in the general population who may be deemed risky to others and who are unlikely to have a mental disorder, e.g. careless drivers, greatly exceeds those with a mental disorder deemed risky; yet these people are not eligible for involuntary detention under mental health law. Therefore, detention on the grounds of risk discriminates against people who have a mental disorder. This situation should sit uneasily in democratic societies with strong civil libertarian principles enshrined in law. Detaining people with a mental disorder who are assessed as a risk to self or others, even when they have no history of having committed a harmful act, amounts to preventive detention; society seems willing to accept this when applied to people thought to be mentally ill but not to others including people whose behaviours are clearly harmful to themselves and others. Therefore, having a mental illness invites socially approved discrimination that is endorsed by (mental health) law and is ethically dubious.

Another ethical concern raised about risk assessment is that people who are assessed as low risk find it difficult to access care than those classified as high risk (Large et al. 2008). Risk assessment may also undermine people's choice of treatment (Mossman 2006) and damage providers' attempts to work collaboratively with people seeking mental health-care (Langan 2010).

A significant pitfall in risk assessment and management concerns the use of the predictive efficacy algorithm. At the heart of risk prediction of harm research is using instruments to predict the likelihood that harm may occur. Even with the application of sophisticated statistical modelling techniques the relationship between the instrument and the likelihood of future harm is essentially one of correlation. Correlations show the strength of relationship between two variables, but one cannot infer causation from this relationship.

If researchers, clinicians, managers, and policymakers are serious about reducing or preventing harm, they will need to identify the likely causes, develop interventions to address these causes, and evaluate these interventions in well-designed studies (Buchanan 2008; Wong and Gordon 2006; Yang et al. 2010). As Yang et al. (2010) illustrate, we could take steps to reduce harm with more confidence if we knew that A (e.g. substance use) causes B (harm) and taking steps to reduce A leads to a reduction in B. Therefore, only a thorough understanding of what causes harm will allow the discovery of causal risk predictors that can then be addressed to reduce or prevent harm.

The conclusions that Yang et al. (2010) and Singh et al. (2011) draw from their impressive meta-analyses of risk assessment measures differ. Yang et al. (2010) (p. 759) conclude: 'It is not possible to say that any one tool predicts harm consistently and significantly better than any others'. Conversely, Singh et al. (2011) conclude: 'The present meta-analysis found that the predictive validity of commonly used risk assessment measures varies widely'. The differences in these conclusions may arise from the application of different statistical modelling. Also, although both reviews studied the same measures, Yang et al. (2010) included measures not present in Singh et al. (2011) and vice versa. This could also account for the different conclusions. But one important similarity in both reviews is the reliance on the predictive efficacy algorithm reporting pooled estimates of predictive accuracy drawn from relationships of correlation, not causation.

The predictive efficacy of risk assessment measures is shown to be vulnerable to the measures of actual harm being predicted (Buchanan 2008; Dolan and Doyle 2000; Mossman 1994; Singh et al. 2011; Yang et al. 2010) and this is another pitfall. The harm that confronts clinicians in health settings comes in many shapes and sizes from verbal abuse through threats to actual, sometimes serious, assaults (NHS SMS 2010). If a particular measure is to be adopted routinely into practice by increasingly busy clinicians it must be capable of addressing the different forms that harm takes in practice. It is not clear from the evidence reviewed thus far what such a measure might look like as some focus on static predictors, others (Historical, Clinical and Risk Management Harm Risk Assessment Scheme [HCR-20], for example) have dynamic/interchangeable predictors whilst the PCL-R is designed for a particular personality variable. Those like the HCR-20 may have more value in general psychiatric wards.

Harm risk measures have been shown across studies and time to perform consistently above chance when testing their predictive efficacy (Buchanan 2008; Dolan and Doyle 2000; Mossman 1994; Singh et al. 2011; Yang et al. 2010). This lends them a degree of clinical utility, but given that routine clinical assessments of risk appear better than chance (Cole-King and Lepping 2010), the added value of risk assessment measures is questionable. The potential value of NND was discussed previously, to add to the clinical utility of risk measures in detention decisions, but outside this realm of decision making around risk, their clinical utility is diminished. Clinical utility is a crucial issue of whether research knowledge can translate easily into practice. Acceptable measures of clinical utility are effect sizes, odds ratios, NNT, and confidence intervals. The limitations of the predictive efficacy algorithm have been discussed. One aspect of attempting to show the clinical utility of risk measures is to consider how the AUC scores compute to measures of clinical utility.

Rice and Harris (2005) calculated effect size equivalents for AUC scores using Cohen's (1992) d statistic – a measure of the size of the effect in outcomes achieved when comparing one intervention with another or with treatment as usual. Using Rice and Harris' (2005) approach the effect sizes are calculated from the AUC scores for the common risk measures shown in Table 12.1.

Effect sizes are often reported as small, medium or large. In Cohen's estimates an effect size of around 0.20 is small, 0.50 medium and 0.80 large. Using these estimates, all of the

Table 12.1 Common actuarial measures and their predictive efficacy (Abderhalden et al. 2008; Singh et al. 2011; Yang et al. 2010).

Measure	AUC
SVR-20 – Sexual Harm Risk 20	0.78
SORAG – Sexual Offender Risk Appraisal Guide	0.75
VRAG – Harm Risk Assessment Guide	0.74
SAVRY – Structured Assessment of Harm Risk in Youth	0.71
OGRS – Offender Group Reconviction Scale	0.71
HCR-20 – Historical, Clinical and Risk Management Harm Risk Assessment Scheme	0.71
RM2000V – Risk Matrix 2000 for Harm	0.70
SARA – Spousal Assault Risk Assessment	0.70
Static-99 –	0.70

Table 12.2 Common actuarial risk measures and their effect sizes.

Measure	Cohen's d
SVR-20 – Sexual Harm Risk 20	1.12
SORAG – Sexual Offender Risk Appraisal Guide	1.06
SAVRY – Structured Assessment of Harm Risk in Youth	1.00
OGRS – Offender Group Reconviction Scale	1.00
HCR-20 – Historical, Clinical and Risk Management Harm Risk Assessment Scheme	1.00
RM2000V – Risk Matrix 2000 for Harm	0.99
SARA – Spousal Assault Risk Assessment	0.99
Static-99 –	0.99
VRAG – Harm Risk Assessment Guide	0.94

AUC scores of the measures shown in Table 12.1 equate to large effect sizes as shown by the data in Table 12.2, suggesting a high degree of clinical utility. Computing pooled determination of risk (DOR) as an indicator of clinical utility, Singh et al. (2011) reported pooled DOR for many of the common risk measures shown in Tables 12.1 and 12.2. These data suggest that the risk measures cited were less likely to produce false positive results. Although these results suggest that risk measures might have more clinical utility than AUC scores show, they do not eliminate the limitations around correlation inherent in the predictive efficacy algorithm.

Harm around mental health issues is linked to environmental factors such as the use of physical restraint and seclusion, overcrowding or overoccupancy as it is sometimes called, staff–patient ratios, ward rules, and staff characteristics like the frequency, nature, and characteristics of interactions staff has with service users. Yet, risk measures seldom include such factors; they are almost without exception individual centric. This person-centric approach helps explain why many service users do not engage with risk assessment, consider the process stigmatising and disempowering (O'Rourke and Bird 2001), and may conceal information during risk assessment interviews to effect the least aversive consequences to themselves. A consequence of this approach is that risk assessment measures lack credibility in the eyes of many service users for whom risk is something that is done to them and violates the principle of current UK health and social care policy that there should be 'no decision about me without me' (Department of Health 2011).

A major pitfall in risk assessment is that assessments are seldom followed by effective risk management approaches (Department of Health 2011; O'Rourke and Bird 2001). Where risk management is apparent, it is often through simplistic restrictive methods with the least effective impact such as locking ward doors (Cole-King and Lepping 2010).

The discourse surrounding risk assessment measures has been subject to social and political critique. It is argued that risk assessments are seldom linked to improved therapeutic outcomes and are designed largely to further marginalise disenfranchised groups and label people (low, moderate or high risk) rather than understanding and helping to resolve their difficulties. It acts as a social surveillance device more concerned with identifying and controlling problems instead of resolving them (Silver and Miller 2002). Actuarial measures offer the promise of reducing deviance and crime without effecting change in individuals or their social circumstances (Garland 1996), justified on the grounds that assessments of risk can lead to variations in coercive responses when they should be secured by a desire to improve, reintegrate, retrain, provide employment, and foster recovery (Feeley and Simon 1992). Marginalised groups such as those with mental illness are further burdened as they often live in communities associated with recurrent harm and crime (Silver 2001) and promote stigma by classifying individuals as risky thus giving society's prejudices and fear the stamp of scientific approval (Walker 1998). Clinicians using risk assessment measures usually have benevolent intentions, but history has shown that such intentions do not always lead to benevolent outcomes (Cohen 1985; Foucault 1979; Rothman 1980).

A considerable pitfall in using risk assessment is that it fails to deliver on what it promises. The vast majority of evidence citing the 'efficacy' of risk assessment is from studies testing the predictive efficacy algorithm, which, as has been shown, does not establish a causal association between assessment and harm reduction. There are few exceptions. In one such exception using a clustered randomised controlled trial of the effect of a structured risk assessment on violent incidents in nine acute psychiatric wards in Switzerland, Abderhalden et al. (2008) reported a significant reduction in the number of violent incidents in the intervention wards. But the failure to match the intervention and control wards for baseline harm levels weakens the impact of these findings. Also, the reduction in harm was not sustained beyond the end of the study. In another study, Kling et al. (2011) reported that risk assessment had little impact on harm reduction levels in a mental health acute care hospital in British Columbia, Canada. If the purpose of risk assessment is to identify risk with a view to preventing or minimising it, there is little evidence that this is being achieved.

Other researchers have taken to investigate the effect of other interventions in reducing harm. For example, Haddock et al. (2009) compared cognitive behaviour therapy (CBT) with social activity therapy (SAT) and reported CBT to be superior in reducing harm, delusions, and risk in people with severe mental illness using mental health services in North West England.

A simple way to address many of the pitfalls in risk assessment is to focus on the issue of safety. The language of risk punishes and stigmatises; in some cases it may traumatise. The language of safety nourishes and protects. A combined approach to safety assessment that uses actuarial measures and sound clinical judgement is recommended. Given that discussing safety issues is a sensitive topic, it is strongly recommended that this discussion does not come at the beginning or end of an assessment interview but is integrated into the middle section of the interview.

Gamble and Brennan (2006) also suggest the following be incorporated into a comprehensive mental health assessment:

physical and mental health status
social need and functioning
symptomatology and coping skills
quality of life and its effects on others
safety
housing and money
social support
medication and its effects
work skills and meaningful daily activity.

An assessment of mental health status may also focus on the following:

- appearance and behaviour – physical appearance, reaction to situation
- mood – mood, affect
- speech – rate, form, volume and quantity of information, content
- form of thought – amount and rate of thought, continuity of ideas
- thought content – delusions, suicidal thoughts, other
- perception – hallucinations, other perceptual disturbances
- sensorium and cognition – level of consciousness, memory, orientation, concentration, abstract thoughts
- insight – understanding of illness
- sexual health – sexual activity, contraceptive use, substance use, cervical screening, testicular examination, HIV status
- person's perception of their needs – ask the person what are their views of their mental health needs

Rating scales may be used with interviews as part of a mental health assessment. Some commonly used rating scales in mental health assessment are as follows:

- The Short Form-12 (SF-12) (Ware et al. 1996) – a measure of general mental and physical health
- The Health of the Nation Outcome Scale (HoNOS) (Wing 1994) – a measure of 12 categories of behaviour and mental state linked to mental health status
- Brief Psychiatric Rating Scale (BPRS) (Ventura et al. 1993) – a measure of psychiatric symptoms
- Edinburgh Post Natal Depression Scale (EPNDS) (Cox et al. 1987) – a measure of depressive symptoms associated with childbirth
- Beck Depression Inventory (BDI) (Beck et al. 1961) – a measure of depressive symptoms
- Side Effects Checklist (SEC) (Andrews and Jenkins 1999) – a measure of side effects of drugs commonly used in psychiatry
- Suicide Assessment and Management (SAM) (Fremouw et al. 1990) – a measure of suicidal intent and previous self-harming behaviour
- Risk Assessment and Management – Clinical Risk Management Tool (CRMT) (Morgan 2005) – a measure of the likelihood of a potentially harmful incident happening, or that has possible beneficial outcomes for the person and others

General Rules in Assessing Mental Health Status

- Be nonjudgemental.
- Be alert to phenomena that are observed.
- Do not jump to conclusions about what the person is saying.
- Clarify with gentle enquiry:
  - 'Please tell me more about that'.
  - 'I'd like to hear of a recent example'.
  - 'When did that last happen?'
  - 'What did you do about it?'
  - 'How often/how long have you experienced that?'

Appearance and Behaviour (Observation)

- Describe in simple terms:
  - unkempt appearance
  - bewildered, agitated, restless, aggressive, tearful, sullen:
    - appropriate to setting?
    - reduced activity in *depression*
    - overactive and intrusive in *mania*
    - tense and reassurance seeking with *anxiety*
  - able to respond to questions
  - evidence of responding to voices and their impact
  - smell of alcohol
  - evidence of drug misuse (e.g. needle marks)

Mood (Part Observation, Part Enquiry)

Mood is a subjective state and is mainly judged by the impression conveyed during the history, although examination gives further clues.

- Ask:
  - 'How have your spirits been recently?'
  - 'To what extent have you been feeling your usual self?'
  - 'Is this how you usually feel?'

    Depressed – depression disorder or an adjustment reaction (see questions under 'Mental Health' in Chapter 1).

    Elevated – manic disorder or intoxication, e.g. ethanol, drugs, delirium.

    Anxious – anxiety disorder or reaction to situation.

    Angry – delirium or reaction to situation.

    Flat – depressed or no emotional rapport, i.e. *schizophrenia* (Phillips and Callaghan 2009).
- If evidence for depression, worry, agitation, irritability – record current nature and severity.
  - if depressed, explore safety issues around suicide and self-harm that the Suicide Research Centre at Oxford University recommends:
    1. Are you feeling hopeless, or that life is not worth living?
    2. Have you made plans to end your life?
    3. Have you told anyone about these plans?
    4. Have you carried out any acts in anticipation of your death, e.g. putting your affairs in order?

5. Do you have access to means to take your own life, e.g. access to pills, firearms, poisons, insecticides, etc.?
6. What support is available to you, e.g. from family, friends, carers?
- Also ask for other clinicians' and relatives' comments.

Speech (Observation)
Describe speech in simple terms and record verbatim typical remarks.

- Rate:
  - fast in *mania*
  - slow in *depression*
- Form:
  - are there abnormalities of grammar or flow? (record examples)
    Disordered thought processes can occur in *schizophrenia, mania, acute organic states, dementia*.
  - are there abnormal sequences of words?
    - non sequiturs with disordered logic in *schizophrenia* – 'word jumble'
    - loosely connected topics in *mania* – 'flight of ideas'
- Content (observations, elaborate with enquiry):
  - 'You said you … Tell me more about that'.
  - 'When you feel sad, what goes through your mind?'

Form of Thought (Form and Content – Largely Inferred from Speech)
- Record person's main thoughts or preoccupations:
  - negative pessimistic in *depression* – ask about suicidal intentions
  - grandiose in *mania*
  - catastrophizing in *anxiety*
    Obsessions – intrusive thoughts or repetitious behaviours that the patient cannot resist although knwoing they are not sensible.
  - perseveration – repetition of a word or phrase; can occur in *anxiety, depression, mania, delirium*, or *dementia*

Thought Content ('Odd Ideas', Thoughts, Beliefs, Delusions)
- Ask person to describe; be nonjudgemental.
- Ask why the person thinks that – may reveal psychotic thoughts or harmful hallucinations.
  - Delusions are fixed, false beliefs without reasonable evidence, e.g. I've got AIDS/cancer.
  - 'Did it ever seem to you that people were talking about you?'
  - 'Have you ever received special messages from the television, radio, or newspaper?'
  - 'Do people seem to be going out of their way to get at you?'
  - 'Have you ever felt that you were especially important in some way or that you had special powers?'
  - 'Do you ever feel you have committed a crime or done something terrible for which you should be punished?'

Perception (Hallucinations and Illusions – Usually Apparent from History)

- Ask:
  - 'Have you had any unusual experiences recently?'
  - 'Do they seem as if they are in the real world or as if they are "inside" your head?'
    Hallucinations are false perceptions without a stimulus (e.g. pink elephants – experienced as real).
    - They can occur in any sensory modality.
    - Visual hallucinations may be suggestive of an organic state.
    - Third person ('he' or 'she') auditory harmful hallucinations are often suggestive of *schizophrenia*.
    - 'Do you ever hear things that other people can't hear such as the voices of people talking?'
    - 'Do you ever have visions or see things that other people can't see?'
    - 'Do you ever have strange sensations in your body or skin?'

Illusions are misinterpreted perceptions (e.g. the person thinks you are a policeman). They are common in psychotic episodes

Sensorium and Cognition (Observations Supplemented by Specific Enquiry)

- Impairment of concentration can occur in:
  - *depression*
  - *anxiety states*
  - *dementia*
  - *confusional state*
- Orientation, thought processes, memory, and logic. These aspects must be tested as part of a mental health assessment.

Insight (Understanding of Condition)

- 'What do you think is wrong with you?'
  - 'Is there any illness that you are particularly worried about?'
  - 'What treatment do you feel is appropriate?'
  - 'Are there any treatments you are frightened of?'
    It is important to ask all persons these questions. If the person appears to lack insight into unusual beliefs or behaviour, this could suggest a psychotic illness.
  - The person's perception of his or her needs and problems

General History and Examination

Mental illness can be the presentation of a physical illness and a full history and examination should be carried out for all patients (USDHHS 2014).

Physical illnesses that may masquerade as mental illnesses include:

- *hypothyroid, hyperthyroid*
- *hypercalcaemia* or *hypokalaemia*
- *cerebral tumour*
- *other causes of increased intracranial pressure*
- *chronic, occult infection*

- *drugs*
- *porphyria*

There is some evidence that mental illnesses may be linked to a physical imbalance of transmitters/receptor function in the brain, and the division of illness into physical and mental is often spurious. In any case, all people, whatever the nature of their experience, should be treated nonjudgementally and with respect.

Challenging Behaviour

Anger and Hostility

- Inordinate anger is often symptomatic of another problem.
- Assess whether the grievance is justified and whether it can be resolved.
- 'Is there anything else that is upsetting you?'
- If the antagonism is directed against you, enquire whether the person would prefer to see somebody else.

Harm and Aggression

- Do not take unnecessary risks (have help nearby).
- Attempt to defuse the situation.
- Ensure person is not armed.
- Determine orientation and whether intoxicated or deluded.
- Fear often underlines aggression – what is the fear?

Self-Injury Behaviour

- Assess intent and history of previous attempts (if any):
  - planning and likelihood of discovery
  - perceived dangerousness of method
  - intention at time
- Assess current intent (see suicide safety assessment questions above)

Sexual Disinhibition

- Often associated with manic disorders.
- Protect person's privacy and dignity.
- Work with person to agree boundaries of acceptable behaviour.
- Agree contract with person and operate within terms of contract.
- Take person into private space.
- Minimise others' ridiculing of the person.

Summary of Common Mental Disorders

Depression

- low mood, tearfulness (not always present)
- lack of interest and self-care
- poor concentration
- negative thought content
- low self-esteem
- wakes up early
- depressed facies

- slow movements and speech
- weight loss
- negative speech content

Anxiety

- generally worried
- thought focuses on catastrophes
- cannot get to sleep
- tense lined face, furrowed brow
- sweaty palms
- shaky
- hyperventilation
- tachycardia

Anorexia Nervosa

- thin, little body fat
- increased, fine body hair
- sees self as fat even if thin
- thoughts dominated by food

Bulimia Nervosa

- often normal weight
- binges followed by self-induced vomiting
- thoughts dominated by food
- erosion of teeth from vomiting

Schizophrenia

- hallucinations
- delusions
- thought disturbances
- disordered thinking
- negative symptoms

Bipolar Disorder – Mania

- rapid speech with 'flight of ideas'
- overactive, cannot keep still
- normal activities disrupted
- overly cheerful or irritable
- stands close and is argumentative

Bipolar Disorder – Depression

- depressed affect
- slow movements and speech
- negative thoughts and delusions, e.g. brain is rotting
- suicidal thoughts
- loss of interest or pleasure in usual activities
- poor concentration

Case Study of a White Heterosexual Male with Paranoid Schizophrenia

The patient describes himself:

'I am a 38-year-old, white, heterosexual male, married with two children. Since February 2007, when I was in my late 20s, I have had periods when I can see and hear three evil men. These men torment me and they conduct painful experiments on me – they implant a chip in my hand to monitor my movements and to give me electric shocks in a bid to control me, and they implant maggot eggs in my head, which hatch and eat away at my brain. The men steal my thoughts – I can feel thoughts being painfully extracted from my head, leaving blanks behind. And I become suspicious of strangers, believing that people are conspiring with the men against me, maybe poisoning my food or reporting my movements. The men try to break me and go into detail about how I should kill myself and end it all. At the beginning of each episode the men feel overwhelming, and on five occasions I've been so distressed that I've gone into hospital for periods ranging from two weeks to three months. I lose insight and believe that all of this is real and have been given a diagnosis of paranoid schizophrenia. After trying a few antipsychotic medications, I was put on medication, which has given me some stability, but with troublesome side-effects. I've also learnt some techniques to help me engage with "the men." My experiences are episodic and when I'm not having a psychotic episode I do not have any residual symptoms. The episodes are triggered by stress and anxiety, and I do really suffer with anxiety when well, which often manifests itself in flare-ups of IBD' (inflammatory bowel disease).

Illustration of Assessment Approaches Discussed in this Chapter

Personal, Family, Social, and Medical History

David is the eldest of two sons and recalls a settled but lonely childhood and adolescence. He describes his father as an 'alcoholic' with episodes of violence towards objects but not people. His parents divorced when David was aged 12 and his mother remarried. At age 17 he was adopted by his stepfather. He reported a good relationship with his mother and stepfather initially, which later became strained owing to his 'dominant, overbearing' stepfather and his mother's sense of personal betrayal because of David's desire to have contact with his biological father, with whom he had a 'physically and emotionally distant' relationship. His father died when David was aged 15.

David achieved A Levels at secondary school and achieved a bachelor's degree in theology at a leading university, graduating with a 2nd-class honours upper division. Married with two young daughters. David works as a research associate at the same university where he undertook his higher education.

David experienced 'depression' in his final year at university, for which his general practitioner prescribed antidepressants. Whilst working towards his master's in philosophy (theology) at the same university in his late 20s he experienced his 1st 'psychotic' episode; the overwhelming, intrusive, threatening, intimidating, and tormenting men. This led to the 1st of several involuntary admissions to acute psychiatric services during a 10-year period initially in the care of early intervention services, and latterly, Community Mental Health Teams. His treatments have consisted mainly of various medication regimes, CBT and recently 'sense making' psychological interventions. He has also used voice dialogues to help him live better with the intrusive voices of the men. He has no family history of mental health problems, save for one cousin who is diagnosed as agoraphobic. His older daughter experiences episodic anxiety.

Physical and Mental Health Status

David describes his physical health as good with no diagnosed illnesses, but he alludes to 'IBD' like symptoms when anxious. He recognises challenges in maintaining a healthy weight associated with the appetite stimulant effects of antipsychotic medication. He was hospitalised with what appeared to be clozapine withdrawal syndrome in 2012. He has a family history through his father's line of coronary heart disease, which caused his father's death. David reports drinking approximately 6–8 units of alcohol per week, mostly at weekends, 'walks most places', once dabbled briefly with smoking, sleeps 'well' most nights, usually skips breakfast, has a light lunch, and eats dinner with his family each evening. He has a yearly physical health check. His mental health status is compromised by the intrusive, tormenting, and harmful presence of seeing and hearing the voices of three evil men with consequent suspicion of strangers and feelings of being persecuted and threatened by harm to self and family.

Social Need, Social Support, and Functioning

David describes himself as shy, introverted, personable, and able to get on well with others; a bit 'geekish' or 'geek chic'. He recalls having difficulty making friends when younger and being bullied at school. He has a robust marriage of 13 years and describes a good relationship with his wife and children, a superficial one with his parents and a distant relationship with his brother. He has excellent working relationships with colleagues and has achieved many successes in his current job. David's level of social support stems from his immediate family, wife and children, his circle of friends, and his church involvement.

Personal Strengths and Coping Skills

David identifies a strong socially supportive network (see above) as being central to his well-developed coping skills. David identifies several personal strengths that help him cope with day-to-day challenges. These include his interest in evidence-based facts. David enjoys weighing up evidence in helping him make decisions; having a bachelor's and master's degree helps him in these endeavours. His social support network and his satisfaction with the quality of this support add to his resilience, which strengthens his resolve in challenging situations.

Quality of Life and Its Effects on Others

Notwithstanding the symptoms that David has experienced recently, he reports his quality of life and life satisfaction as high; 'Life is really good' he states.

Safety

Safety issues were explored using the questions that the Oxford Suicide Centre recommends.

1. Are you feeling hopeless, or that life is not worth living? – Yes
2. Have you made plans to end your life? – David reports concrete ideas of jumping in front of a train as a relief from the tormenting voices and visions.
3. Have you told anyone about these plans? – David reported sharing these plans with his wife and psychologist.
4. Have you carried out any acts in anticipation of your death, e.g. putting your affairs in order? – David reported he had not carried out any such acts or made such plans.

5. Do you have access to means to take your own life, e.g. access to pills, firearms, poisons, insecticides, etc.? – David reported he had access to medication that he could use to take his life.
6. What support is available to you, e.g. from family, friends, carers? – David reported he has strong support available from his wife and church friends.

David reported he sought voluntary admission owing to concerns about the safety of his family.

Housing and Money
David has safe, secure accommodation in the form of a rented house and reports no financial concerns.

Medication and Its Effects
David is currently prescribed a 2nd-generation antipsychotic nightly, an anxiolytic as required and used periodically, and an antimuscarinic to treat salivary secretions.

283

Work Skills and Meaningful Daily Activity
As reported previously, David works as a research associate in a leading university and is enjoying great success in this job. He also has an active social life outside work.

Summary Statements Following Assessment
Following the assessment, the practitioner worked with David on formulating/summarising his main needs/problems that need addressing. This took the form of asking him to write each statement and agreeing with him the specific issues/problems/needs, the impact of the issues, and any relevant safety issues. He developed two statements. The specific issues are highlighted in red, the impact of these are highlighted in green, and safety issues are highlighted in blue.

1. From time to time I am tormented by three evil men who issue commands that I should end my life – I find them so intimidating and all powerful that there are safety concerns that I will follow through on their demands.
2. I am very suspicious of staff, believing that they are conspiring with the men against me; this leads me to disengage and to withdraw from others.

The summary statements bring the assessment to an end.

Conclusions
Assessment is an important part of the process of mental healthcare and, when done in collaboration with the service user, allows for a meaningful narrative of a person's history and situation and an agreed identification of the person's specific issues that need addressing, the impact of the issues on their life, and the recognition of any safety issues for the person or those in their orbit. A comprehensive assessment contains several linked components and is central the mental healthcare process and allows for further planning, implementation, and review of evidence-based interventions.

Acknowledgements

I am indebted to Andrew Grundy at the University of Nottingham for his assistance with this chapter.

References

Abderhalden, C., Needham, I., Dassen, T. et al. (2008). Structured risk assessment and violence in acute psychiatric wards: randomised controlled trial. *British Journal of Psychiatry* 193 (1): 44–50.

Andrews, G. and Jenkins, R. ed. (1999). *Management of Mental Disorders*, U.K. edition. Sydney: WHO Collaborating Centre for Mental Health and Substance Misuse.

Attenborough, J. (2006). Motivational interviewing. In: *The Oxford Handbook of Mental Health Nursing* (ed. P. Callaghan and H. Waldock), 98. Oxford: Oxford University Press.

Barker, P. (2004). *Assessment in Psychiatric and Mental Health Nursing. In Search of the Whole Person*. Surrey: Nelson Thornes.

Beck, A., Ward, C., Mendelson, M. et al. (1961). Inventory for measuring depression. *Archives of General Psychiatry* 4: 561–571.

Buchanan, A. (2008). Risk of violence by psychiatric patients; beyond the 'Actuarial Versus Clinical' assessement debate. *Psychiatric Services* 59 (2): 184–190.

Budde, S. and Schene, P. (2004). Informal social support interventions and their role in violence prevention: an agenda for future evaluation. *Journal of Interpersonal Violence* 19 (3): 341–355.

Burke, B.L., Arkowitz, H., and Menchola, M. (2003). The efficacy of motivational interviewing: a meta-analysis of controlled clinical trials. *Journal of Consulting and Clinical Psychology* 71 (5): 843–861.

Callaghan, P., Khalil, E., and Morres, I. (2010). A prospective evaluation of the transtheoretical model applied to exercise in young people. *International Journal of Nursing Studies* 47: 3–12.

Cohen, S. (1985). *Visions of Social Control*. Cambridge: Polity Press.

Cohen, S. (1992) Confidence Intervals, Effect Size, and Statistical Power. https://quizlet.com/161223313/confidence-intervals-effect-size-and-statistical-power-flash-cards (accessed 28 August 2018).

Cole-King, A. and Lepping, P. (2010). Will the new Government change our approach to risk? *British Medical Journal* 341: c3890. doi:10.1136/bmj.c3890.

Cox, J., Holden, J., and Sagovsky, R. (1987). Detection of postnatal depression: development of the 10-item Edinburgh Post Natal Depression Scale. *British Journal of Psychiatry* 150: 782–786.

Department of Health (2011). *No Health Without Mental Health: Delivering Better Mental Health Outcomes for People of all Ages*. London: Department of Health.

Dolan, M. and Doyle, M. (2000). Violence risk prediction. *British Journal of Psychiatry* 177: 303–311.

Felley, M.M. and Simon, J. (1992). The new penology: notes on the merging strategy of corrections and its implications. *Criminology* 30: 449–474.

Foucault, M. (1979). *Discipline and Punish: The Birth of the Prison*. New York: Vintage.

Fremouw, W., de Perczel, M., and Ellis, T. (1990). *Suicide Risk Assessment and Response Guidelines*. New York: Pergamon Press.

Gamble, C. and Brennan, G. (2006). *Working with Serious Mental Illness. A Manual for Clinical Practice*, 2e. London: Bailliere Tindall.

Garland, D. (1996). The limits of the sovereign state. *British Journal of Criminology* 36: 445–470.

Haddock, G., Barrowclough, C., Shaw, J. et al. (2009). Cognitive-behavioural therapy v. social activity therapy for people with psychosis and a history of violence: randomised controlled trial. *British Journal of Psychiatry* 194 (2): 152, eScholarID:1d18415 |–157. doi:10.1192/bjp.bp.107.039859.

Hettema, J., Steele, J., and Miller, W.R. (2005). Motivational interviewing. *Annual Review of Clinical Psychology* 1: 91–111.

Katona, C., Cooper, C., and Robertson, M. (2008). Mental health legislation in Northern Ireland. In: *Psychiatry at a Glance*, 4e (ed. C. Katona, C. Cooper and M. Robertson), 90–91. London: Blackwell Publishing.

Kling, R.N., Yassi, A., Smailes, E. et al. (2011). Evaluation of a violence risk assessment system (the alert system) for reducing violence in an acute hospital: a before and after study. *International Journal of Nursing Studies* 48 (5): 534–539.

Langan, J. (2010). Challenging assumptions about risk factors and the role of screening for violence risk in the field of mental health. *Health, Risk and Society* 12: 85–100.

Large, M.M. and Nielssen, O.B. (2011). Probability and loss: two sides of the risk assessment coin. *The Psychiatrist* 35: 413–418.

Large, M.M., Nielssen, O., Ryan, C.J., and Hayes, R. (2008). Mental health laws that require dangerousness for involuntary admission may delay the initial treatment of schizophrenia. *Social Psychiatry and Psychiatric Epidemiology* 43 (3): 251–256.

Maneesakorn, S., Robson, D., Gournay, K., and Gray, R. (2007). An RCT of adherence therapy for people with schizophrenia in Chian Mai, Thailand. *Journal of Clinical Nursing* 16: 1302–1312.

Miller, W.R. and Rollnick, S. (2002). *Motivational Interviewing: Preparing People for Change*, vol. 2. New York: Guidlford.

Morgan, S. (2005). *Clinical Risk Management: A Clinical Tool and Practitioner Manual*. London: Sainsbury Centre for Mental Health.

Mossman, D. (1994). Assessing predictions of violence: being accurate about accuracy. *Journal of Consulting and Clinical Psychology* 62 (4): 783–792.

Mossman, D. (2006). Critique of pure risk assessment or, Kant meets Tarasoff. *University of Cincinnati Law Review* 75: 523–609.

NHS Security Management Services (2010). *Violence Against Frontline NHS Staff*. London: NHS SMS.

O'Rourke, M. and Bird, L. (2001). *Risk Management in Mental Health*. London: The Mental Health Foundation.

Phillips, P. and Callaghan, P. (2009). Working with people with substance misuse problems. In: *Mental Health Nursing Skills* (ed. P. Callaghan, J. Playle and L. Cooper), 203–212. Oxford: Oxford University Press.

Rice, M.E. and Harris, G.T. (2005). Comparing effect sizes in follow-up studies: ROC area, Cohen's d, and r. *Law & Human Behavior* 29: 615–620.

Rogers, C.R. (1961). *On Becoming a Person: A Therapist's View of Psychotherapy*. New York: Houghton-Miflin.

Rothman, D.J. (1980). *Conscience and Convenience: The Asylum and Its Alternatives in Progressive America*. Boston: Little Brown.

Silver, E. (2001). Race, neighbourhood disadvantage and violence among persons with mental disorders: the importance of contextual measurement. *Law and Human Behaviour* 24: 449–456.

Silver, E. and Miller, L.L. (2002). A cautionary note on the use of actuarial risk assessment tools for social control. *Crime and Delinquency* 48 (1): 138–161.

Singh, J.P., Grann, M., and Fazel, S. (2011). A comparative study of violence risk assessment tools: analysis of 68 studies involving 25,980 participants. *Clinical Psychology Review* doi: 10.1016/j.cpr.2010.11009.

Szmukler, G. (2010) How Mental Health Legislation Discriminates Unfairly against People with Mental Illness. http://www.gresham.ac.uk/lectures-and-events/how-mental-health-law-discriminates-unfairly-against-people-with-mental-illness (accessed 3 December 2015).

University of Manchester (2015) The National Confidential Enquiry into Suicide and Homicide by People with Mental Illness. *Annual Report 2015*: England, Northern Ireland, Scotland and Wales July 2015.

USDHHS (2014) Healthy People 2020. www.healthypeople.gov (accessed 25 January 2018).

Ventura, M., Green, M., Shaner, A., and Liberman, R. (1993). Training and quality assurance with the brief psychiatric rating scale: 'The drift buster'. *International Journal of Methods in Psychiatric Research* 3: 221–244.

Walker, S. (1998). *Sense and Nonsense About Crime and Drugs. A Policy Guide*. Belmont, CA: Wadsworth Publishing.

Ware, J., Kosinski, M., and Keller, S. (1996). A 12-item short-form health survey: construction of scales and preliminary tests of reliability and validity. *Medical Care* 34: 220–233.

Wing, J. (1994). *Health of the Nation Outcome Scales: HoNOS Field Trials*. London: Royal College of Psychiatrists Research Unit.

Wong, S.C.P. and Gordon, A.E. (2006). The validity and reliability of the violence risk scale: a treatment friendly violence risk assessment tool. *Psychology, Public Policy, and Law* 12 (3): 279–309.

Yang, M., Wong, S.P., and Coid, J. (2010). The efficacy of violence prediction: a meta-analytic comparison of nine risk assessment tools. *Pyschological Bulletin* 136 (5): 740–767.

Chapter 13

Examination of the Musculoskeletal System

Daniel Apau, Michael Babcock, and Nicola L. Whiteing

General Examination

Introduction

The musculoskeletal assessment constitutes an essential aspect in evaluating the patient's health. Functions of the musculoskeletal system involve a functional relationship between the muscles and bones of the body (Martini et al. 2012). Changes in the musculoskeletal system affect other systems.

Anatomy and Physiology

The musculoskeletal system performs several essential functions: supports and maintains body shape, supports and protects internal organs, enables movement, stores calcium and phosphate in bone, and is involved in hematopoiesis. The musculoskeletal system is made up of inert and contractile tissues andis composed of bones, muscles, ligaments, joints, and cartilage. Martini et al. (2012) and Tortora and Derrickson (2013) indicate even though most of the skeletal muscle fibres contract and shorten at similar rates, microscopic changes/variations can affect to a significant extent the power, range, and speed of movement. Therefore, issues such as the aging process, lack of exercise, and injury, for example, can have a significant impact on overall health and sense of well-being.

Fascicles

Muscle fibres in skeletal muscles form bundles. The fibres run parallel and their organisation varies in association with a tendon. Fascicle arrangement is correlated to muscle strength, power, and range of motion (ROM). Based on the pattern of the fascicles, muscles can be categorised into parallel muscles, convergent muscles, pennate muscles, or circular muscles. For example, parallel muscles (biceps brachii muscles) are found in the arms, convergent muscles (pectoralis muscles) are found in the chest, bipennate muscles (rectus femoris muscles) are found in the leg, multipennate muscles (deltoid muscles) are found in the arms, and circular muscles (orbicularis oris muscles) are found in the mouth and anus.

Physical Assessment for Nurses and Healthcare Professionals, Third Edition. Edited by Carol Lynn Cox.
© 2019 John Wiley & Sons Ltd. Published 2019 by John Wiley & Sons Ltd.

Parallel Muscles

Most of the muscles in the body are composed of parallel muscles. This means the fascicles run parallel to the long axis of a bone. Some are flat bands with broad attachments (aponeuroses) whereas others are cylindrical with tendons on one or both ends. Those that are cylindrical are generally plump and the muscle has a spindle-shaped appearance. Its central body is known as a 'belly'. The biceps brachii muscle is an example. When the elbow bends, the muscle shortens and gets larger. You can see the bulge of the belly.

Convergent Muscles

In convergent muscles, the muscle fascicles extend over a broad area and converge on a single attachment. This type of muscle pulls on a tendon, or a slender band of collagen fibres (raphe). These muscles pull and spread out similar to a fan or triangle with a tendon at the apex. It is important to note that convergent muscles pull in different directions rather than pulling in the same direction (Martini et al. 2012; Tortora and Derrickson 2013).

Pennate Muscles

In pennate muscles (penna – meaning 'feather') fascicles form a common angle with a tendon. Because these muscles pull at an angle, the muscles do not pull as far as parallel muscles. Pennate muscles contain far more muscle fibres than parallel muscles, so they produce more tension when contracted (Martini et al. 2012; Tortora and Derrickson 2013). When all of the muscle fibres are attached to the same side of a tendon they are considered to be unipennate. If they have fibres on both sides of a tendon they are considered to be bipennate. If a tendon branches within a pennate muscle, it is considered to be multipennate. For example, the triangular muscle of the shoulder (deltoid muscle) is considered to be multipennate.

Muscle Efficiency

There are three classes of levers that increase muscle efficiency: 1st, 2nd, and 3rd class. Skeletal muscles work in collaboration with other muscles. They do not work in isolation. The nature and site of attachment of the muscles determines their force, speed, and the ROM that can be produced. Their characteristics are interdependent. Attaching a muscle to a lever (rigid structure), such as bone, modifies the force, speed, and direction of movement when the muscle contracts. The lever moves on a fixed point (called a fulcrum). Each joint is a fulcrum. Levers can change the direction of an applied force, distance, speed of movement, and effective strength.

In a 1st-class lever, the fulcrum lies between the applied force and the load. The human body has few 1st-class levers. An example in the body is the neck. In a 2nd-class lever, the load is between the applied force and the fulcrum. Here, load is the weight and the force is an upward lift. An example in the body is ankle extension. Third-class levers are the most common. Here the force is applied between the load and the fulcrum. The affect is the reverse of a 2nd-class lever. An example is the biceps brachii muscle which flexes the elbow.

Origins and Insertions

In the human body the ends of muscles are attached to structures. The structures limit their movement. Generally, one end is in a fixed position and during contraction the other end moves towards the fixed end. The place where the muscle is fixed in considered to be the origin and the place where the movement end attaches is the site of insertion.

Actions

When a muscle moves a part of the human skeleton the movement will involve one of the following: flexion, extension, adduction (moving inwards), abduction (moving outwards or away), protraction, retraction, elevation, depression, rotation, circumduction, pronation, supination, inversion, eversion, lateral flexion, opposition, or reposition. Based on the muscle's action it is described as an agonist (prime mover), an antagonist (opposes action), or a synergist (helps a larger agonist work more efficiently).

Support and Movement

There are 206 bones in the human body. A small portion of the human population have an extra bone, which occurs in the form of an extra rib. The bones that form the longitudinal axis of the body are the skull and associated bones, the thoracic cage, and the vertebral column. The axial skeleton contains 40% of the bones in the human body, 80 in total. It is the axial skeleton that provides the framework for supporting the brain, the spinal cord, and the organs in the subdivisions of the ventral body (Martini et al. 2012; Tortora and Derrickson 2013). The axial skeleton provides the surface area for the attachment of muscles that maintain and change the position of the head, neck, and trunk; perform respiratory movements; and stabilise or position parts of the appendicular skeleton. Joints in the axial skeleton permit limited movement only. These structures are strong and reinforced with ligaments which aid in the protection of internal structures. The appendicular system consists of the remaining 60% of bones that make up the skeletal system. The appendicular skeleton is composed of the bones of the arms and legs and their supporting elements or 'girdles' that connect them to the trunk. The appendicular skeleton lets you 'manipulate objects and move from place to place' (Martini et al. 2012: 233).

Assessment/Examination

Musculoskeletal disorders are common and major cause of ill health accounting for over 21 million general practitioner consultations alone in the United Kingdom in 2015 (MKS Toolkit 2015) and 50% (126 million in ages 18 and over) of primary care consultations in the United States of America in 2014 (Bone and Joint Initiative 2014). In Europe, musculoskeletal conditions are the most common cause of severe long-term pain and disability (22%) (EU Report v5.0 2010). Musculoskeletal conditions lead to significant healthcare and social support costs and are a major cause of work absence and incapacity. In addition, they have a significant economic cost through lost productivity and can seriously affect the quality of life of those with the conditions and that of their families, friends, and carers (EU Report v5.0 2010).

For the patient presenting with a musculoskeletal problem the primary complaint is likely to be that of pain or a decrease in functional ability. These are symptoms that the patient is unlikely to ignore. Therefore musculoskeletal complaints make up a large amount of the primary care or minor injury practitioners caseload. The aim of the musculoskeletal assessment is to determine the degree to which the patient's activities of living are affected, through a systematic assessment. The musculoskeletal assessment is closely linked with the neurological assessment as bone and muscle functioning is directly coordinated by the central nervous system (Ball et al. 2014a, b; Barkauskas et al. 2002; Bickley and Szilagyi 2007, 2013; Dains et al. 2012, 2015; Epstein et al. 2008). You should read the neurological assessment in Chapter 10 in conjunction with this chapter.

Frequent Musculoskeletal Complaints

Sprains and Strains

Sprains and strains are the most common musculoskeletal complaint the practitioner might encounter in either urgent care, a primary care setting, or minor injury unit. Careful consideration must be given when using above terms to convey the exact nature of injury. Strain refers to an injury of tendons or tearing of muscle fibres as a result of overstretching. Sprain, on the hand, refers to ligamental injuries resulting from overstretching a unit over its functional ROM (Ball et al. 2014a, b; Bickley and Szilagyi 2007, 2013; Dains et al. 2012, 2015; Japp and Robertson 2013; Jarvis 2008, 2015; Seidel et al. 2006, 2010; Swartz 2006, 2014; Talley and O'Connor 2006, 2014; Tallia and Scherger 2013).

Osteoarthritis

A degenerative joint disease due to a progressive breakdown of the joint surfaces. Direct and indirect trauma to the articular cartilage and infection can all lead to osteoarthritis. Osteoarthritis primarily affects weight-bearing joints (hips, knees) with patients presenting to their medical provider with increased pain and a decrease in their functional ability. The end result is often a joint replacement. However in many instances, symptoms can be managed/reduced through a range of pharmacological and nonpharmacological means.

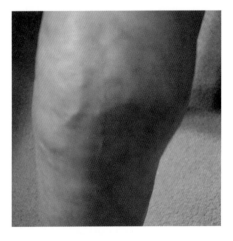

Osteoarthritis in the knee

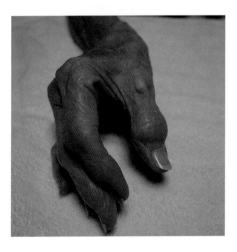

Osteoartiritis

Rheumatoid Arthritis

This is the most common chronic inflammatory disease of joints. A systemic disease causing many different structures to be affected. Unlike osteoarthritis, which invariably affects one joint in isolation, treatment aims to control the pain associated with synovitis and maintain as much function as possible.

Osteoporosis

Because of a lack of oestrogen in postmenopausal women, a reduction in the amount of collagen in bones occurs. The bone becomes thin and a kyphosis of the spine is often seen with pain over the spinous processes. Fractures of the femoral neck and crush fractures of the vertebrae are common after a fairly minor trip or fall.

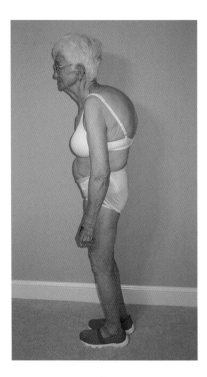

Kyphosis

Fractures

Fractures are usually caused by trauma either significant, or minor and repeated. Pathological fractures occur as a result of disease, e.g. tumours, osteoporosis, Paget's disease, and osteomalacia. There are many types of fracture. However, the principles behind their management remain the same.

Key Principles of Musculoskeletal Assessment

- Consider the nature of presenting complaint to align and focus your assessment bearing in mind other systemic causes. In general, the nature of the presenting complaint could be pain, swelling, crepitus, locking, wasting, fasciculation, or cramps.
- The nature of symptom onset whether trauma related, insidious, or episodic is vital in establishing severity.
- The ROM and limiting factors will establish effects on activities of living.
- Ascertain possible nonmusculoskeletal origin of pain including referred pain.

Practical Considerations

- In order that a comprehensive musculoskeletal assessment is undertaken, the patient will have to be exposed.
- The patient should be allowed to redress as the examination proceeds or be covered as appropriate to ensure privacy and dignity.
- The musculoskeletal assessment has two stages: inspection and palpation. Unlike other systems examinations, you should work through the two stages together rather than inspecting all joints and then returning to palpate.
- Always ask whether the patient has any pain and if so, assess the pain-free side first.
- Arrange your assessment by examining each area in relation to patient comfort, allowing the joint/extremity to be supported.
- Always compare each side.
- Organise your examination of the bones, muscles, and joints in a head-to-toe method. This will help avoid omissions.
- Certain situations will require you to perform a movement so the patient can emulate
- Always start each part of the examination from the neutral position (Figure 13.1).

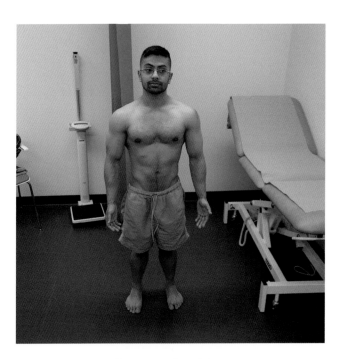

The neutral position

Assessment Consideration

Your assessment should seek to elicit the source and tissue type involved in the presentation. The two tissue types for consideration are:

- Inert tissues: bony cartilage, capsule and ligament, bursa
- Contractile tissues: muscle, musculotendinous junction, body of tendon, bone at insertion of tendon.

Different assessment techniques are required for the type of tissue involved in the presentation (see ROMs below).

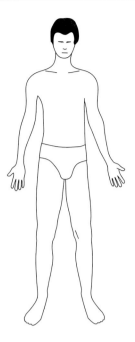

Figure 13.1   The neutral position.

Legal Consideration

Because of the increasing litigation culture careful consideration should be given to any potential litigation following musculoskeletal assessment. With this in mind, the traditional assessment of look, feel, and move can be modified in suspicious circumstances. It is important at times to consider and document limitations of active movements by the patient prior to any passive movement or manipulation by the practitioner (Thomas and Monaghan 2007; Walsh 2006).

Inspection

For a comprehensive assessment, inspection should commence as patient walks into consulting room observing for gait and body alignment. Inspection should be carried out observing from anterior, posterior, and lateral views. Inspection should assess for:

- size
- contour
- symmetry
- involuntary movements (tremors, fasciculations)
- deformities (subluxation, dislocation, varus, valgus)
- swelling/oedema (effusions, haematoma)
- discolouration (vascular insufficiency, bruising, haematoma)
- hypertrophy/atrophy of muscles (steroid use, malnutrition, spinal cord lesion)
- posture and body alignment
- structural relationships
- scars indicating any previous surgery or trauma
- condition of skin (pressure ulcers, necrosis, scarring)

Palpation

- Palpate joints, bursal sites, bones, and surrounding muscles.
- Assess the patient for both verbal and nonverbal cues of pain.

- Ask the patient, 'Does the pain radiate elsewhere from the initial region?'
- Palpation should assess for the following:
  - increased temperature (use the back of the hand above, below, and on the joint and compare with the other side)
  - swelling/oedema
  - tenderness
  - crepitus (loose cartilage [etc.], listen for crepitus as well as feeling)
  - consistency and tone of muscle

Range of movement (ROM)

- Assess the degree of deviation away from the neutral position.
- A goniometer should be used to obtain an accurate ROM (Japp and Robertson 2013; Jarvis 2008, 2015).
  - Active ROM involves the patient moving the joint himself. Active movements test:
    - Inert and contractile tissues
    - Test for pain, power, and range
  - Movement should be smooth and pain free.
  - Passive ROM involves you providing motion in order to move the joint. Passive movements:
    - Test inert (eliminates muscle, tendon, and tenoperiosteal junction)
    - Test for pain, range, and feel
    - Test for passive stretch or squeezing
- Resisted involves the practitioner initiating the movement with the patient opposing the movement. Resisted movement:
  - Test contractile tissues if no movement of joint, e.g. 'I am going to push foot up; don't let me'
  - Assess for pain and weakness
  - Isometric contraction
  - Stress testing involves:
  - Passive stretching of ligaments to detect injury

Question whether:

- Active ROM is less than passive ROM – focus on true weakness, joint stability, pain, and malignancy.
- Active and passive ROM is limited – determine whether there is any excess fluid or any loose bodies in the joint (e.g. cartilage), joint surface irregularity (e.g. osteoarthritis, contracture of muscle, ligaments, or capsule).

Limb Measurement

- Ensure limbs are in the neutral position.
- Ensure the patient is lying straight – many discrepancies in limb length are due to inaccurate positioning.
- Full length upper limb – measure from the acromion process to the end of the middle finger.
- Upper arm only – acromion process to the olecranon process.
- Lower arm only – olecranon process to the styloid process of the ulna.
- Full length lower limb – lower edge of the ileum to tibial malleolus.
- Upper leg only – lower edge of the ileum to the medial aspect of the knee.
- Lower leg only – medial aspect of the knee to the tibial malleolus.

Establish whether shortening is due to a loss of bone length or a deformity at the joint, e.g. a hip dislocation.

Bones

Examine for:

- deformity
- tumours

  - pain – is the pain focal (fracture/trauma, infection, malignancy, Paget's disease, osteoid osteoma), or diffuse (malignancy, Paget's disease, osteomalacia, osteoporosis, metabolic bone disease)?
  - consider character, onset, site, radiation, severity, periodicity, exacerbating and relieving factors, diurnal variation.

Joints

Always compare each joint bilaterally to make a comparison. Examine for:

- pain – causes include inflammatory (e.g. rheumatoid arthritis), mechanical (e.g. osteoarthritis), infective (e.g. pyogenic tuberculosis), or traumatic (e.g. fractures).
- questions to ask:
  - Where is the maximal site of pain?
  - Does the pain change during the course of the day?
  - Has the pain been there for a short or long time?
  - Does the pain get better or worse as the patient moves about?
- tenderness
- swelling
- partial or complete loss of mobility
- stiffness
- deformity
- weakness
- fatigue
- warmth
- redness
- lesions or ulcers

Pitting of nails is present in 50% of cases of joint disease.

Muscles

Assess:

- size
- contour
- tone
- strength/weakness
  - questions to ask:
    - Is the weakness global or focal?
    - Is the weakness secondary to a painful limb?
    - Does the weakness fluctuate in degree?
    - Is the weakness increasing in severity?
    - Is the weakness associated with sensory symptoms or signs?
    - Is there a family history of muscle disease?
    - Is the weakness symmetrical?
    - Is the weakness predominantly proximal or distal?
- pain – causes include inflammatory (e.g. polymyalgia rheumatica), infective (e.g. pyogenic cysticercosis), traumatic, or neuropathic (e.g. Guillain-Barré syndrome).

The Examination

When asking the patient to perform active ROM, instruct them in a way that will be understood. It may be necessary for you to perform the movement first so that the patient can then copy it.

GALS Screen

The GALS (gait, arms, legs, spine) screen provides a useful rapid screen of the overall integrity of the locomotor system. It is felt that the general survey (described next) followed by a regional joint examination is necessary for the patient presenting with a musculoskeletal complaint; however, the GALS screen may be used to make a quick 'screening' examination of the whole locomotor system in order to identify an abnormality in the absence of symptoms (Doherty et al. 1992; Thomas and Monaghan 2007).

General Survey

The general survey should start as soon as you meet the patient. Call the patient into the examination room and look at how they move. You can gain an accurate assessment of the patient's pattern of gait as they enter the room – once you ask the patient to walk for you the gait may change. Watch the patient throughout the examination. Observe how they get on and off the examination couch and up from a chair. Look at the speed of manoeuvres and any pain elicited.

Shake the patient's hand and gain an idea of muscle strength.

Observe the patient's gait anteriorly and posteriorly, with and without shoes on:

- Does the patient trip?
- Is there a limp present? – Look at the patient's shoes and see if one side of the heel is worn more than the other.
- Alignment of the pelvis and shoulders during walking.
- Does the patient stagger to one particular side?
- Does the patient, despite apparently severe ataxia, seldom sustain injury?
- If a Trendelenburg gait pattern is suspected, ask the patient to stand on one leg; if the hip abductors are weak, the pelvis will tilt towards the non-weight-bearing side.
- For examples of abnormal gait patterns, refer to Chapter 10.

General inspection:

- Posture
- Body alignment
- Hypertrophy/atrophy of the muscles – dominant side is usually slightly bigger than the nondominant. Hypertrophy can be seen in young men using steroids. Atrophy of the muscles can be due to malnutrition, lack of use of muscles due to joint disease, or a spinal cord lesion due to the lack of neural input to the muscle. May need to measure the circumference of muscle bulk and document on each visit to assess any decrease. Differences of > 1 cm noted at different times are not significant.
- Genu valgum/genu varum
- Hyperextension of the knees – will often indicate hypermobility of all joints; however, hypermobility could be due to ligament ruptures, intraarticular fractures, or connective tissue disruption, e.g. Marfan's syndrome.
- Carrying angle – elbows should be at approximately 5–15° in an adult (see Figure 13.1).
- Spine – scoliosis, kyphosis, lordosis, gibbus
- Symmetry
- Contour
- Size
- Involuntary movements
- Gross deformities
- Limb measurement

Regional Examination

Jaw

The temporomandibular joint (TMJ) – the articulation between the temporal bone and the mandible.

- Place fingertips over the TMJ, anterior to the external meatus of the ear.
- Palpate whilst the patient goes through the ROMs:
  - open and close the mouth – extension
  - project the lower jaw – flexion
  - move the jaw from side to side – abduction and adduction
  - is there any crepitus?
- Ask the patient to bite down hard – palpate the muscle strength of the masseter muscles.
- Ask the patient to clench teeth whilst you push lightly on the chin – also tests the motor function of cranial nerve V.

Spine

- Normal curvatures at the spine are concave at the cervical region, convex at the thoracic region, and concave at the lumbar region.

I Cervical spine

The sternoclavicular joint – the articulation between the sternum and the clavicle.
The cervical vertebrae – C1–C7, most mobile of all spinal vertebrae.

- Using thumbs, palpate all spinous processes.
- Palpate along the clavicles and manubrium of the sternum.
- Observe patient as they go through the ROMs (Figure 13.2):
  - chin to chest – flexion
  - raise the head back to the neutral position – extension
  - bend the head backwards – hyperextension
  - turn head to each side – lateral rotation
  - place each ear to each shoulder – lateral bending
- To test the muscle strength of the trapezius and sternocleidomastoid muscles, the above ROMs should be performed to resistance.

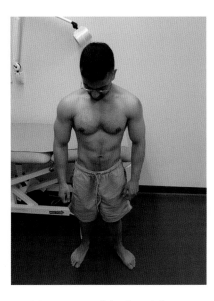

Movement of the head down

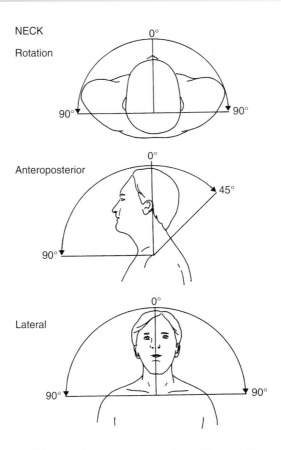

NECK

Rotation

Anteroposterior

Lateral

Figure 13.2   Movements of the neck. *Source*: Reproduced from Talley and O'Connor (1998). © 1998, Elsevier, Sydney.

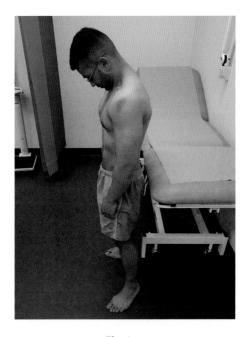

Flexion

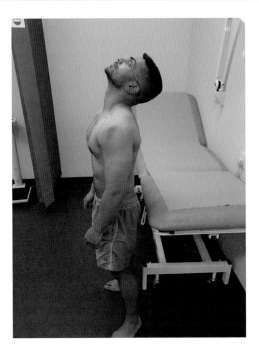

Hyperextension

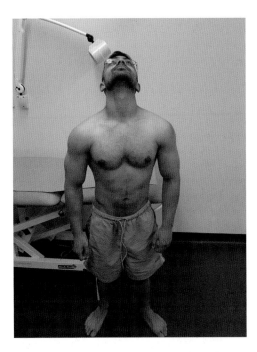

Movement of the head backward

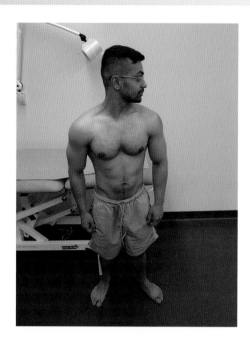

Lateral rotation 1

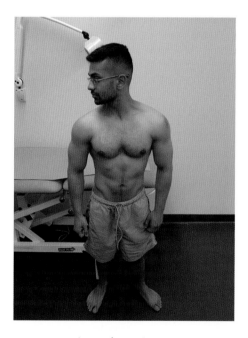

Lateral rotation 2

II Thoracic and lumbar spine

Thoracic vertebrae – T1–T12.
Lumbar vertebrae – L1–L5.

- Look at equality of height at the shoulders and the iliac crests.
- Using your thumbs, palpate along all spinous processes – if no pain is elicited, but malignancy or osteoporosis is suspected, light percussion of the spinous processes using the ulnar aspect of your fist may prove a useful technique.

- Palpate around the scapulae and assess for equality in height.
- Have the patient stand with feet 15 cm apart and ask them to bend forwards slowly as if touching toes. Observe for any abnormal curvatures of the spine (Figure 13.3a and b):
  - scoliosis – a lateral curvature of the spine
  - lordosis – an exaggerated lumbar curvature (can be normal during pregnancy, in the obese or women of Afro-Caribbean origin)
  - kyphosis – a rounded thoracic convexity (commonly known as the 'Dowager's hump'); common in osteoporotic women
  - gibbus – when a defect is of a sharp angle, the spinous processes are seen more prominently on the back forming an apex

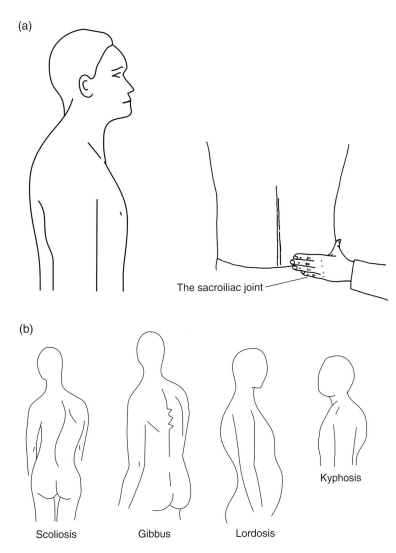

(a)

The sacroiliac joint

(b)

Scoliosis   Gibbus   Lordosis   Kyphosis

Figure 13.3 (a) Thoracolumbar spine and sacroiliac joint. *Source*: Reproduced from Talley & O'Connor (1998). © 1998, Elsevier, Sydney. (b) Changes in the thoracolumbar spine.

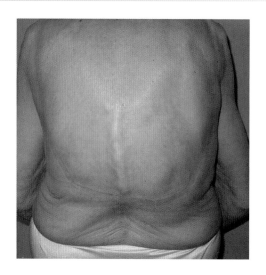

Gibbus

- list – the spine is tilted to one side with no compensation
- If the patient is able to stay in a flexed position, it is useful for you to palpate the patient's spinous processes whilst in this position. An early scoliosis may be detected through palpation, which may be missed upon inspection in the upright position.

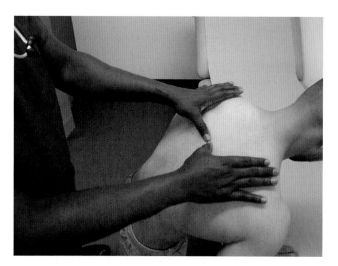

Palpate the vertebra

- A spinal curvature may have an effect on the patient's respiratory function, thus, attention may also need to be paid to a respiratory assessment.

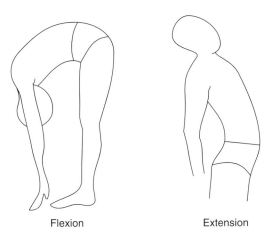

Flexion   Extension

Figure 13.4   Flexion and extension of the spine.

- Observe the patient as they go through the ROMs (Figure 13.4):
  - ○ Bend forwards to touch toes – flexion.

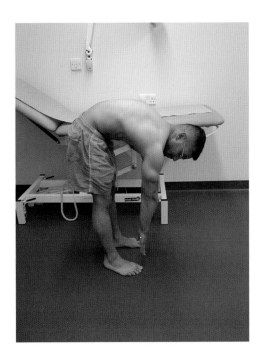

Flexion of the spine

  - ○ Stand back up into the neutral position – extension.
  - ○ Bend back as far as possible running hands down the back of the thighs – hyperextension.

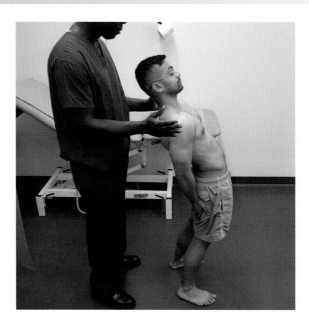

Support the patient if you suspect the patient may fall when assessing specific movements

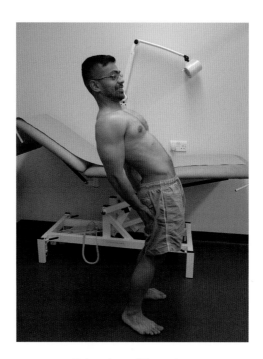

Extension of the spine

○ Run a hand down each leg laterally – lateral bending.

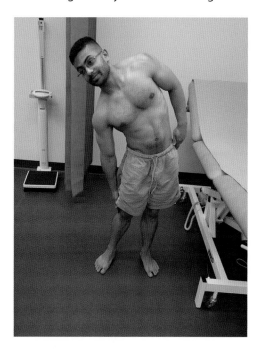

Lateral movement of the spine 1

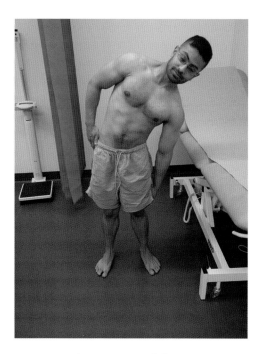

Lateral movement of the spine 2

- Turn to the right and left in a circular motion – rotation*.

*Internal rotation or medial rotation and external rotation or lateral rotation

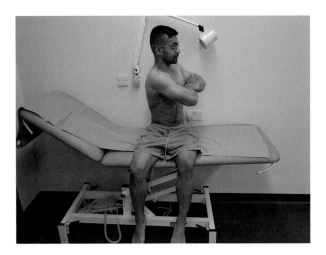

Assess spinal rotation 1

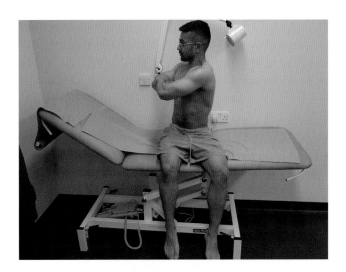

Assess spinal rotation 2

It is important that you stabilise the patient's pelvis during this ROM, or the movement will come from the pelvis and not the spine. You should have the patient sitting in a chair or on an examination couch/table with arms crossed to assess this movement.

- To assess the muscle strength of the trapezius and paravertebral muscles, the above should be performed to resistance.

Stretch tests

- If a patient presents with a history of lower back pain, you should assess ability to straight leg raise (SLR) with the Lasegue Test (Figure 13.4) If Lasegue Test is positive then the Bragard test (Figure 13.5) should be included as an extra manoeuver

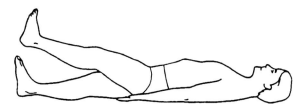

Figure 13.5   Straight leg raise with pain increased on dorsiflexion of the foot (Bragard's Test).

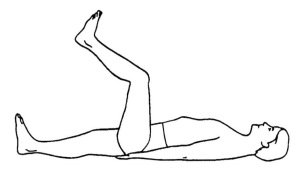

Figure 13.6   Further extension of the nerve root increases pain when the knee is extended (Lasegue's Test).

- ○ The patient should lie supine with the leg as relaxed as possible. You should slowly raise the foot, keeping the knee straight until the patient complains of pain, then dorsiflex the foot.
- ○ You should make a note of the ROM obtained before a complaint of pain and whether the pain intensifies upon dorsiflexion of the foot.
- ○ A positive SLR test includes pain before 70° is reached in an L5 or S1 distribution, increased pain on dorsiflexion of the foot along the sciatic nerve trajectory, and relief of pain on flexion of the knee (Barkauskas et al. 2002; Seidel et al. 2006, 2010; Walsh 2006).
- ○ A positive test is indicative of a herniated lumbar disc.
- • If it is felt that a lumbar disc may have prolapsed higher (L2–L4) a stretch test for the femoral nerve should be performed (Figure 13.6).
- ○ The patient should lie prone and extend the hip with the knee in a flexed position.
- ○ Note the point at which the patient complains of pain.
- ○ Pain will be elicited in the lumbar region as the femoral nerve roots are tightened.
- ○ Lying prone may not be possible for all patients, so an alternative test can be performed with the patient lying laterally with knees bent. This position produces a stretch of the femoral nerve. The stretch is enhanced as the patient bends the head towards the chest.
- • Patella and achilles reflexes should also be tested.

Upper Limb
Shoulder
The acromioclavicular joint – the articulation between the acromion process of the scapula and the clavicle.

The glenohumeral joint – the articulation between the glenoid fossa and the humerus.
The sternoclavicular joint – the articulation between the sternum and the clavicle.

- Inspect the shoulder from anterior and posterior views.
- Look at the shape of the shoulders – anterior dislocation of the shoulder can be seen as a flattening of the lateral aspect. Check for altered sensation laterally as the axillary nerve may have been damaged by the dislocation.
- Look for swelling at the joint.
- Observe the equality of shoulder height.
- Look for muscle wasting – may be present in arthritic joints when the patient does not use the arm.
- Palpate each of the shoulder joints and the bursal sites (subacromial bursa and subscapular bursa).
- Assess the temperature of the joint and note any colour changes in conjunction with an increased temperature.
- Palpate the clavicles, scapulae, acromion process and biceps groove.
- Palpate the associated muscles – particularly those of the rotator cuff.
- Observe the patient as they goes through the ROM:

    - extend both arms forwards – flexion
    - back to the neutral position – extension

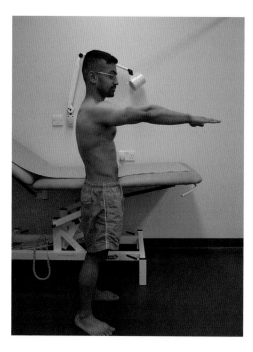

Flexion

- extend both arms backwards – hyperextension

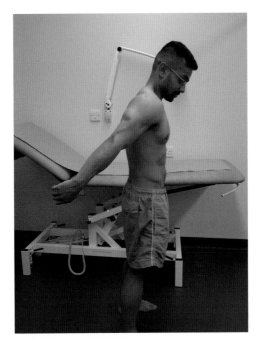

Hyperextension

- put an arm out to the side – abduction

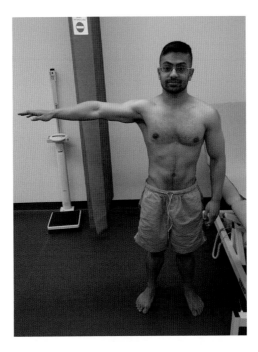

Abduction

- put an arm across the body – adduction
- roll arms forwards and backwards in a circular motion – circumduction
- put an arm behind the back and touch the opposite shoulder blade – internal rotation

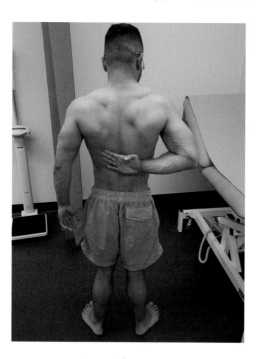

Internal rotation

- put an arm behind the head – external rotation

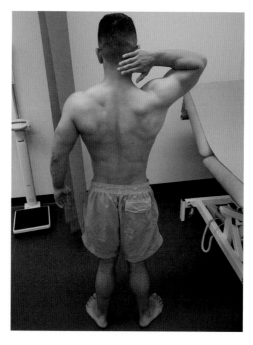

External rotation

- draw shoulders upwards – elevation
- draw the shoulders downwards – depression
- draw the shoulders forwards – protraction
- draw the shoulder back – retraction – gives a good view of the equality of scapula height (Figures 13.7 and 13.8)

Elbow

The articulation between the humerus, radius, and ulna.

- Inspect and palpate with the elbow in a flexed and extended position.
- Inspect for swelling, redness, and increased temperature.
- Inspect for tracking marks and any associated cellulitis in the cubital fossa region – drug misuse.
- Palpate the olecranon bursa, the distal humerus, medial and lateral epicondyles, the olecranon process, coronoid process of the ulna and the radius.

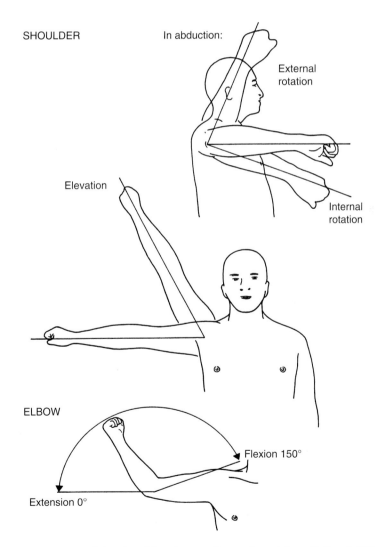

Figure 13.7 Movements of the shoulder. *Source*: Reproduced from Talley & O'Connor (1998). © 1998, Elsevier, Sydney.

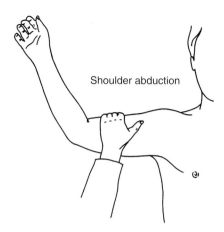

Shoulder abduction

Figure 13.8 Shoulder abduction. *Source*: Reproduced from Talley & O'Connor (1998). © 1998, Elsevier, Sydney.

- Assess for any pain or tenderness over the annular ligament.
- Assess for any joint swelling in the grooves either side of the olecranon process.
- Observe the patient as he goes through the ROM:
  - bend the arm – flexion
  - straighten the arm – extension
  - turn the hand palm up – supination
  - turn the hand palm down – pronation

Ensure that the elbow is flexed to 90° and is locked against the side of the body when testing supination and pronation; otherwise the movement will come from the glenohumeral joint and not that of the elbow (Figures 13.9 and 13.10).

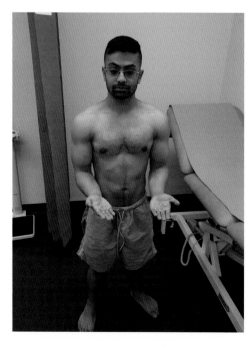

Supination (Note the elbows are held next to the body so that the lower arms move and not the shoulders)

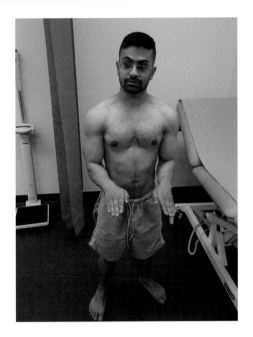

Pronation

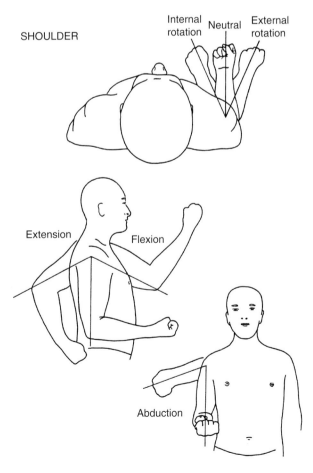

Figure 13.9 Movements of the elbows and shoulders. *Source*: Reproduced from Talley & O'Connor (1998). © 1998, Elsevier, Sydney.

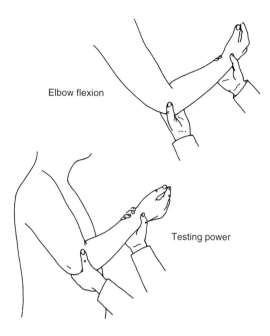

Elbow flexion

Testing power

Figure 13.10 Flexion and testing power of the elbow. *Source*: Reproduced from Talley & O'Connor (1998). © 1998, Elsevier, Sydney.

Wrist

The articulation between the distal radius and the proximal portions of the carpus.

- Inspect both wrists for symmetry, contour, swelling, atrophy, and smoothness.
- Because of little tissue covering the dorsal aspect of the wrist joint, swelling is clearly visible.
- Use thumbs and index fingers to palpate the wrist and proximal portions of the carpus.
- Apply pressure in the anatomical snuff box – fractures of the scaphoid are not clearly visible on plain A–P and lateral X-rays and scaphoid views are needed. Pain in the anatomical snuff box is a good indicator of a fracture. If not diagnosed and treated quickly, the patient is at risk of avascular necrosis, particularly if the fracture is through the highly vascular proximal pole.
- Palpate the ulna tip for any pain and across the underlying bones of the carpus – scaphoid, lunate, pisiform, trapezium, trapezoid, hamate, and capitate.
- Observe the patient as they go through the ROMs (Figure 13.11):
  - bend hand down – flexion
  - bend hand upwards – extension
  - with the hand pronated, turn it towards the right – radial deviation
  - with the hand pronated, turn it towards the left – ulna deviation
- If carpal tunnel syndrome is suspected, one of two tests can be carried out:
  - Phalen's test – ask the patient to maintain palmar flexion for one minute. This will produce numbness. When hands are brought back to the normal position the numbness disappears.
  - Tinel's test – lightly tap the median nerve. This will produce a tingling which will stop when tapping is ceased.

Fingers

Metacarpophalangeal joints – the articulation between the distal portions of the carpus and the metacarpal bones.

Proximal interphalangeal joints – the articulation between the metacarpal and the proximal phalanges.

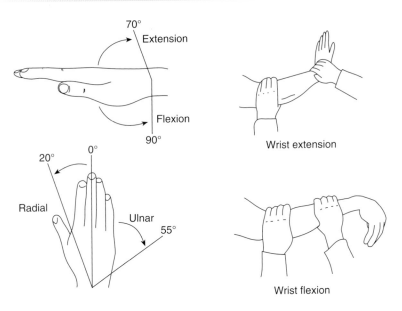

Figure 13.11 Movements of the wrist. *Source*: Reproduced from Talley & O'Connor (1998). © 1998, Elsevier, Sydney.

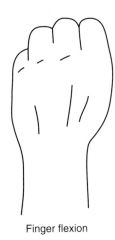

Finger flexion

Figure 13.12 Flexion of the fingers. *Source*: Reproduced from Talley & O'Connor (1998). © 1998, Elsevier, Sydney.

Distal interphalangeal joints – the articulation between the proximal and distal phalanges.

- Inspect each of the fingers and each of the joints – rheumatoid arthritis is particularly evident in the joints of the fingers.
- Look at the condition of the nails.
- Using the thumb and index finger, palpate each of the metacarpophalangeal and interphalangeal joints.
- Observe the patient as they goes through the ROMs:
  - make a fist – full finger flexion (Figure 13.12)
  - open a fist – full finger extension
  - spread fingers out – abduction (Figure 13.13)
  - bring fingers in together from abduction – adduction
  - push fingers forwards – hyperflexion

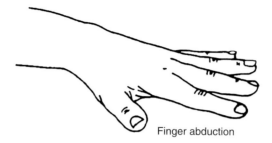

Finger abduction

Figure 13.13   Abduction of the fingers. *Source*: Reproduced from Talley & O'Connor (1998). © 1998, Elsevier, Sydney.

- ○ push fingers backwards – hyperextension
- ○ little finger to thumb – opposition
- ○ thumb to little finger – opposition
- Carry out ROM with wrist flexed as well as in neutral to test for tendon shortening.

Lower Limb

Pelvis and Hips

The sacroiliac joints – the articulation between the sacrum and the ileum.

The symphysis pubis – The articulation bilaterally between the inferior and superior pubic rami.

The hip joint – the articulation between the acetabulum and the femur.

- Inspect the iliac crests for symmetry and equality of height.
- Look at the number and level of gluteal folds.
- Look at the size of the buttocks.
- Inspect the femoral area for signs of tracking and associated cellulitis – drug misuse.
- In supine position, inspect the body alignment looking for external rotation of the hips and inequality of leg length – often seen in osteoarthritis, fractures, or dislocations of the hip.
- Gait – (refer to the general survey in this chapter and Chapters 2 and 10).
- Palpate bursal sites.
- In supine position, palpate hips and pelvis for tenderness, increased temperature, or crepitus.
- Rock the pelvis from side to side whilst holding the iliac crests to test for stability at the sacroiliac joints.
- With the patient lying prone, apply slight pressure to the sacrum to test for stability at the symphysis pubis – this joint can become lax in women carrying and/or following the birth of large babies.
- Observe the patient as they go through the ROMs:
  - ○ in supine position:
    - — raise the leg above the body keeping the knee in extension – flexion
    - — raise the leg above the body and then flex the knee and bring it towards the chest – flexion (Figure 13.14)

Hold the iliac crest as the patient goes through the movement and feel when the pelvis takes over from the hip joint. This will enable an accurate measurement of range (Figure 13.15).

HIP

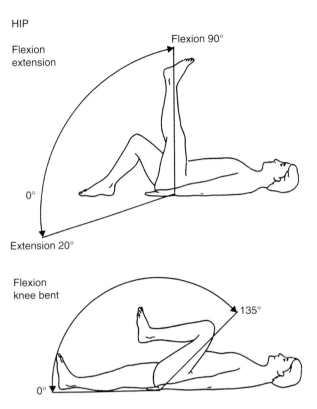

Flexion
extension

Flexion 90°

0°

Extension 20°

Flexion
knee bent

135°

0°

Figure 13.14 Movements of the hip, flexion and extension. *Source*: Reproduced from Talley & O'Connor (1998). © 1998, Elsevier, Sydney.

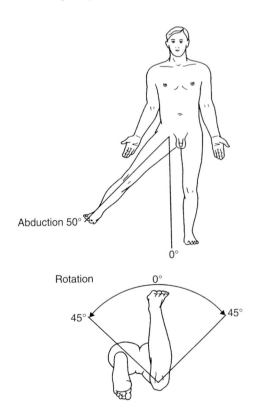

Abduction 50°

0°

Rotation

0°

45°   45°

Figure 13.15 Movements of the hip, abduction and rotation. *Source*: Reproduced from Talley & O'Connor (1998). © 1998, Elsevier, Sydney.

- swing the leg across the body – adduction
- swing the leg outwards – abduction
- place the side of the patient's foot on the opposite knee and move the flexed knee towards the side of the examination couch – external rotation

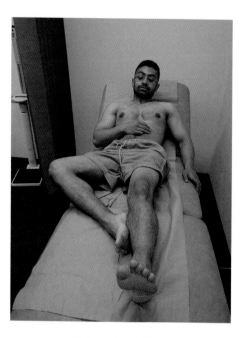

External rotation

- place the side of the patient's foot on the side of the examination couch with the knee flexed and let the patient's leg fall inwards – internal rotation

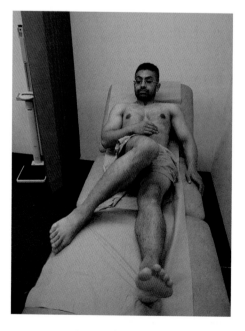

Internal rotation

○ in prone or standing position:
— ask the patient to swing the straightened leg behind the body – hyperextension

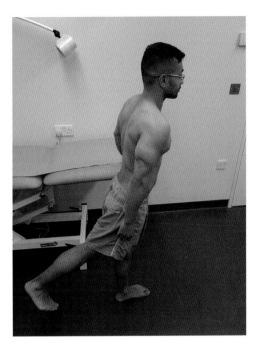

Hyperextension

Knees

The articulation between the femur, patella, and tibia. The preferred position for knee examination is patient positioned supine on a couch.

- Inspect the knee in flexion and extension.
- Inspect for swelling, contour, and symmetry.
- Inspect the popliteal region for swelling with the knee in extension.
- Inspect the patella, particularly as the knee is flexed. Ensure that the patella tracks in a straight line and the quadriceps femoris tendon is not pulling it laterally because of the muscle being lax.
- During walking, observe for any locking of the knee or giving way – ligament injuries, loose bodies within the joint, meniscal tears.
- Palpate the suprapatella pouch, and bursae of the knee – suprapatella, prepatella, infrapatella, and semimembranous.
- Palpate the medial and lateral collateral ligaments for any pain and the cruciate ligaments.
- Palpate the patella, holding at the apex of the patella, ensure that it moves freely.
- Palpate the head of fibula and tibial tuberosity for any pain or tenderness.
- Palpate the medial and lateral joint surfaces.
- If swelling is present to the knee, test for an effusion – 'bulge sign'. Milk up the medial side of the swelling so that it disappears behind the patella, lightly tap the lateral side and the bulge will reappear. A positive bulge sign may be absent in large effusions.
- Observe the patient as they go through the ROMs:
  ○ bend the knee – flexion
  ○ straighten the knee – extension (Figure 13.16)

Flexion to 135° ↓

Extenion to 5° ↑

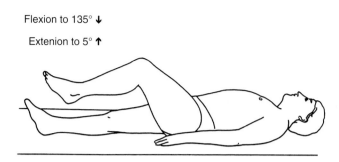

Figure 13.16   Movements of the knee. *Source*: Reproduced from Talley & O'Connor (1998). © 1998, Elsevier, Sydney.

- in supine position; place your hand under the patient's knee and ask him to press down against your hand – hyperextension; if a patient has hyperextended knees, you will not be able to place your hand between the patient's knee and the examination couch
- if ligament injury is suspected, ligament instability or drawer tests should be performed; these tests are beyond the scope of this chapter; refer to texts that address sports injury

Ankles

The articulation between the tibia, fibula, and talus.

The subtalar joint – The articulation between the calcaneum and the talus.

- Inspect the ankle during weight bearing and nonweight bearing.
- Inspect the achilles tendon for ulcers or necrosis – damage to the achilles tendon can result in a *foot drop*; thus the patient's foot should be inspected for plantar flexion and adduction at rest.
- Inspect the condition of the medial and lateral malleoli.
- Inspect the condition of the calcaneum.
- Inspect the ankle for swelling and contour – particularly over the anterior aspect of the ankle where swelling is more visible.
- Palpate the ankle for oedema, pain, or tenderness.
- Palpate the achilles tendon for any pain – to test if the achilles is intact, have the patient either kneeling or with legs hanging over the edge of an examination couch. Apply pressure just below the fullest part of the calf, if the achilles tendon is intact the foot will plantarflex. If it does plantarflex but with pain it is the gastrocnemius muscle that is causing the problem rather than the achilles tendon. If the achilles tendon is ruptured, the foot will not plantarflex.
- Palpate the calcaneum for any pain.
- If spinal cord compression is suspected assess for ankle clonus.
- Observe the patient as he goes through the ROMs:
  - point the foot downwards – plantar flexion
  - point the foot upwards – dorsiflexion
  - rotate the foot laterally – abduction
  - rotate the foot medially – adduction
  - point the medial side of the foot towards the floor – eversion
  - point the lateral side of the foot towards the floor – inversion

Toes

The tarsometatarsal joint – the articulation between the distal portions of the talus and the metatarsal bones.

The metatarsophalangeal joints – the articulation between the metatarsal bone and the proximal phalanx.

The interphalangeal joint – the articulation between the distal and proximal phalanx bones.

- Inspect each toe for calluses, corns, hammer toes and general condition of the skin.
- Inspect the hallux for evidence of valgus deformities (bunions).
- On weight bearing, inspect for the presence of an arch.
- Inspect the condition of the plantar aspect of the foot.
- Palpate each of the toes for pain or tenderness.
- Palpate for any pain on the plantar, lateral, and medial aspects of the foot.
- Provide passive movement to each of the metatarsalphalangeal and interphalangeal joints to assess for flexion, extension, and hypertension using the index finger and thumb. Assess for any bogginess of the joints or pain elicited during movement.
- Observe the patient as he goes through active ROMs:
  - curl up the toes – full flexion
  - straighten the toes – full extension
  - spread the toes out – abduction

Muscle Strength Tests
Upper Limb

- With elbows flexed, ask the patient to hold their arms above the head. You should apply pressure to the palms of their hands – deltoids.
- With arms in extension ask the patient to flex elbows; you should try and hold their arms in extension – biceps.

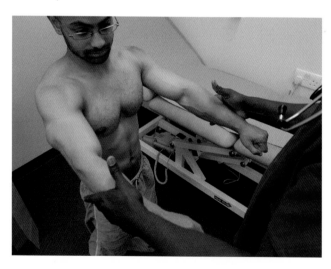

Assess muscle strength

- With the arms flexed, ask the patient to extend them whilst you try to hold them in a flexed position – triceps.
- Ask the patient to shrug shoulders against resistance from you – trapezius. (This test will also assess the motor function of cranial nerve 11.)
- Ask the patient to maintain wrist flexion whilst you try to extend the wrist – wrist flexors.
- Ask the patient to maintain the wrist in extension as you try to flex it – wrist extensors.
- Ask patient to squeeze your 1st two fingers bilaterally to assess his grip strength.

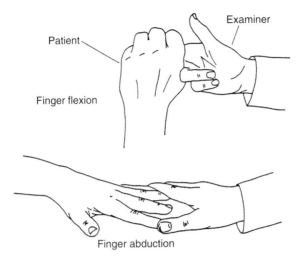

Patient

Examiner

Finger flexion

Finger abduction

Figure 13.17 Testing power in the hand. *Source*: Reproduced from Talley & O'Connor (1998). © 1998, Elsevier, Sydney.

- Ask the patient to maintain a fist whilst you try to extend the fingers.
- Ask the patient to keep fingers in extension as you try to flex them into a fist.
- Ask the patient to spread fingers out whilst you try to push them together.
- Ask the patient to put fingers together as you try to pull them apart (Figure 13.17).

Lower Limb

In supine position:

- Ask the patient to raise their extended leg whilst you try to hold it down – gluteals.

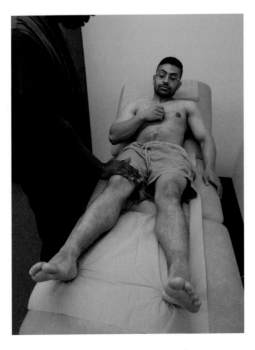

Assess muscle strength

- Ask the patient to push their extended knees outwards against your hands – gluteals and tensor fascia lata.
- Ask the patient to push their extended knees inwards against your hands – gluteals and adductors.

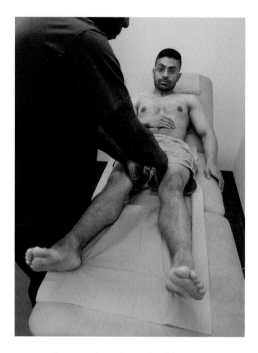

Assess gluteals and adductors

- Ask the patient to extend their knee as you try to flex it – quadriceps.
- Ask the patient to flex their knee you try to extend it – hamstrings.
- Ask the patient to dorsiflex their foot against your hand – tibialis anterior and extensors.

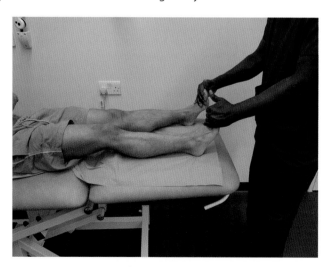

Assess dorsiflexion

- Ask the patient to plantarflex their foot against your hand – tibialis posterior, flexors, gastrocnemius, and soleus.

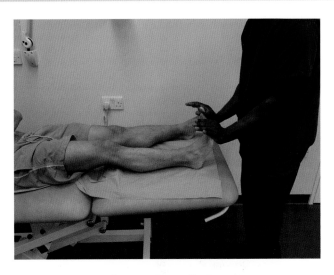

Assess plantar flexion

- Ask the patient to push the side of his foot against your hands.
- In sitting position (with legs hanging):
- Ask the patient to cross his legs alternately – hamstrings, gluteals, hip abductors, and hip adductors.

Terms of Location

Anterior	The front of the body.
Posterior	The back of the body.
Medial	Towards the midline of the body.
Lateral	Away from the midline of the body.
Inferior	Below, or in the direction of the bottom of the body.
Superior	Above, or in the direction of the top of the body.
Proximal	Towards the midpoint of the body, or another structure.
Distal	Away from the midpoint of the body, or another structure.
Dorsal	On, or in the direction of the back of the hand, or top of the foot.
Plantar	On, or in the direction of the sole of the foot.
Palmar	On, or in the direction of the palm of the hand.

Terms Used to Describe ROM

Flexion	To make the inner angle of the joint smaller.
Extension	To make the inner angle of the joint larger.
Abduction	To move away from the midline of the body.
Adduction	To move towards the midline of the body.

Lateral bending	Side bending.
Internal rotation	Rotating around a long axis, inwardly.
External rotation	Rotating around a long axis, outwardly.
Circumduction	Circular movement.
Dorsiflexion	To bend the ankle with the foot moving upwards.
Plantar flexion	To bend the ankle with the foot moving downwards.
Eversion	Turning the sole of the foot out.
Inversion	Turning the sole of the foot inwards.
Pronation	To rotate the forearm with the palm turning inwards.
Supination	To rotate the forearm with the palm turning outwards.
Elevation	Draw up.
Depression	Draw down.
Protraction	Draw forwards.
Retraction	Draw backwards.
Radial deviation	With palm facing down, hand moves towards from the body.
Ulnar deviation	With palm facing down, hand moves away the body.

325

Case Study of a 35-Year-Old Man with Lower Back Pain

Presenting Problem/History

Chief Complaint
'My lower back and right arm hurts'
   A 35-year-old man comes to your clinic complaining of terrible lower back pain for the last two days. He is worried because on waking up this morning he had a 'funny feeling' in his left big toe. He is moderately overweight (body mass index 28).

History (Interview including a review of systems)
The patient woke up with a sore back two days ago. The pain is in the lower back, bilateral. He explains he cannot remember any precipitating factors except he has been going to gym and using most of the machinery in the gym. The pain in the lower back radiates down into the left buttock, thigh, and knee with a funny feeling in the left big toe. He feels better when moving around during the day but this morning he seems to be stamping his left foot slightly when walking. He does not seem to use his left big toe to grip properly when walking. He indicates it is uncomfortable to sit down and prefers to stand as much

as possible. Walking is bearable apart from the stamping. However, climbing stairs or any twisting movements are 'agony'. He felt a little better after the warm shower he took this morning. He has been using simple painkillers (ibuprofen 400 mg three times daily for the last day) but it is not helping. He sleeps on a double bed with a new orthopaedic mattress. He says the left big toe 'feels funny', but denies any pins and needles or numbness and has no problems with bowel/bladder. He states he has no neck pain or pain in other joints.

Past Medical History

- Appendicectomy (aged 18 years)
- Back pain. Spine X-ray (no abnormalities detected [NAD]) (five years ago)
- Depression - treated with paroxetine (since six years ago)

Medication: None apart from ibuprofen as above
Allergies: No known allergies

Social History

IT technician – He has an 'ergonomic' work station. Nonsmoker, moderate alcohol. Has been going to the gym for the past three months to try and lose some weight. He has started a weight loss programme but has an erratic diet. Moderately overweight. Lives with wife and two young children.

Family History

Mother suffered from osteoarthritis

Sexual History

Current partner known for 10 years. Wife on 'the pill'.

Review of Systems

As above Nil Remarkable

Differential Diagnosis

Low back strain, ankylosing spondylitis, cauda equina syndrome, herniated disc, sequestered disc, malignancy, tumour

Assessment Including Labs/Other

Vital signs: Pulse 85 regular, Respiratory Rate 16, Blood Pressure 155/92, T 36.4°C
   Inspection:

- Examine the patient's gait and posture as walking into consulting room to elicit any signs of weakness, instability, or abnormal gait
- Inspect along the spine for any obvious deformities or swelling
  - Results: The patient walked slowly into room; stamping left foot slightly. Difficulty in sitting down on chair. Sitting stiffly. Looks in pain. Nil muscles wasting to legs. Nil obvious deformity, swelling, or inflammation.

Palpation:

- Palpate along the spinal column and interconnecting muscles to assess for tenderness, warmth indication signs of inflammation, masses, or spasms.
  - Results: Slight tenderness on palpation along L3, L4, and L5.

ROM and special tests:

- Active ROM should elicit flexion, extension, right and left lateral flexion. The angle of flexion is important as flexion less than 90°, extension less than 30° and lateral flexions less than 35° indicates reduced ROM.
  - Results: Spine and lower back: Flexion, extension, lateral bending, and rotation limited by pain.

- Lasegue's Sign Test:
- The patient was asked to (SLR) his leg up on the affected site whilst supine. The angle at which pain was elicited was documented. He was asked to SRL the opposite leg for pain to the affected site.
  - Results: Lasegue's sign. SLR of left leg pain elicited on left lower at 60° exacerbated with dorxiflexion of left foot. SLR of right leg pain elicited lower to left lower back.

Neurological examination of lower limbs:

- Sensation tests:
  - Global and specific sensory test are undertaken of lower limbs to delineate any alterations in sensation.
- Reflexes:
  - Deep tendon reflexes of limbs are conducted to elicit any deficits.
- Results: Global sensation grossly intact to both limbs. Specific test using tuning fork, sharp and blunt touch elicited reduced sensation to left big toe.

Laboratory tests:

- Full blood count, erythrocyte sedimentation rate, HLA-B27 gene, C-reactive protein

Special tests:

- Magnetic resonance imaging lower spine

Diagnosis

Lumbar disc problem at possible L4/L5 with possible nerve impingement due to sensory problems of left big toe and JA stamping left foot when walking.

Stamping of left foot indicates reduced ability to grip with big toe when walking.

Treatment Plan

Specialist referral.

Case Study of a 48-Year-Old Man Complaining of 'Pain in My Right Shoulder'

Presenting Problem

48-year-old male presents with 'pain in my right shoulder'

Subjective

Patient complains of right anterolateral shoulder pain for the past year. The pain is aggravated by reaching movements and seems to be getting worse over time. He complains that the pain is now interfering with his work as an automobile mechanic and that the pain often bothers him whilst trying to sleep. The pain is somewhat alleviated by ibuprofen. He denies any history of trauma, falls, or previous shoulder injury. He denies weakness, numbness, or tingling. The patient is otherwise healthy and has no chronic medical conditions.

Objective

Vitals: Temp. 98.5 °F, Pulse 78, Respiratory rate 14, Blood pressure 133/75, O_2 sat. 99% on room air

Patient is alert, oriented, and in no acute distress. Inspection reveals no gross deformity, atrophy, or asymmetry. Palpation reveals R subacromial tenderness. Active abduction of the R humerus is slightly limited due to pain, with otherwise full active ROM. Full passive ROM of the upper extremities bilaterally. Strength is 5/5 in the upper extremities bilaterally. The pain is reproduced by the Neer test (passive shoulder flexion whilst preventing the shoulder from shrugging), Hawkins-Kennedy test (passive internal rotation of the humerus with the shoulder and elbow flexed at 90°), and 'empty can' test (with the patient's straightened arm held out in front in complete internal rotation, as if emptying a can, the clinician attempts to adduct the arm whilst the patient resists).

Differential Diagnosis

Shoulder impingement syndrome, rotator cuff tear, adhesive capsulitis ('frozen shoulder')

Assessment

This patient has shoulder impingement syndrome, potentially with rotator cuff tendinopathy and/or subacromial bursitis. The lack of shoulder weakness on exam makes rotator cuff tear unlikely, which would result in significant weakness with resisted shoulder abduction (supraspinatus), external rotation (infraspinatus, teres minor), and/or internal rotation (subscapularis). The patient's full passive ROM rules out adhesive capsulitis ('frozen shoulder'), the major feature of which is markedly decreased ROM. With shoulder impingement syndrome, active ROM may be limited due to pain but passive ROM should be preserved. Shoulder impingement syndrome is marked by a narrowing of the space between the humeral head and the underside of the acromion of the scapula, which can cause compression of the subacromial bursa (resulting in subacromial bursitis) and supraspinatus tendon (resulting in rotator cuff tendinopathy). The Neer test, Hawkins-Kennedy test, and 'empty can' test reproduce the pain of shoulder impingement syndrome by moving the greater tubercle of the humerus into the subacromial space, further narrowing the space and compressing the structures (subacromial bursa, supraspinatus tendon) within.

Plan
Rest and ice to reduce inflammation and swelling
Short course of NSAIDs to reduce inflammation and provide analgesia
Physical therapy referral (strengthening of rotator cuff muscles can prevent upward translation of the humeral head, thereby widening the subacromial space)
Subacromial glucocorticoid injections may provide symptomatic relief and increase patient compliance with physical therapy
If conservative therapies are ineffective, referral to an orthopaedic specialist may be indicated.

Reference Grid for Examination

Joint	Position	Flexion	Hyperflexion	Extension	Hyperextension	Internal rotation	External rotation	Lateral rotation	Adduction	Abduction	Supination	Pronation	Dorsiflexion	Plantarflexion	Eversion	Inversion	Lateral bending	Circumduction	Radial deviation	Ulna deviation	Opposition	Depression	Elevation	Protraction	Retraction
Jaw	Sitting	X		X					X	X															
Neck	Sitting	X		X	X			X									X								
Shoulder	Standing	X		X		X	X		X	X								X				X	X	X	X
Elbow	Sitting	X		X							X	X													
Wrist	Sitting	X		X															X	X					
Fingers	Sitting	X		X																	X				
Hips	Supine / Prone / standing	X	X	X	X	X	X		X	X															
Knees	Supine	X		X	X				X	X															
Ankles	Supine												X	X	X	X									
Toes	Supine	X		X																					
Spine (thoracic and lumbar)	Standing	X		X	X			X									X								

References

Ball, J., Dains, J., Flynn, J. et al. (2014a). *Seidel's Guide to Physical Examination*, 8e. St. Louis: Mosby.

Ball, J., Dains, J., Flynn, J. et al. (2014b). *Student Laboratory Manual to Accompany Seidel's Guide to Physical Examination*, 8e. St. Louis: Mosby.

Barkauskas, V., Baumann, L., and Darling-Fisher, C. (2002). *Health and Physical Assessment*, 3e. London: Mosby.

Bickley, L. and Szilagyi, P. (2007). *Bates' Guide to Physical Examination and History Taking*, 9e. Philadelphia: Lippincott.

Bickley, L. and Szilagyi, P. (2013). *Bates' Guide to Physical Examination and History Taking*, 11e. New York: Wolters Kluwer/Lippincott Williams & Wilkins.

Bone and Joint Initiative (2014) The Burden of Musculoskeletal Diseases in the United States http://www.boneandjointburden.org/2014-report (accessed 27 January 2018).

Dains, J., Baumann, L., and Scheibel, P. (2012). *Advanced Health Assessment and Clinical Diagnosis in Primary Care*, 4e. St. Louis: Elsevier.

Dains, J., Baumann, L., and Scheibel, P. (2015). *Advanced Health Assessment and Clinical Diagnosis in Primary Care*, 5e. St. Louis: Mosby.

Doherty, M., Dacre, J., Dieppe, P., and Snaith, M. (1992). The 'GALS' locomotor screen. *Annals of the Rheumatic Diseases* 51 (10): 1165–1169.

Epstein, O., Perkin, G., de Bono, D., and Cookson, J. (2008). *Clinical Examination*, 4e. London: Mosby.

EU Report v5.0 (2010) Musculoskeletal Health in Europe. http://www.eumusc.net/myUploadData/files/Musculoskeletal%20Health%20in%20Europe%20Report%20v5.pdf (accessed 27 January 2018).

Japp, A. and Robertson, C. (2013). *Macleod's Clinical Diagnosis*. Edinburgh: Churchill Livingstone, Elsevier.

Jarvis, C. (2008). *Physical Examination and Health Assessment*, 5e. St. Louis: Saunders.

Jarvis, C. (2015). *Physical Examination and Health Assessment*, 7e. Edinburgh: Elsevier.

Martini, F., Nath, J., and Bartholomew, E. (2012). *The Musculoskeletal System in Fundamentals of Anatomy & Physiology*, 9e. San Francisco, CA: Pearson Benjamin Cummings.

MSK (2015) Musculoskeletal Health in the Workplace: a Toolkit for Employers. https://wellbeing.bitc.org.uk/sites/default/files/business_in_the_community_musculoskeletal_toolkit.pdf (accessed 28 August 2018).

Seidel, H., Ball, J., Dains, J., and Benedict, G. (2006). *Mosby's Physical Examination Handbook*. St. Louis: Mosby.

Seidel, H., Ball, J., Dains, J., and Benedict, G. (2010). *Mosby's Physical Examination Handbook*, 7e. St. Louis: Mosby-Year Book.

Swartz, M. (2006). *Physical Diagnosis, History and Examination*, 5e. London: W. B. Saunders.

Swartz, M. (2014). *Physical Diagnosis: History and Examination*, With Student Consult Online Access, 7e. London: Elsevier.

Talley, N. and O'Connor, S. (2006). *Clinical Examination: A Systematic Guide to Physical Diagnosis*, 5e. London: Churchill Livingstone.

Talley, N. and O'Connor, S. (2014). *Clinical Examination: A Systematic Guide to Physical Diagnosis*, 7e. London: Churchill Livingstone, Elsevier.

Tallia, A. and Scherger, J. (2013). *Swanson's Family Practice Review*, 6e. St. Louis: Mosby.

Thomas, J. and Monaghan, T. (2007). *Oxford Handbook of Clinical Examination and Practical Skills*. Oxford: Oxford University Press.

Tortora, G. and Derrickson, B. (2013). *Principles of Anatomy and Physiology*, 14e. Oxford: Wiley.

Walsh, M. (2006). *Nurse Practitioners Clinical Skills and Professional Issues*, 2e. Edinburgh: Elsevier.

Chapter 14

Assessment of the Child

Carol Lynn Cox

General Examination

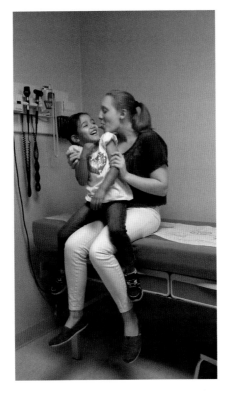

Children at play

Physical Assessment for Nurses and Healthcare Professionals, Third Edition. Edited by Carol Lynn Cox.
© 2019 John Wiley & Sons Ltd. Published 2019 by John Wiley & Sons Ltd.

Introduction

The child health assessment and physical examination are aimed at promoting the health of the child and preventing illness and disability through early identification of actual and potential problems. As a practitioner, your anticipatory guidance can be used to help parents deal with physical and developmental issues before they become problems as well as providing early intervention for healthcare needs (Altdoeffer and Maley 2017; Ball et al. 2014a, b; Bickley 2016; Bickley and Szilagyi 2007, 2013; Dains et al. 2015; Department of Health 2004; Duderstadt 2014; Epstein et al. 2008; Japp and Robertson 2013; Jarvis 2015; Sawyer 2012; Seidel et al. 2010; Talley and O'Connor 2014).

Approaching the Patient

- Approach the infant/child/young person from the perspective of wellness. (The term 'young person' is used throughout this text to represent the outdated term 'adolescent', and the term 'young people' is used for 'adolescents'.)
- Greet the parent/carer and the infant/child/young person using a gentle/normal tone of voice. It is important to use age-appropriate and developmentally appropriate language when talking to infants/children/young people.
- State your name and your clinical status (e.g. advanced practice nurse, physician assistant, or other).
- Make sure the patient is comfortable.
- Explain that you wish to ask questions to find out about the health history of the infant/ child/young person or what happened to the infant/child/young person.

  Appropriate consent for this should be obtained from both the parent/carer and child/ young person, remembering that different guidance pertains to a child/young person refusing to consent.

  Inform the parent/carer and patient how long you are likely to take and what to expect. For example, that after discussing the infant's/child's/young person's history or what has happened to the infant/child/young person, you would like to examine the infant/child/ young person.
- Use gentle touch.

General Considerations

You will see the infant/child frequently, generally every two to three months during infancy when growth changes are the most rapid and dramatic.

Assess the quality of the parent/carer–infant/child/young person relationship.

This along with other signs could raise issues of safeguarding children.

Give recognition and praise for parenting/caring skills.

Ask neutral questions.

The history will follow the same sequence as for the adult. Keep in mind physiological differences between infants, children, young people, and adults. The format that is generally followed is:

- Biographical information
- Chief complaint
- Present illness or health status
- Past medical history
- Developmental data
- Nutritional data (e.g. breastfeeding, if so when started/stopped and bottle augmentation)
- Family history
- Review of systems (physical, sociological, and psychological)
- Anticipatory guidance

The physical examination will generally follow the same sequence as for the adult. For example, the physical examination of an infant less than five months is relatively straight-forward and can proceed cephalocaudally (Barnes 2003; Bickley 2016; Duderstadt 2014; Talley and O'Connor 2014). In the examination you should be prepared for the following:

- *Infant: Respect the parent/carer relationship. Stranger and separation anxiety is important in infants older than six months. This peaks at nine months.*

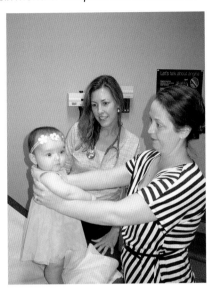

Assess relationship of parent and infant

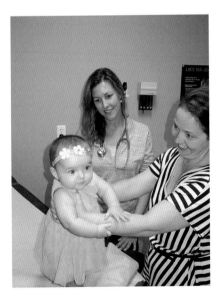

Assess whether the infant interacts with others

- Toddler: Independence is developing. Separation and stranger anxiety makes social interaction challenging. Modify the examination.
- Preschool child: Fear of bodily harm is an issue. Allow for play with the equipment on a doll or on you/parent/carer. This reduces fear.

- School-age child: Willing participants and curious about what is going on around them. Encourage questions.
- Young person: A period of tremendous growth. Behaviours are not predictable. Young people have a strong orientation towards independence and peer group. Young people will be starting to question authority. They may be primarily concerned about themselves and egocentric. Older young people will be goal oriented. Encourage relevant conversation, be nonjudgemental. Request opinions/thoughts regarding life/health decisions. Privacy is important. Give the option of an interview with or without the parent/carer present. Talk with the young person alone as well as with the parent/carer. Examine older young people without the parent/carer present but with a chaperone if necessary (Ball et al. 2014a, b; Bickley 2016; Bickley and Szilagyi 2007, 2013; Dains et al. 2015; Department of Health 2004; Duderstadt 2014; Engle 2002; Epstein et al. 2008; Japp and Robertson 2013; Jarvis 2015; Sawyer 2012; Seidel et al. 2010; Talley and O'Connor 2014).

Usual Sequence of Events

1. History
2. Examination
3. Problem list
4. Differential diagnosis
5. Investigations
6. Diagnosis confirmed
7. Treatment

Approach to the Assessment of the Child

Well infant/child/young person visit:

- Biographical data: date of birth, address, phone, nickname, birthplace, ethnicity, primary provider, name of school, last well visit
- Source of data: accompanied by whom, reliability of historian, use of translator or other special circumstances.
- Chief complaint/reason for visit: well child versus episodic visit.
- Past medical history: prenatal care/exposures, birth history, postnatal period, milestones, childhood illnesses, accidents/injuries, chronic illness, operations/hospitalizations, immunizations, allergies, medications. (In an infant assessment consider gestational age at birth, birth weight, prenatal care, intrauterine exposures, any problems during labour, delivery, and/or the neonatal period.) (Barnes 2003; Todd and Barnes 2003)
- Interval history: current status with regard to nutrition, growth and development, elimination, and sleep.
- Review of systems: any special concerns or worries (systems based).

Episodic visit:

- History of present illness: location, character/quality, quantity/severity, timing, setting, aggravating/relieving factors, associated factors, parent/child's perception, any other people sick at home, does illness awaken from sleep; is child playing, eating, sleeping: what has already been done to treat illness, coping of family with illness.

Note: young people will not require as much depth with regard to prenatal, birth history, and early developmental history (see Table 14.1) (Altdoeffer and Maley 2017; Ball et al. 2014a, b; Bickley 2016; Bickley and Szilagyi 2007, 2013; Daines et al. 2015; Department of Health 2004; Duderstadt 2014; Epstein et al. 2008; Japp and Robertson 2013; Jarvis 2015; Sawyer 2012; Seidel et al. 2010; Talley and O'Connor 2014).

Table 14.1   Approach to history taking – age-related history.

Infant (birth–12 months)

- Parent's/carer's perception of infant
- Parent/carer comfort with handling/care
- Condition of parent/carer
- Parent's/carer's perception of growth and development
- Breast versus bottle feeding
- Introduction of solids
- Night waking
- Food intolerances
- Parent's/carer's plans to return to work
- Possible childcare plans
- Siblings/rivalry

Toddler (1–2 years)

- Parent's/carer's reaction to increasing independence
- Struggles/tantrums
- How discipline is managed
- Problems with negativity, autonomy, and egocentrism
- Family stressors
- Parent's/carer's perception of growth and development
- Language acquisition
- Feeding/diet
- Sleeping patterns

Preschool (3–5 years)

- School readiness
- Discipline
- Childcare
- Family stressors
- Sibling relations
- Toileting/potty training
- Bladder control
- Bowel control

School-age (6–11 years)

- School performance

(Continued)

Table 14.1 *(Continued)*

- Friends/peers

- Extracurricular activities

- Discipline

Young person (12–18 years)

- Home environment: parents/carers, employed, with whom living, parental/carer relationship, other adult relationships

- Education or employment: school performance, favourite subjects, plans after completing school, truant or expelled, employment

- Activities: after-school activities, spare time interests, who young person spends time with

The points that follow are important to discern, if possible. It is extremely difficult to gain information on these points, especially in front of parents/carers, and even when young people are alone they may not answer these questions honestly for fear that their parents would be told. Use discretion when approaching these issues:

- Drugs/alcohol/smoking: use or sale of illicit and over the counter/natural drugs, use of steroids or other prescription drugs, friends using or selling drugs (it is useful to acknowledge that many young people experiment with drugs, alcohol, or smoking and then proceed to ask about the young person's and friends' use)

- Sexual activity/sexuality: sexual orientation, sexually active (age of 1st encounter, condom use/birth control, number of partners), history of sexual or physical abuse

- Suicide/depression: unhappy, sad or tearful, tired/unmotivated, feelings of worthlessness, wish/plan for self-harm

- Safety: access to guns, seat belt use, helmet use, risk taking/high-risk situations (joy riding/car theft, shoplifting, arrests)

Source: Adapted from Barnes and Smart (2003). Additional information contributing to adaptation from Gill and O'Brien (2007) and Engle (2002).

Differences in Anatomy and Physiology (Table 14.2)

Table 14.2 Differences in anatomy and physiology.

Infant

- Head and neck comprise ~ 45% of total body surface area (TBSA)

- Higher % of body composition is water (65–75% at birth)

- Infant head is 25% of body length and 1/3 of weight

- Rapid brain growth reflected in head circumference

- Presence of fontanelles

- Palpable sutures (newborn to 6 months)

- Skin thinner and eccrine (sweat) glands not functioning until 1 to 2 months

- Unstable/decreased ability to control temperature due to immature hypothalamus

- Poor protection from cold; cannot contract skin/shiver and SQ layer ineffective at insulation

- Melanocytes inefficient at birth

Table 14.2 *(Continued)*

- Well-developed system of lymphoid tissue that grows rapidly after birth
- Dramatic growth and development of nervous system during year 1 of life
- Motor activity under control of spinal cord and medulla; little cortical control
- Peripheral neurons not yet myelinated
- Movements are primarily reflexive (for the 1st few months)
- Development of cerebral cortex inhibits reflexes with subsequent disappearance of primitive reflexes
- Development proceeds in cephalocaudal and proximodistal directions, paralleling spinal cord myelination
- Rapidly improving visual acuity
- Nasolacrimal duct system not functioning until 3 months
- Tongue is larger in proportion to the mouth
- Ethmoid, maxillary, and sphenoid sinuses present but small
- External auditory canal relatively short and straight
- Eustachian tubes shorter, wider, more horizontal
- Heart is more horizontal and higher in the thoracic cavity (apex 4th ICS)
- Smaller/narrower airways
- Supporting structures of respiratory tree not fully developed
- Respiratory efforts are largely abdominal due to reliance on the diaphragm for breathing
- Chest wall much thinner with little musculature; sounds easily transmitted
- Obligate nose breathers (up to 6–12 weeks); nasal obstruction can be dangerous
- Prominent abdomen with poor muscle tone.
- Stomach capacity is small but increases rapidly with age, whilst gastric emptying time is faster.
- Proportionately longer gastrointestinal tract is a source of greater fluid loss
- Liver takes up proportionately more space in the abdomen
- Bladder located higher in the abdomen (between symphysis pubis and umbilicus)
- C-shaped curvature of the spine

Toddler

- Continues to have disproportionately large head
- 40% TBSA composed of head and trunk
- By the end of the 1st year of life, the brain has reached approximately 2/3 of its adult size and 90% complete by 2 years of age
- Chest circumference surpasses head circumference by 18 months
- Myelination of the spinal cord almost complete by 2 years of age
- Ear canals narrow with upwards slope

(Continued)

Table 14.2 (*Continued*)

- Ethmoid and maxillary sinuses slightly more developed (no frontal and sphenoid is minute)
- Lymphoid tissue develops with rapid growth rate
- Heart continues to be more horizontal and higher in the thoracic cavity (apex 4th ICS and S3 may be heard)
- Thin chest wall; sounds easily transmitted
- Weak abdominal musculature gives appearance of a pot belly
- Erect posture develops anterior curve to lumbar spine
- Voluntary movement under cortical control
- Development of gross motor skills parallels distal myelination

Preschool

- Face tends to grow proportionally
- Most physiologic systems mature
- Elongation of the limbs
- TBSA of head and trunk ~38%
- Neck with adult proportions by 4 years of age
- Hypertrophied lymph tissue (reaches adult size by 6 years of age)
- Superficial lymph nodes often palpable as normal variant
- Ethmoid and maxillary sinuses slightly more developed (no frontal and sphenoid still minute)
- Heart is more horizontal and higher in the thoracic cavity (reaches adult position at 7 years of age)
- Thin chest wall; sounds easily transmitted
- Adult proportions

School-age

- Adult proportions
- Ethmoid sinus grows rapidly between 6 to 8 years of age
- Frontal sinus develops ~ 7 years of age; sphenoid minute until puberty
- Jaw widens for eruption of permanent teeth
- Heart reaches adult position in thoracic cavity by 7 years of age
- Under age 7 respiratory movement is primarily abdominal or diaphragmatic
- Lymph tissue hypertrophied to greater than adult size and are at the peak of their development (regression of tissue to adult size occurs during adolescence)
- Continued growth and development of nervous system

Young person

- Rapidly accelerating physical growth (reaches peak at 11–14 years of age)
- In females, an increase in total body fat content is associated with pubertal development
- Growth decelerates in females by 14–17 years of age

Table 14.2   (*Continued*)

- Males become more muscular with a peak deceleration in the rate of fat accumulation at the time of growth spurt
- In general females reach maturity about 1.5–2 years earlier than males
- Testosterone stimulates growth of thyroid and cricoid cartilages and laryngeal muscles, resulting in deepening of the male voice
- Major organ systems mature with orderly development of musculoskeletal system from distal to proximal parts of the body
- Increased size and strength of the heart
- Lungs increase in diameter and length with concomitant increase in respiratory volume, vital capacity and respiratory functional efficiency
- Gastrointestinal development leads to increase in size and capacity which assume adult levels at about 14 years of age
- Development of secondary sex characteristics as a result of puberty
- Menarche closely related to the peak of the weight velocity curve and the deceleration phase of the height velocity curve and genetic and nutritional factors
- Neurophysiological structures and function completely developed by the end of middle adolescence
- Slight atrophy of lymph tissue to adult size

341

Source: Adapted from Todd and Barnes (2003), and Barnes (1998). Additional information contributing to adaptation from Gill and O'Brien (2007) and Engle (2002).

Developmental Considerations Affecting the Physical Assessment (Table 14.3)

Table 14.3   Developmental considerations affecting the physical assessment.

Infant
• Most dramatic and rapid period of growth and development
• Attachment and trust to parent/carer is important
• Stranger anxiety appears ~ 6 months of age
• Object permanence not developed until ~ 10–12 months of age
• Separation anxiety starts to effect social interactions at about 9 months of age
• Safety is paramount as gross and fine motor development progress rapidly
Toddler
• Separation and stranger anxiety continue to influence social interactions
• Autonomy, egocentrism and negativism are major developmental issues
• Parent/carer is home-base for explorations
• Knows 6–8 body parts by 30 months
• Fears bodily harm

(*Continued*)

Table 14.3   *(Continued)*

• Verbal communication skills limited
• Safety continues to be paramount
Preschool
• Development of sense of initiative is important
• Able to 'help', participate, and cooperate
• Knows most body parts and some internal parts
• Fears bodily harm
• Verbal communication skills more advanced
• Cognition characterised by egocentricity, literal interpretations, and magical thinking
School-age
• Sense of industry is important
• Articulate and active participant in care
• Increased self-control
• Understands simple scientific explanations (cause and effect) although thinking still concrete
Young person
• Increasing independence
• Time of tremendous growth and change
• Older young people have an orientation to the future
• Separates easily from parents/carers
• Peer group important
• Knows basic anatomy and physiology
• Has own opinions/ideas
• Active and articulate participant in care

Source: Adapted from Barnes and Smart (2003). Additional information contributing to adaptation from Gill and O'Brien (2007) and Engle (2002).

Developmental Approach to the Physical Assessment (Table 14.4)

Table 14.4   Developmental approach to the physical assessment.

Infant
• Keep parent/carer in view
• Before 6 months of age examine on table; after 6 months examine in parent's/carer's lap
• Undress fully in warm room
• Careful with nappy removal

Table 14.4 (*Continued*)

- Distract with bright objects/rattles
- Soft manner, avoid loud noises and abrupt movements
- Have bottle or dummy handy
- Vary examination sequence with activity level (if asleep/quiet auscultate heart, lungs, and abdomen first)
- Proceed in a cephalocaudal sequence
- Elicit reflexes during the examination
- Save the traumatic procedures for last (ears and temperature, for example)

Toddler

- Most difficult group to examine
- Approach gradually and minimise initial physical contact
- Leave with parent (sitting or standing if possible)
- Allow toddler to inspect equipment (demonstration usually not helpful)
- Start inspection distally through play (toes/fingers)
- Praise the toddler
- Parent removes clothes gradually as needed (toddlers do not like being undressed or touched)
- Describe examination in short phrases
- Save ears, mouth, and anything lying down for last

Preschool

- Allow close proximity to parent/carer
- Usually cooperative; able to proceed head to toe
- Request self-undressing (bit by bit exposure – modesty important)
- Expect cooperation
- Allow for choice when possible
- If uncooperative start distally with play
- Allow brief inspection of equipment with demonstration and brief explanation
- Use games/stories for cooperation
- Paper-doll technique very effective*a*
- Praise, reward, and positive reinforcement
- Examine the genitalia last

School-age

- Usually cooperative
- Child should undress self, privacy is important; provide gown if possible

(*Continued*)

Table 14.4 (*Continued*)

• Explain purpose/function of equipment; spare equipment is useful for them to hold/look at and use on a doll, paper doll[a] or on you or parent/carer
• Examination can be an important teaching exercise
• Examine in a head to toe direction
• Examine the genitalia last
• Praise and feedback regarding normalcy is important
Young person
• Give option of parent/carer being present during the examination
• Undress in private; provide gown
• Expose one area at a time
• The examination can be an important teaching exercise
• Examine in head to toe sequence
• Examine genitalia last
• Feedback regarding normalcy is important
• Anticipatory guidance regarding sexual development (use Tanner staging)
• Matter of fact approach to history and examination
• Encourage appropriate decision-making skills

Source: Adapted from Barnes and Smart (2003). Additional information contributing to adaptation from Gill and O'Brien (2007) and Engle (2002).
[a] Draw doll on examination table paper. Point out/draw where body parts are located on the doll.

The examination of infants, children, and young people requires flexibility.

- Allow the infant's/child's/young person's developmental level to guide your history taking and physical examination.
- The atmosphere and environment are important. (The room should be warm with appropriate decoration and the use of toys. Take into consideration the special needs of young people including an unhurried social environment. Always limit the number of people in the room.)
- Remain organised. (Things can easily slip into chaos, particularly with children.)
- Exercise care in the use of equipment and remember safety. (Little hands can grab equipment. Do not leave the child unattended on the examination table. Maintain safety with outlets and equipment.)
- The assessment, whether comprehensive or episodic, is always head to abdomen.
- Incorporate health education and growth and development anticipatory guidance into the examination.
- Move from the easy/simple to more distressing; use positive reinforcement and 'prizes'.
- Use demonstration and play to your advantage.
- Expect an age-appropriate level of cooperation.

Physical Examination of the Infant and Toddler

System	Normal variants	Abnormal variants
General appearance • Parent/carer/child interaction • Posture, position, movement • Hygiene • Nutrition • Weight • Height • Head circumference	• Pink, well-nourished, well-dressed, bright-eyed, and alert infant in no apparent distress, positive parent/carer/child interaction, moving all four extremities • 0–6 months: weight gain = 140–210 g week^{-1} (35–57 oz); increase in length = 1.25 cm (0.5 inches month^{-1} – PLOT – Plot out the child's length vs. age and compare to the average) • Head is ~2 cm > chest until 6–24 months when chest > head – PLOT • Birth weight regained by 7–10 days • Birth weight doubled by 4–6 months • Birth weight tripled by 1 year • Height at 2 years about half adult height • Growth can be characterised by 'spurts'	• Parent/carer displays disinterested attitude towards infant and/or lack of attachment • Dysmorphic features, facies, and/or movements • Foul or unusual odour from child • Rapidly growing or nongrowing head • Weight loss or failure to gain weight (after 10 days of age) • Wide discrepancy between height, weight, and head percentiles

Vital signs (observations)
• Temperature
• Apical pulse
• Respiratory rate
• Blood pressure (auscultate, palpate, or flush methods)
	• Vital signs within expected range:
	  ○ Count apical pulse for 60 seconds – sinus arrhythmic normal (rate increases on inspiration)
	  ○ Respiratory pattern in infants can be erratic – count for 60 seconds and watch abdomen as breathing is more diaphragmatic than thoracic
	  ○ Palpation yields systolic pressure, flush yields mean blood pressure (BP)
		• Vital signs outside of expected range

Skin, nails, and hair	• Warm skin with pink undertones • Mongolian spots common (especially in Black, Latino, and Asian infants) • Café-au-lait spots common • Haemangiomas common (stork bite/salmon patch, cherry angioma, and strawberry haemangioma) • Neonatal acne, milia, erythema toxicum, seborrhoea of the scalp are common • Mottling/reticulated pattern over extremities in response to cold room (cutis marmorata) • Jaundice in newborn (3rd–4th day of life) requires investigation (assess in natural light) • Assess turgor on abdomen • Pink nail beds with good capillary refill • Infant hair may be patchy especially at temples and occiput • Newborn with lanugo (downy hair)	• Poor colour or cyanosis • 6 or > 6 café-au-lait spots require evaluation (neurofibromatosis) • Cavernous haemangioma or nevus flammeus (port-wine stain) • Unfamiliar rash • Persistent mottling/cyanosis • Jaundice on 1st day of life or after two weeks of age • Bruising • Poor turgor/lack of subcutaneous fat • Discoloured nail beds of clubbing • Hair tufts/dimples/break in skin on spine requires investigation

(Continued)

System	Normal variants	Abnormal variants
Head, neck, lymph nodes, eyes, ears, nose, mouth, and throat	• Palpate suture lines in newborn: frontal, coronal, saggital, lamboidal • Sutures may overlap at birth with moulded appearance to head • Newborn: bogginess (bleeding into the periosteum) evidenced by swelling that does not cross the suture line (cephalohaemotoma) or oedematous swelling of the superficial tissues of the scalp evidenced by generalised soft swelling not bounded by suture lines (caput succedaneum) • Frontal bossing (prominence of the forehead) characteristic of premature infants • Anterior fontanelle begins to close at ~ 9 months; closes ~18 months (soft but firm, slightly concave, may pulsate slightly and will tense slightly with crying) • Posterior fontanelle closes ~ 1–2 months (may be closed/absent at birth) • Supple neck that moves easily, symmetrical alignment of head and clavicles • Short neck • An infant < 4 months of age may show head lag when pulled to a sitting position • Lymph glands not normally palpable in infants • Cervical lymph nodes difficult to examine in toddlers: soft, round, slightly boggy, nontender (diffuse cervical nodes common) • Inguinal nodes often palpable • Epitrochlear and axillary nodes usually not palpable • Pupils Equal, Round, Reactive to Light (PERRL) • Newborn blinks when bright light is introduced • Tilt to open eyes and turn head to one side whilst holding upright: assess for fixation (tests vestibular function reflex), red reflex and white reflex (cataract or retinoblastoma) • At two weeks fixates on bright object • At one month fixates on object and follow to midline • Six months fixates and follows 180° • Symmetry of corneal light reflex □ six months • Bright clear eyes, white sclera, no discharge • Tiny dark flecks in sclera of Black and Asian children is common • Grey blue or 'muddy' colour of sclera in Black children • Newborn may have residual chemical inflammation s/p eye drops (< or = 24h); sclera may have blue tint; lacrimal glands not functioning at birth, eye colour not confirmed until nine months of age • Tip of pinna at height of outer corner of eye and 10° from vertical (posteriorly) • Canal with some soft cerumen	• Palpable sutures □ 6 months • Marked asymmetry of the head that persists (investigate) • Absence of or markedly enlarged (> 2.5 or 2.6 cm) anterior fontanelle • Bulging or sunken anterior fontanelle • Resistance or pained crying with range of motion (ROM) of neck and/or head tilt • Webbed neck/congenital torticollis (investigate) • Poor head control or marked lag □ 4 months • Firm/hard warm, red, tender, enlarged nodes • Prominent supraclavicular node (investigate) • Lack of papillary or blink reflex/response • Lack of vestibular function reflex • Absence of red reflex (retinal disorders) and presence of white reflex • Inability to fixate and follow objects • Asymmetry of corneal light reflex • Purulent discharge from eyes • Swelling of lachrymal duct with discharge • Low set ears or deviation in alignment (mental retardation or genitourinary [GU] problem), foul or sweet odour from canal • TM: abnormal light reflex, contour, lack of landmarks or movement; red/purple • Nasal flaring • Cleft or notched palate (hard or soft) • White nonremovable plaques on tongue or buccal mucosa (thrush) • No teeth by 12–15 months of age • 3+ to 4+ tonsils

Category	Normal/findings	Variations/abnormal
	• Tympanic membrane (TM) difficult to see before one month of age • Pearly TM with sharp landmarks, cone of light, and gentle movement • TM will redden with crying (fades on inspiration) • Patent nares (check for breath on stethoscope with one naris blocked) • Ethmoid, maxillary, and sphenoid sinuses present at birth, however quite small (sphenoid is minute) • Sucking tubercle possible finding in older infants (salivation starts ~ three months) • Newborn: fused palate, pink gingivae with raised ridge, pearls on palate/gum • Moist pink membranes • Eruption of lower centrals at ~6months (to estimate dentition in children □ 2 years subtract '6' from the child's age in months) • Throat is clear and pink • Tonsils not visible in newborn • Toddler: 1+ to 2+ common	
Breasts and chest	• Rounded symmetrical thoracic cage that is smaller in circumference than head (at nipple line ~ 2 cm smaller than head until about 2 years of age) • 2nd rib attaches at sternal angle (angle of Louis) • Anteroposterior measurement is equal to side-to-side (lateral) measurement giving chest a circular or 'barrel' shape • Symmetrical nipples placed (slightly lateral of mid-clavicular line between 4th or 5th ribs) with flat nipple and slightly darker pigmentation to areola • Newborn may have a slight enlargement of breast tissue with clear or white fluid from nipple (witch's milk) – resolves within a few days/weeks	• Variations in shape, symmetry or movement • Supernumerary nipple(s)
Pulmonary (respiratory)	• Count rate for full minute (easiest to count when sleeping) • Common for respiratory pattern to be irregular (patterns of apnoea for 10–15 seconds not unusual) • Abdominal bulge with respiration with little chest movement • May have slight flaring of lower costal margins normal • Palpation yields no masses or lumps • Percussion is not very useful in infants • Crying can enhance auscultation of breath sounds (listen closely on expiration) • Auscultate all fields systematically and symmetrically from apices to bases • Bronchovesicular sounds throughout lung fields • Transmission of upper airway sounds common • Breath sounds may sound louder/harsher due to thinness of chest wall • Upper airway sounds easily transmitted (listen at nose, sounds will be louder) • Paediatric stethoscope makes auscultation easier (less 'noise' because diaphragm is smaller)	• Rate not within normal limits for age • Nasal flaring, sternal/intercostal retractions or grunting • Adventitious sounds: • Discontinuous sounds (crackles) or continuous sounds (wheezes = high-pitched hissing or shrill quality and rhonchi = low pitched and have a snoring quality) • Diminished or absent breath sounds, tubular sounds over lung fields/prolonged expiratory phase (indicating consolidation)

(Continued)

System	Normal variants	Abnormal variants
Cardiovascular	- Inspect nail beds (hands and feet) = pink with brisk capillary refill - Note any extracardiac signs (pallor, cyanosis, distress) - Palpate the precordium and locate the point of maximal impulse (PMI) (higher up on the thorax – 4th intercostal space [ICS] lateral of midclavicular line [MCL]) - Auscultate as for adult, one sound at a time; follow systematic approach - Sinus arrhythmic normal (accelerates with inspiration) - Heart sounds louder due to thin chest wall - Infant – difficult to separate S_1 and S_2 (S_2 higher pitch and louder at the base) - Soft murmurs (e.g. S_3) grade 1/6 or 2/6 systolic murmur in newborn for 1st 2–3 days or continuous 'machinery' murmur (patent ductus arteriosis) within 1st 2–3 days in new-born - If newborn has a murmur at birth, reevaluate after day 3 of life	- Poor refill or absence of pink undertones - Infant or toddler with signs and symptoms of congestive heart failure (CHF) (respiratory distress, wet lungs, enlarged liver, and tachycardia) - Murmurs persisting after 3 days of life in newborn (although S_3 may remain present and is not considered pathological) - Very loud holosystolic (pansystolic) or diastolic murmurs
Abdomen	- Contour of abdomen is protuberant but symmetrical - Fine superficial venous pattern - Inspect umbilical cord in newborn - ☐ bowel sounds - Tympani over stomach with dullness at liver edge and bladder - Assess turgor over abdomen - Soft abdomen (flex knees up by holding feet frog-legged; feed or use dummy if crying) - Umbilical hernia common (increased incidence in Black infants) with increased prominence when crying (can be up to 2.5 cm) - Diastasis recti common (increased incidence in Black infants) – separation of rectus muscle causing a visible bulge - Caecum easily palpable in right lower quadrant (RLQ) and sigmoid colon (soft sausage in left inguinal area that moves) - Infant liver fills right upper quadrant (RUQ) with border ~ at right costal margin or 1–2 cm below - May feel spleen tip 1–2 cm below left costal margin (roll onto left side) - Palpate for femoral pulses (strong and equal bilaterally) - Palpate for femoral hernia (3 fingers spread medially from pulse)	- Scaphoid shape - Dilated veins - Inflammation or drainage at umbilicus or cord - Absent or diminished bowel sounds - Tethering or poor recoil of skin - Crying or obvious pain with palpation - Masses or lumps (check epigastric area for olive-shaped mass = pyloric stenosis and pyloric regurgitation may be auscultated) - Umbilical hernia ☐ 2.5 cm - Diastasis recti after 3 months of age - Masses - Enlarged liver - Enlarged spleen (feels like a water balloon) - Full, bounding, or absent femoral pulses - Femoral hernia

| Musculoskeletal | • Observe movement, general symmetry and muscle strength/tone
• Count fingers and toes
• Slight tremulousness in hands/feet of newborn normal
• Start at feet and work up
• Toddlers: wide-based gait with arms out for balance
• Check flexibility of heel cords (angle of foot to tibia 80° or less)
• Feet often appear flat (pes planus) due to fat pads and nonweight bearing
• Palpate forefoot for mobility and positioning relation to hindfoot (flexible metatarsus adductus – concave medial border and convex lateral border of foot – acceptable up to age 3 although position and stretching exercises may be done)
• Bow-legged (genu varum) stance of toddlers (< 2.5 cm between knees when medial malleoli are together)
• Check for tibial torsion: with knees bent place fingers on malleoli (all 4 malleoli should be parallel or less than 20° out of straight with medial malleolus anterior to lateral malleolus)
• Check hips for Galeazzi or Allis sign
• Unequal thigh folds

• Ortolani's sign (check every visit until 1 year of age) – With the infant supine, put your thumbs on the inner aspect of both thighs and your fingertips resting over the trochanter muscles, flex both hips and knees; abduct each knee until the lateral aspects of the knees touch the examining table; note that this test is reliable until the child is 1 year of age; in the older infant it is less reliable (use ROM of hips after 1 year)
• Barlow's test (this test is less reliable in the neonate) – with the infant supine, flex and slightly adduct both hips; at the same time, lift the femur and apply pressure to the trochanter
• Check arms, hands, and palmar crease
• Palpate clavicles in newborn and arm ROM: smooth, even, regular
• C-shape to spine of infant; lumbar lordosis in toddler
• Inspect spine: smooth without dimples, tufts, cyst, or mass | • Hyper/hypotonia and scissoring
• Extra digits
• Marked tremors
• Abnormal gait
• Tight heel cords or foot rigidity
• Fixed adduction of forefoot with inversion (metatarsus varus – not able to be brought to neutral position with passive ROM)
• Talipes equinovarus (clubfoot) fixed metatarsus varus with downwards pointing of foot (equinus)
• Tibial torsion (lateral malleolus anterior to medial malleolus)
• Click/clunk during manoeuvre ☐ DDH (developmental dysplasia of the hip)
• Uneven knees – Galeazzi or Allis sign
• Uneven gluteal folds (investigate)
• Limited abduction (investigate)
• Lack of symmetry, simian crease, or webbing of fingers/toes
• Fractured clavicle or irregularity
• Tufts, dimples, cysts, masses along spine |

(Continued)

System	Normal variants	Abnormal variants

Neurological	• A large part of the examination is observational: smoothness of movement and spontaneous activity
	• Bright, active, and alert appearance unless asleep
	• Strong cry and suck in newborn
	• Cranial nerves (CN) assessment for newborn:
	  ○ CN II, III, IV, VI: optic blink reflex to bright light
	  ○ CN V: rooting and sucking reflex
	  ○ CN VII: facial movements
	  ○ CN VIII: Moro (startle reflex) or acoustic blink reflex
	  ○ CN IX, X: swallowing, gag reflex, coordinated suck
	  ○ CN XII: pinch nose and mouth will open with tongue rise in midline
	• Note/monitor newborn reflexes (rooting, Moro, sucking, plantar and palmar grasp, Babinski, tonic neck, placing, stepping Galant)
	• Note developmental milestones: fix/follow, head lag/head control, sitting, loss of primitive reflexes, fine motor development
		• Jerkiness, tremors, flaccidity
		• Altered level of consciousness
		• Weak cry and/or poor suck
		• Hyper/hyporeflexive newborn
		• Absence or poor response
		• Persistence of primitive reflexes
		• Lack of milestone achievement

Genitourinary	• **Male:** keep warm with nappy on before exam (cremasteric reflex is strong) • Inspect penis (size, circumcised/noncircumcised) • Meatus at midline and at tip slightly voiding in straight stream (by history) • Foreskin tight until 3 months of age (DO NOT RETRACT) • Testicles descended bilaterally (block inguinal canal) • Have toddler sit cross-legged to block canals (migratory testes common due to strength of cremasteric reflex) • Fluid in scrotum in children < 2 years of age is common (transilluminate for hydrocele) • Palpate for inguinal hernia • **Female:** external genitalia may be engorged at birth (and for a few weeks following birth) with slight sanguineous drainage from maternal oestrogen effect • Inspect external genitalia for position, intact structures, and presence of vagina • Smooth, shiny mucosa without excoriation/irritation	• **Male:** red inflamed or oozing penile tip • Ambiguous genitalia • Poor stream, pinpoint meatus and/or hypospadias or epispadias • Phimosis/paraphimosis • Cryptorchidism • Hydrocele □ age 2 or if accompanied by pain, nonillumination, or increase in size • Inguinal hernia • **Female:** ambiguous genitalia • Anatomical/structure abnormality • Excoriation, irritation, foul odour, or discharge or signs/symptoms of abuse
Rectum/anus	• Patency • Anal reflex • Absence of fissure, redness, lesions • Nappy dermatitis common	• Imperforate anus • Lack of sphincter tone • Fissure, redness, lesions, signs/symptoms of sexual abuse • Severe nappy dermatitis, candidiasis, or staphylococcal superinfection

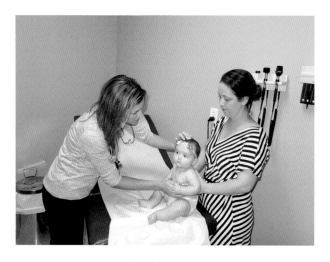

Assess the shape of the head

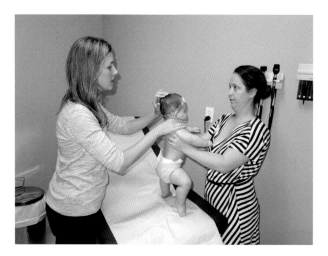

Assess the fontanels

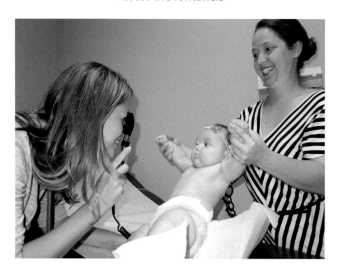

Check for the red reflex with the ophthalmoscope

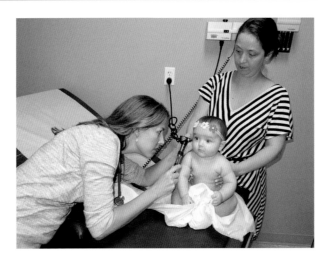

Check the ears with an otoscope

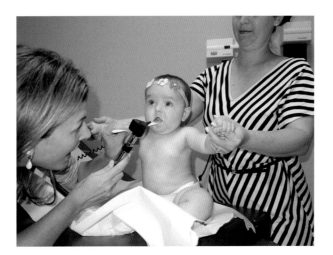

Check the mouth

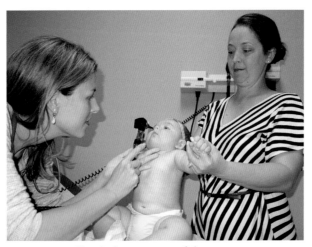

Check the patency of the nose

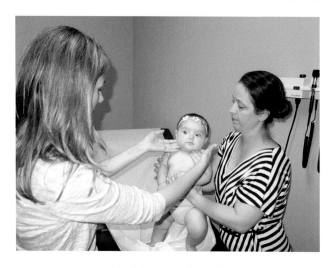

Check the lymph nodes

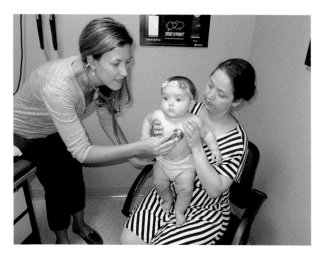

Auscultate the heart

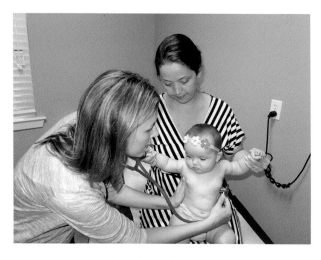

Auscultate the lungs

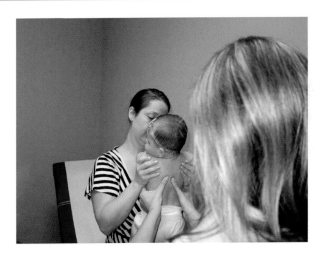

Assess diaphragmatic excursion

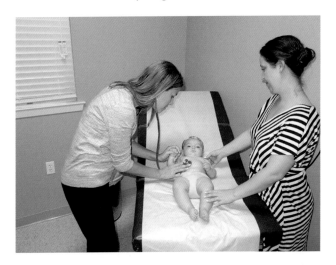

Auscultate the abdomen

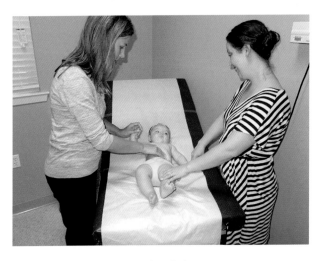

Palpate the abdomen

Physical Examination of the Child

System	Normal variants	Abnormal variants
General appearance • Parent/carer/child interaction • Behaviour • Mobility • Gross/fine motor skills • Speech • Hygiene • Nutritional status • Weight • Height	• Well-nourished, well-developed, bright-eyed, and active child in no apparent distress; positive parent/carer/child interaction • Weight gain: 2 kg year^{-1} from 1 to 10 years of age – PLOT • Height gain: 6–8 cm year^{-1} (height at 2 years of age ~ half adult height) – PLOT • Growth can be characterised by steady gains along predictable trajectory	• Disinterested attitude of parent/carer, lack of mutual response between child and parent/carer • Dysmorphic features, facies, and/or movements • Foul or unusual odour from child • Rapidly growing or nongrowing child • Weight loss of failure to gain weight • Wide discrepancy between height and weight
Vital signs (observations) • Temperature • Apical pulse • Respiratory rate • BP	Vital signs within expected range: • Axillary or tympanic temperature measurement • Count apical pulse for 60 seconds – sinus arrhythmic normal (rate accelerates on inspiration) • Use palpation or flush techniques if uncooperative	• Vital signs outside of expected range
Skin, nails, hair, head, neck, lymph nodes, eyes, ears, nose, mouth, and throat	• Warm skin with pink undertones • Skin slightly dry without rashes, hyperpigmentation, or lesions • Café-au-lait spots common • Assess turgor on abdomen • Pink nail beds with good capillary refill • Shiny, firm elastic hair • No lice • Head has rounded shape and is held erect • No discomfort on palpation of sinuses • Supple neck that moves easily • Cervical lymph nodes often normally palpable in children: soft, red, slightly boggy nontender (diffuse cervical nodes common) • Inguinal nodes often palpable • Epitrochlear and axillary nodes usually not palpable • Bright clear eyes, white sclera, no discharge • Tiny dark flecks in sclera of Black and Asian children is common	• Poor colour or cyanosis • Excessive sweating in children may accompany hypoglycaemia, heart disease, or hyperthyroidism • 6 or > 6 café-au-lait spots require evaluation (neurofibromatosis) • Bruising/unusual marks • Poor turgor/lack of subcutaneous fat • Discoloured nail beds or clubbing • Exceptionally dry or brittle hair (nutritional deficiencies) • Lice • Asymmetry with swelling or bruising • Head consistently held to one side (investigate vision/strabismus) • Tenderness over sinuses

(Continued)

System	Normal variants	Abnormal variants
	• Grey blue or 'muddy' colour of sclera in black children • Pupils Equal, Round, Reactive to Light and Accommodation (PERRLA) • Eyeball reaches adult size by 8 years of age (vision 6/9 by 4 years and 6/6 by 7) • Symmetry of corneal light reflex • Negative cover test • Optic disc creamy yellow/orange with sharp margins • Sharp vessels • Palpebral conjunctivae pink and glossy • Tip of pinna at height of outer corner of eye and 10° from vertical (posteriorly) • Canal with some soft cerumen • Pearly TM with sharp landmarks, cone of light, and gentle movement • TM will redden with crying (fades on inspiration) • Patent nares (check for breath on stethoscope with one naris blocked) • Firm pink membranes • Moist, pink, firm, and smooth oral mucosa • Teeth in good repair/condition; appropriate number and alignment • Tonsils usually large and may have crypts • Uvula at the midline	• Resistance or pained crying with ROM of neck and/or head tilt • Firm/hard, warm, red, tender, enlarged nodes • Supraclavicular node (investigate) • Purulent discharge from eyes • Lack of papillary response • Vision outside of age-appropriate norms • Asymmetry of corneal light reflex • No movement of uncovered eye and steadiness of covered eye • Pallor to disc, opacities, irregular shape or blurred margins of disc • Congested/dilated vessels • Cobblestone appearance in allergic children • Pallor of outer eye canthus in anaemia • Low set ears with deviation in alignment • Foul or sweet odour from canal • Excoriated or inflamed canal • Abnormal light reflex, contour, lack of landmarks or movement, red/purple colour • Nasal flaring • Boggy, pale, or grey mucosa = allergy • Red, inflamed mucosa = infection • Bleeding, lesions, swelling of gums • Dry mucous membranes • Dental caries
		• Poor hygiene • Red, swollen inflamed tonsils with white membrane or plaques • 3+ to 4+ tonsils • deviation of uvula (? upper motor neuron lesion) or absence of movement (investigate)

	Assessment	Variations/abnormal
Breasts/chest	• Symmetrical thoracic cage that is wider than it is thick • After 7 years of age, breathing is largely thoracic in females but remains abdominal in males • 2nd rib attaches at sternal angle (angle of Louis) • Symmetrical nipples placed (slightly lateral of midclavicular line (between 4th or 5th ribs) with flat nipple and slightly darker pigmentation to areola	• Variations in shape, symmetry, or movement • Supernumerary nipple(s)
Pulmonary (respiratory)	• Count rate for 30 seconds • Palpation yields no masses or lumps • Percussion helpful only in older children (dullness is heard over liver and heart) • Crying can enhance auscultation of breath sounds (listen closely on expiration) • Auscultate all fields systematically and symmetrically from apices to bases • Bronchovesicular sounds throughout lung fields • Transmission of upper airway sounds common • Breath sounds may sound louder/harsher due to thinness of chest wall • Upper airway sounds easily transmitted (listen at nose, sounds will be louder) • Paediatric stethoscope makes auscultation easier ('less 'noise' since diaphragm is smaller)	• Rate within normal limits for age • Nasal flaring or sternal/intercostal retractions • Adventitious sounds: discontinuous sounds (crackles) or continuous sounds (wheezes = high-pitched hissing or shrill quality and rhonchi = low pitched and have a snoring quality) • Diminished or absent breath sounds, tubular sounds over lung fields/prolonged expiratory phase (indicating consolidation)

Cardiovascular	• Inspect nail beds (hands and feet) □ pink with good capillary refill
	• Note any extracardiac signs (pallor, cyanosis, distress)
	• Inspect and palpate the precordium
	• Palpate the apical impulse (PMI) = roll onto left side
	  ○ 4th ICS lateral to MCL at age 4
	  ○ 4th ICS at MCL age 4–6 years
	  ○ 5th ICS medial to MCL > age 7
	• Auscultate one sound at a time (S_1 or S_2) for quality, rate, intensity, and rhythm
	• Auscultate in 'Z' pattern over thorax
	• Auscultate supine and sitting (left lateral, standing, squatting, standing after squatting = useful positions in evaluation of murmurs)
	• Innocent murmurs common (soft, short, systolic, vibratory, heard best at left sternal border without radiation)
		• Poor refill or absence of pink undertones
		• Thoracic bulging or thrills
		• Signs and symptoms of CHF (respiratory distress, wet lungs, enlarged liver, tachycardia, and poor growth)
		• A_2 moves laterally with cardiac enlargement
		• Abnormal sounds and/or S_4
		• Very loud, holosystolic (pansystolic) or diastolic murmurs
		• Murmurs without innocent qualities

(Continued)

System	Normal variants	Abnormal variants
Abdomen	• Functional murmurs (physiological murmurs) common with fever • Sinus arrhythmic normal (accelerates with inspiration) • Heart sounds louder due to thin chest wall • Contour of preschool abdomen may be slightly protuberant when standing but flat when supine • School age with slim abdominal shape as potbelly lost • Slight peristaltic waves may be visible in thin children • Positive bowel sound (all 4 quadrants) • Tympani over stomach with dullness at liver edge • Liver span changes with age/growth • Soft abdomen (use child's hand to start if ticklish) • Caecum easily palpable in RLQ and sigmoid colon (soft sausage in left inguinal area that moves) • May feel spleen tip 1–2 cm below left costal margin (roll onto left side) • Palpate for femoral pulses (strong and equal bilaterally) • Palpate for femoral hernia (3 fingers spread medially from pulse)	• Scaphoid shape or distended shape • Marked peristaltic waves (obstruction) • Absent or diminished bowel sounds • Engorged or enlarged liver • Crying or obvious pain with palpation • Masses or lumps or bulges (umbilical hernia closed by 4 years of age) • Enlarged spleen (feels like a water balloon) • Full, bounding, or absent femoral pulses • Femoral hernia
Musculoskeletal	• Observe movement, general symmetry, and muscle strength/tone • Note gait (base narrow, arms by sides, shoes with wear on outside of heels and inside of toes) • Note 'plumb line' down back: back of head, along spine to middle of sacrum • Shoulders level and scapulae even • Preschool child: slight genu valgum (< 2.5 cm between medial malleoli when knees together) • Preschool child: may look flat footed (pes planus) until 36 months due to fat pads at arch • Normal Trendelenburg sign (progressive subluxation of the hip): even iliac crests when weight is shifted from one leg to the other • Full ROM of remaining joints • Check for tibial torsion: with legs hanging over exam table place fingers on malleoli (all 4 malleoli should be parallel or less than 20° out of straight with medial malleolus anterior to lateral malleolus	• Hyper/hypotonia and scissoring • Abnormal gait or limp • Asymmetry of shoulders or unevenness of scapulae • 2.5 cm between medial malleoli • Marked pronation of the foot past 36 months • Subluxation of the hip: uneven iliac crests when weight shifted from one leg to the other (when child stands on 'affected leg' the pelvis drops) • Pain, tenderness, swelling, or restricted movement in any joint • Tibial torsion after 3 years of age

Neurological	A large part of the examination is observational: smoothness of movement, spontaneous activity and behaviour	Jerkiness, tremors, flaccidity, bizarre behaviour
	Bright, interactive	Altered level of consciousness
	Gross and fine motor skills appropriate for age (able to balance on one foot and hop by 4 years of age and accurate finger-to-nose test with eyes open and closed by 5)	Delays in fine or gross motor skills
		Hyperactivity or decreased/absent reflexes
	Deep tendon reflexes (DTRs) difficult to assess in children under the age of 5	Absent or poor response
	CN assessment in older children as adult:	Persistence of primitive reflexes
	○ CN II: fundoscopic	Lack of milestone achievement
	○ CN III, IV, VI: PERRLA and extraocular movements	
	○ CN V: clenching teeth	
	○ CN VII: smile	
	○ CN VIII: hearing screen	
	○ CN IX, X: rise of uvula with 'ahhhh'	
	○ CN XII: clear speech 'light, tight, dynamite'	
Genitourinary	**Male:** keep warm with nappy on before exam (cremasteric reflex is strong)	**Male:** red inflamed or oozing penile tip
	Inspect penis (size, circumcised/noncircumcised)	Poor stream, pinpoint meatus, and/or hypospadias or epispadias
	Meatus at midline and at tip slightly voiding in straight stream (by history)	Phimosis/paraphimosis
	Foreskin retractable by 4–5 years of age	Cryptorchidism
	Testicles descended bilaterally (block inguinal canal)	Inguinal hernia
	Palpate for inguinal hernia	**Female:** abnormal anatomical structures
	Female: inspect external genitalia for position, intact structures and presence of vagina and patent hymen	Excoriation, irritation, foul odour, or discharge or signs/symptoms of abuse
	Smooth shiny mucosa without excoriation/irritation	
Rectum/anus	Absence of fissure, redness, lesions	Fissure, redness, lesions, signs/symptoms of sexual abuse

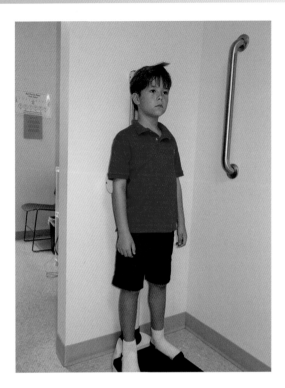

Check the height of the child

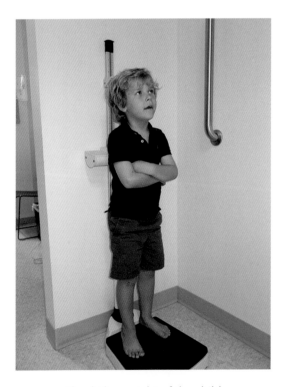

Check the weight of the child

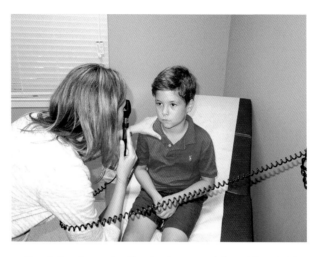

Check for the red reflex in the eye of the older child

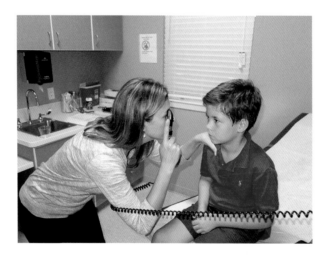

Get ready to 'zoom in'

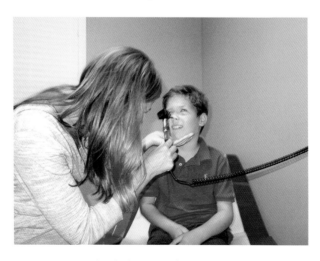

Check the nose for patency

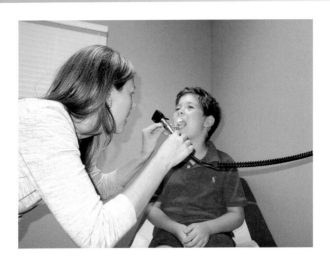

Checking the mouth of the older child

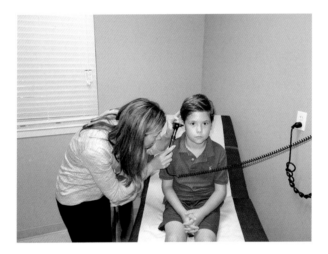

Examination of the tympanic membrane of the older child

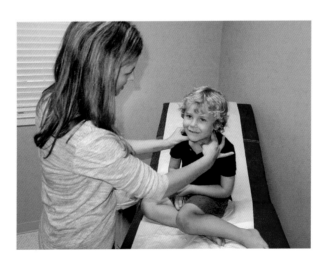

Check the lymph nodes

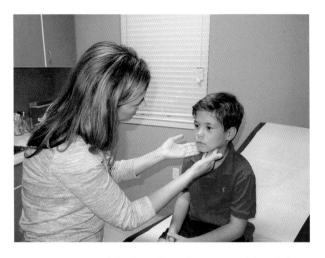

Examination of the lymph nodes in the older child

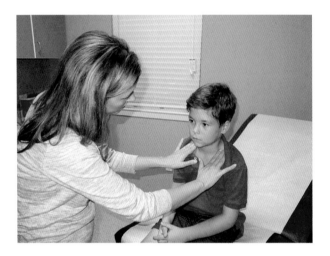

Palpation

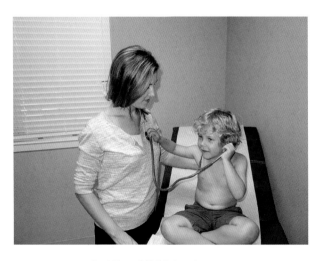

Let the child listen to you

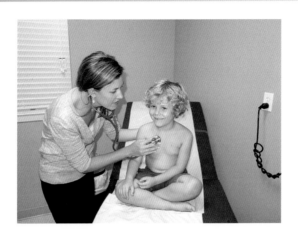

Auscultation of the lungs

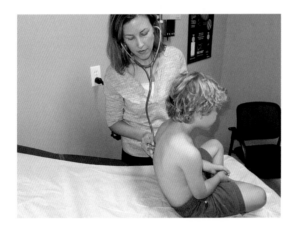

Posterior auscultation of the lungs

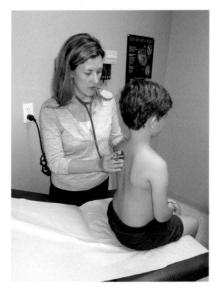

Auscultation of the posterior lungs

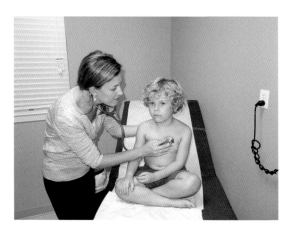

Auscultate the heart

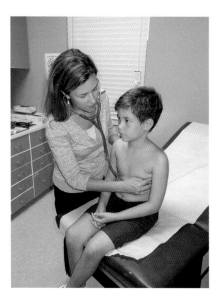

Auscultation of the heart at the apex

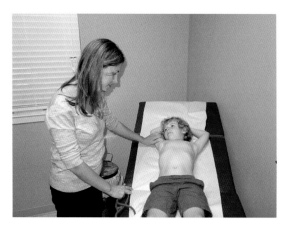

Inspect the abdomen

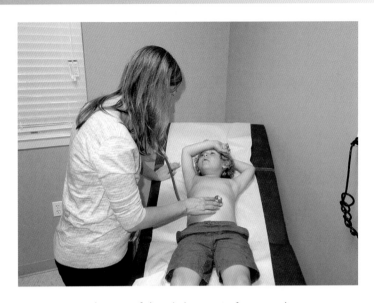

Auscultation of the abdomen in four quadrants

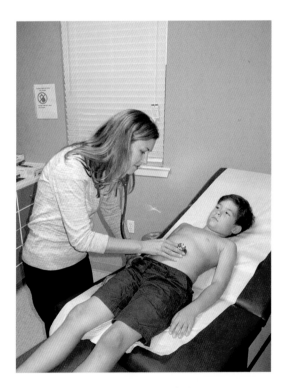

Auscultation of the abdomen

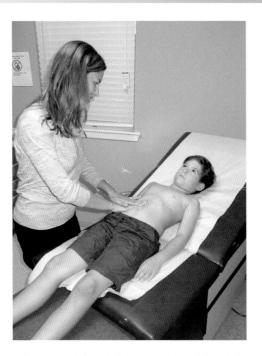

Palpation of the abdomen in the older child

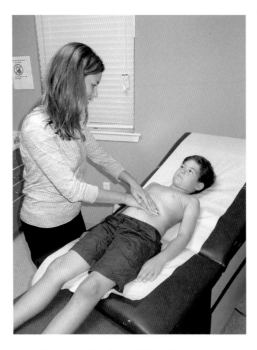

Deep palpation of the abdomen

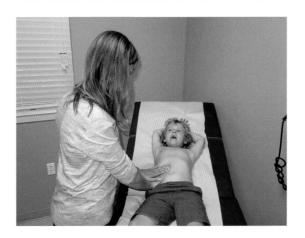

Palpation of the liver

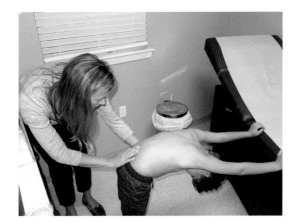

Assess the spine in the older child

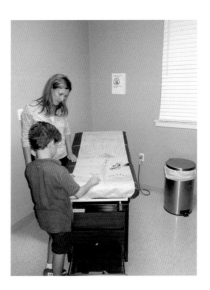

Observe how the child plays

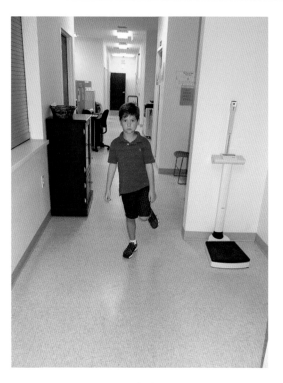

Assess balance

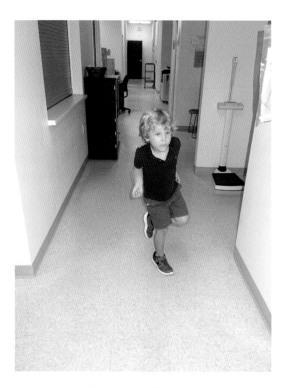

Assess coordination

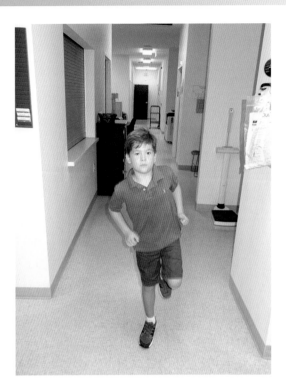

Assess jumping

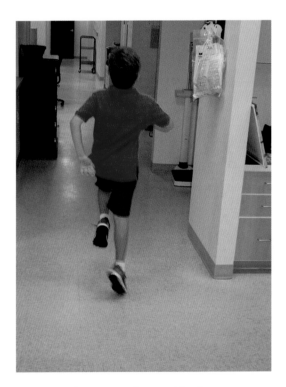

Assess running or skipping

Physical Examination of the Young Person

System	Normal variants	Abnormal variants
General appearance • Hygiene • Dress • Behaviour, mobility • Gross/fine motor skills • Speech • Nutritional status • Weight • Height **Vital signs (observations)** • Temperature • Apical pulse • Respiratory rate • BP	• Well-nourished young person in no apparent distress • Parent/carer may or may not be present (as young person prefers) • Weight gain (females) from age 10 to 14 years ~ 17.5 kg – PLOT • Weight gain (males) from age 12 to 16 years ~ 23.7 kg – PLOT • Height gain (females) from 11 to 15 years height ~ 16 cm; 95% of adult height achieved by menarche – PLOT • Height gain (males) from 12 to 16 years ~ 22 cm; 95% of adult height achieved by 16 years – PLOT • Growth can be characterised by rapid gains with endocrine and hormonal changes, increased bone growth and muscle mass • Females typically double their body weight between 8 and 15 years of age • Males double their body weight between 10 and 17 years of age • Steady gains along predictable trajectory • Vital signs within expected range	• Distressed appearance • Homelessness • Intoxication or under the influence of drugs • Dysmorphic features, facies, and/or movements • Foul or unusual odour from young person • Weight loss or failure to gain weight • Wide discrepancy between height and weight • Vital signs outside of expected range
Skin, nails, hair, head, neck, lymph nodes, eyes, ears, nose, mouth, and throat	• Skin, nails, hair, head, neck, lymph nodes, eyes, ears, nose, and throat as adult • Note: acne: location, severity, extent, type (comedones, pustules, cysts), healing or active and any other lesions (peak at 14–16 for girls and 16–19 in boys) • Mouth – underside of teeth without pitting	• Severe acne: cysts, nodules, severe pustules • Pitting, erosion of enamel related to bulimia (exposure of teeth to stomach acids)
Breasts/chest	• **Male:** gynaecomastia is common finding in young males, often presents as tender nodule and may persist for several years • **Female:** young females may present with cystic changes or fibroadenomas • Tanner staging of female breasts (Sexual Maturity Rating) • Asymmetry in female breast development common	• Variation in shape, symmetry, or movement • Cysts or nodule lesion that persists at midpoint of menstrual cycle may require investigation • Breast development < 8 years of age requires evaluation • No female breast development by 13 years of age requires evaluation

(Continued)

System	Normal variants	Abnormal variants
Pulmonary (respiratory)	• As adult	• As adult
Cardiovascular	• As adult • 20–40% of young people with precordial murmur (evaluate as for children)	• As adult • Murmur without qualities of innocent or functional murmurs
Abdomen	• As adult	• As adult

Musculoskeletal	• As adult
	• Scoliosis screen (standing upright and bent forwards):
	  ○ symmetrical appearance to posterior ribs
	  ○ equal elevation of shoulders, scapulae, and iliac crests
	  ○ no areas of prominence on one side of back
		• As adult
		• Asymmetry of ribs, shoulders, scapulae, or areas of the back

Neurological	• As adult	• As adult

Genitourinary	• **Male:** Sexual Maturity Rating:
	  ○ enlargement of testes
	  ○ pubic hair growth (Tanner staging of pubic hair growth)
	  ○ darkening of scrotal colour
	  ○ roughening of scrotal skin
	  ○ increase in penile length and width
	  ○ axillary hair growth
	• **Female:** Sexual Maturity Rating:
	  ○ presence of pubic hair (Tanner staging of pubic hair growth)
	  ○ axillary hair
	  ○ darkening/dulling of genitalia mucosa
	  ○ –pelvic exam indicated in history of sexual activity
		• **Male:** no development of secondary sex characteristics by 14 years
		• **Female:** no development of secondary sex characteristics by 13 years

Rectum/anus	• As adult (internal examination rarely indicated)	• As adult

Aylott 2007a, b; Aylott 2006a, b; Barnes 2003; Bickley 2016, Bickley and Szilagyi 2007, 2013; Epstein et al. 2008; Japp and Robertson 2013; Jarvis 2015

Case Study of a 24-Month-Old Female with Croup (Laryngotracheobronchitis)

Presenting Problem/History

A 24-month-old female was brought to Urgent Care by her mother who states, 'She has had a cold (runny nose, cough, and low-grade fever) for —three to four days. Last night she would not settle down to go to bed and had to sit up to relax and breathe. The more anxious she got, the more her cough sounded like she was barking.' The mother indicated the patient is a healthy child with no history of asthma or other chronic illnesses and is up to date on her immunizations except that she has not received the flu vaccine. The patient attends day care five days per week whilst her mother works.

Differential Diagnosis

Upper respiratory infection, croup, laryngitis, asthma, partial upper airway obstruction, epiglottitis

Assessment

Vitals: BP: 104/58, P: 130, T: 38.5 °C (rectal), RR: 34, SAO2: 96%; Wt: 12.7 kg

Skin: warm to the touch; moist, pink, with good mobility and turgor; no rashes.

Head, Eyes, Ears, Nose, and Throat (HEENT): Eyes, no redness or drainage. Ears, with no redness, tenderness, or swelling noted. Nose, congested with clear nasal drainage; no nasal flaring noted. Throat, slight erythema present; tonsils normal; tongue, oral mucosa, and lips are pink.

Neck: no lymphadenopathy or tenderness

Cardiovascular: No murmurs

Respiratory: 'barking' cough; some stridor on inspiration, no retractions of the chest wall noted; hoarse voice

Neuro: Appears somewhat anxious, but alert

Gastrointestinal/GU: Abdomen is soft and tender, no guarding. Mother states that patient's appetite has decreased. The patient is wearing a diaper, and mother states no changes noted in urine or stool.

Diagnosis

Croup

Treatment Plan

- CXR to confirm diagnosis
- Patient may need a glucocorticoid or epinephrine to help decrease airway swelling if symptoms do not improve or worsen
- May give acetaminophen or ibuprofen for fever/pain related to cough
- Keep child well hydrated
- Try a steam shower for coughing: sit with child in the bathroom with hot shower running (keep child away from hot water) and have child breathe in the humidified air to help with cough
- Cool-mist humidifier at night
- Important to keep the patient calm, as anxiety can increase/worsen symptoms
- Good handwashing, cover cough, and limit contact with other people
- Clean toys and let day care know.

References

Altdoeffer, K. and Maley, M. (2017). Pediatric and adolescent review (2017). In: *Lippincott Certificatiom Review: Family Nurse Practitioner & Adult-Gerontology Nurse Practitioner* (ed. A. Rundio and W. Lorman), 410–411. New York: Wolters Kluwer.

Aylott, M. (2006a). Developing rigour in observation of the sick child: part 1. *Paediatric Nursing* 18 (8): 38–44.

Aylott, M. (2006b). Observing the sick child: part 2. *Paediatric Nursing* 18 (9): 38–44.

Aylott, M. (2007a). Observing the sick child: part 2b respiratory palpation. *Paediatric Nursing* 19 (1): 38–45.

Aylott, M. (2007b). Observing the sick child: part 2c respiratory auscultation. *Paediatric Nursing* 19 (3): 38–45.

Ball, J., Dains, J., Flynn, J. et al. (2014a). *Seidel's Guide to Physical Examination*, 8e. St. Louis: Mosby.

Ball, J., Dains, J., Flynn, J. et al. (2014b). *Student Laboratory Manual to Accompany Seidel's Guide to Physical Examination*, 8e. St. Louis: Mosby.

Barnes, K. (1998). *Lecture Notes on A Developmental Approach to the Assessment of the Paediatric Patient*. London: City University London.

Barnes, K. (2003). *Paediatrics: A Clinical Guide for Nurse Practitioners*. London: Butterworth Heinemann.

Barnes, K. and Smart, F. (2003). A developmental approach to the history and physical examination in paediatrics. In: *Paediatrics: a Clinical Guide for Nurse Practitioners* (ed. K. Barnes), 3–7. London: Butterworth Heinemann.

Bickley, L. (2016). *Bates' Guide to Physical Examination and History Taking*, 8e. Philadelphia: Lippincott.

Bickley, L. and Szilagyi, P. (2013). *Bates' Guide to Physical Examination and History Taking*, 11e. Philadelphia: Lippincott.

Bickley, L. and Szilagyi, P. (2007). *Bates' Guide to Physical Examination and History Taking*, 5e. Philadelphia: Lippincott.

Dains, J., Baumann, L., and Scheibel, P. (2015). *Advanced Health Assessment and Clinical Diagnosis in Primary Care*, 5e. St. Louis: Mosby.

Department of Health (2004) *The National Service Framework for Children, Young People and Maternity Services Core Standards: Standard 1 Promoting Health and Well-being, Identifying Needs and Intervening Early*. http://www.dh.gov.uk/en/Publicationsandstatistics/Publications/PublicationsPolicyAndGuidance/Browsable/DH_4865614 (accessed 10 June 2016).

Duderstadt, K. (2014). *Paediatric Physical Examination*, 2e. St. Louis: C. V. Mosby Company.

Engle, J. (2002). *Paediatric Assessment*, 4e. London: Mosby.

Epstein, O., Perkin, G., de Bono, D., and Cookson, J. (2008). *Clinical Examination*, 4e. London: Mosby.

Gill, D. and O'Brien, N. (2007). *Paediatric Clinical Examination Made Easy*, 5e. Edinburgh: Churchill Livingstone.

Japp, A. and Robertson, C. (2013). *Macleod's Clinical Diagnosis*. Edinburgh: Churchill Livingstone, Elsevier.

Jarvis, C. (2015). *Physical Examination and Health Assessment*, 7e. Edinburgh: Elsevier.

Sawyer, S.S. (2012). *Pediatric Physical Examination and Health Assessment*. London: Jones and Bartlett Learning International.

Seidel, H., Ball, J., Dains, J., and Benedict, G. (2010). *Mosby's Physical Examination Handbook*, 7e. St. Louis: Mosby-Year Book.

Talley, N. and O'Connor, S. (2014). *Clinical Examination: a Systematic Guide to Physical Diagnosis*, 7e. London: Churchill Livingstone, Elsevier.

Todd, S. and Barnes, K. (2003). Anatomical and physiological differences in paediatrics. In: *Paediatrics: a Clinical Guide for Nurse Practitioners* (ed. K. Barnes), 8–11. London: Butterworth Heinemann.

Chapter 15

Assessment of Disability Including Care of the Older Adult

Carol Lynn Cox and Brandy Lunsford

General Examination

Introduction

It is important, particularly in the older adult, to assess whether the patient has a disability. The older adult requires a lot of attention. Not only is depression a prevalent factor, but, according to Swartz (2006, 2014) and Antimisiaris and Morton (2017), older adults are faced with changes in their self-image and the way they are perceived by others. The nurse must never assume that the older adults' complaints are 'natural for their age' (Swartz 2006: 42). The nurse should question whether the complaint:

- interferes with normal life and aspirations
- makes the patient dependent on others
- requires temporary assistance for specific problems
- occasional or regular assistance long term
  - supervised accommodation
  - assisted living accommodation
- nursing home with 24-hour care

It is necessary to assess the following in a patient:

- ability to do day-to-day functions
- mental ability, including confusion or dementia (consideration should be given to Alzheimer's disease; see Appendix G)
- emotional state and drive
  The descriptive terms used for disability have specific definitions in a World Health Organization Classification (WHO 1980).
- Impairment – any loss or abnormality of anatomical, physiological, or psychological function, i.e. systems or parts of body that do not work.

Physical Assessment for Nurses and Healthcare Professionals, Third Edition. Edited by Carol Lynn Cox.
© 2019 John Wiley & Sons Ltd. Published 2019 by John Wiley & Sons Ltd.

- Disability – any restrictions or lack of ability (due to an impairment) to perform an activity within the range considered normal, e.g. activities that cannot be done.
- Handicap – a limitation of normal occupation because of impairment or disability, e.g. social consequences.

Thus:

- A hemiparesis is an impairment.
- An inability to wash or dress is a disability.
- An inability to do an occupation is a handicap.

It is important to note that disability and handicap are not always given due attention and are the practical and social aspects of the disease process. It is a mistake if the nurse is preoccupied by impairments, because the patient often perceives disability as the major problem.

The impairments, disability, and handicap should have been covered in a normal history and examination, but it can be helpful to bring together important facts to provide an overall assessment.

A summary description of a patient may include the following.

- aetiology
- familial hypercholesterolaemia
- pathology
- atheroma
- right middle cerebral artery thrombosis
- impairment
- left hemiparesis
- paralysed left arm, fixed in flexion
  - upper motor neuron signs in left arm and face
  - hearing loss/deafness
- disability
- difficulty during feeding
- cannot drive car
- handicap
- can no longer work as a travelling salesman
- embarrassed to socialise
- social circumstances
- partner can cope with day-to-day living, but lack of income from occupation and withdrawal from society present major problems (Ball et al. 2014a, b; Bickley and Szilagyi 2007, 2013; Collins-Bride and Saxe 2013; Dains et al. 2012, 2015; Japp and Robertson 2013; Jarvis 2015; Kane et al. 2013; Muché 2017; Reuben et al. 2014; Rundio and Lorman 2017; Talley and O'Connor 2006, 2014; Thompson 2002).

Assessment of Impairment

The routine history and examination will often reveal impairments. Additional standard clinical measures are often used to assist quantification, e.g.:

- treadmill exercise test
- peak flow meter
- Medical Research Council scale of muscle power
- making five-pointed star from matches (to detect dyspraxia in hepatic encephalopathy)

Questionnaires can similarly provide a semiquantitative index of important aspects of impairment and give a brief shorthand description of a patient. The role of the questionnaire is in part a checklist to make sure the key questions are asked (Rhoads and Paterson 2013).

Cognitive Function

In the older adult, impaired cognitive function can be assessed by a standard 10-point mental test score introduced by Hodkinson (1972). The test assumes normal communication skills. One mark each is given for correct answers to 10 standard questions (see Appendix C for questionnaire):

- age of patient
- time (to nearest hour)
- address given, for recall at end of test, e.g. 42 West Street or 92 Columbia Road
- recognise two people
- year (if January, the previous year is accepted)
- name of place, e.g. hospital or area of town if at home
- patient's date of birth
- start of World War I
- name of monarch in United Kingdom UK, president in United States of America (USA)
- count backwards from 20 to 1 (no errors allowed unless self-corrected)
- (check recall of address)

This scale is a basic test of gross defects of memory and orientation and is designed to detect cognitive impairment. It has the advantages of brevity, relative lack of culture-specific knowledge, and widespread use. In the older adult, 8–10 is normal, 7 is probably normal, 6 or less is abnormal.

Specific problems, such as confusion or wandering at night, are not included in the mental test score and indicate that the score is a useful checklist but not a substitute for a clinical assessment. Most dementias are associated with Alzheimer's disease in 50–85% of cases or vascular multi-infarct dementia in 10–20% of cases (Antimisiaris and Morton 2017; Bickley and Szilagyi 2007, 2013). Dementia frequently has a slow insidious onset and families and clinicians may not detect it especially in the early stages of cognitive impairment (see Appendix H). You should look for problems with memory early on and then for changes in cognitive function and/or activities of daily living (ADLs) later on. Take note when a family member mentions or complains about new or unusual behaviour, and investigate any possible contributing factors such as medications, depression, metabolic abnormalities, or other medical and psychiatric conditions (Bickley and Szilagyi 2007, 2013; Seidel et al. 2006, 2010; Swartz 2006, 2014).

Affect and Drive

Motivation is an important determinant of successful rehabilitation. Depression, accompanied by lack of motivation, is a major cause of disability. In older adults depression is often underdiagnosed and undertreated. Asking the question: 'Do you often feel sad or depressed?' is 'approximately 80% sensitive and specific'; therefore positive responses should indicate the need for further investigation' (Bickley and Szilagyi 2007:408–409).

Enquire about symptoms of depression and relevant examination, e.g. 'How is your mood? Have you lost interest in things?'

Making appropriate lifestyle changes, recruiting help from friends or relatives, can be key to increasing motivation. Pharmaceutical treatment of depression can also be helpful.

Assessment of Hearing

According to Bickley and Szilagyi (2007, 2013) more than one-third of adults over the age of 65 have detectable hearing deficits. The Royal National Institute for Deaf People (RNID) indicates that around the age of 50 the proportion of deaf people begins to increase sharply and that by the age of 60, 55% are deaf or hard of hearing RNID (2015). Being deaf or hard of hearing means different things to different people. Many older adults will not notice that their hearing has deteriorated until considerable hearing loss has occurred. Commonly, older adults develop an ability to lip read to a degree as their hearing deteriorates. It has been estimated that there are nine million deaf and hard of hearing people in the UK. This number is rising as the number of people over the age of 60 increases (RNID). Most of the nine million deaf and hard of hearing people in the UK have developed a hearing loss as they have grown older. Presbycusis is the term used for age-related hearing loss. It is the most common type of deafness in older adults (RNID).

There are two primary types of deafness:

- conductive deafness, where sound has difficulty passing through the outer or middle ear
- sensorineural deafness, where the cause of deafness is in the cochlea or hearing nerve.

According to the RNID (2015) some people may have the same type and degree of hearing loss in each ear whilst for others it may be different in each ear. It is recommended that a hearing test is conducted to identify the type of deafness a person has. Older adults who need hearing aids should be told they can get them free of charge on the National Health Service (RNID).

Assessment of Disability

Assessing restrictions to daily activities is often the key to successful management.

- Make a list of disabilities separate from other problems, e.g. diagnoses, symptoms, impairments, social problems.

This list can assist with setting priorities, including which investigations or therapies are most likely to be of benefit to the patient.

Activities of Daily Living (ADL)

These are key functions which in the older adult affect the degree of independence. Several scales of disability have been used. One of these, the Barthel index of ADL, records the following disabilities that can affect self-care and mobility (see Appendix D for questionnaire):

- continence – urinary and faecal
- ability to use toilet
- grooming
- feeding
- dressing
- bathing
- transfer, e.g. chair to bed
- walking
- using stairs

The assessment denotes the current state and not the underlying cause or the potential improvement. It does not include cognitive functions or emotional state. It emphasises independence, so a catheterised patient who can competently manage the device achieves the full score for urinary continence. The total score provides an overall estimate or summary of dependence, but between-patient comparisons are difficult as they may have different combinations of disability. Interpretation of score depends on disability and facilities available.

Instrumental Activities of Daily Living (IADL)

These are slightly more complex activities relating to an individual's ability to live independently. They often require special assessment in the home environment:

- preparing a meal
- doing light housework
- using transport
- managing money
- shopping
- doing laundry
- taking medications
- using a telephone

Communication

In the older adult, difficulty in communication is a frequent problem, and impairment of the following may need special attention:

- deafness (do the ears need syringing? is a hearing aid required?)
- speech (is dysarthria due to lack of teeth?)
- an alarm to call for help when required
- aids for reading, e.g. spectacles, magnifying glass
- adaptation of doorbell, telephone, radio, or television

Analysing Disabilities and Handicaps and Setting Objectives

After writing a list of disabilities, it is necessary to develop a possible treatment plan with specific objectives. The plan needs to be realistic. A multidisciplinary team approach, including social workers, physiotherapists, occupational therapists, nurses, and doctors, is essential in the rehabilitation of older adult patients.

The overall aims in treating the older adult include the following:

- to make diagnoses, if feasible, particularly to treatable illnesses
- to comfort and alleviate problems and stresses, even if one cannot cure
- to add life to years, even if one cannot add years to life

Specific aspects which may need attention include the following:

- alleviate social problems if feasible
- improve heating, clothing, toilet facilities, cooking facilities
- arrange support services, e.g. help with shopping, provision of meals, attendance at day centre
- arrange regular visits from district/public health nurse or other helper
- make sure family, neighbours, and friends understand the situation
- treat depression
- help with sorting out finances
- provide aids, e.g.
- large-handled implements
- walking frame or stick
- slip-on shoes
- handles by bath or toilet
- aids/assistance to keep as mobile as feasible

- facilitate visits to hearing-aid centre, optician, chiropodist, dentist
- ensure medications are kept to a minimum, and the instructions and packaging are suitable

A major problem is if the disability leads to the patient being unwelcome. This depends on the reactions of others and requires tactful discussion with all concerned.

Identifying Causes for Disabilities

Specific disabilities may have specific causes which can be alleviated. In the older adult, common problems include the following:

Confusion

This is an impairment. Common causes are:

- infection, e.g. urinary tract
- drugs
- other illnesses, e.g. heart failure
- sensory deprivation, e.g. deafness, inability to see, darkness

Assume all confusion is an acute response to an unidentified cause.

Incontinence
- toilet too far away, e.g. upstairs
- physical restriction of gait
- urinary infection
- stress incontinence
- faecal impaction
- Parkinson's disease
- stroke
- uterine prolapse
- diabetes

'Off legs'
- neurological impairment
- unsuspected fracture of leg
- depressed
- general illness, e.g. infection, heart failure, renal failure, hypothermia, hypothyroid, diabetes, hypokalaemia (Antimisiaris and Morton 2017; Muché 2017)

Falls
- rugs that are not secure
- dark stairs
- poor vision, e.g. cataracts
- postural hypotension
- cardiac arrhythmias
- epilepsy
- neurological deficit, e.g. Parkinson's disease, hemiparesis
- cough or micturition syncope
- use of alcohol or opiates

References

Antimisiaris, D. and Morton, L. (2017). *Geriatrics, An Issue of Primary Care: Clinics in Office Practice*, 1e. Louisville: Elsevier.

Ball, J., Dains, J., Flynn, J. et al. (2014a). *Seidel's Guide to Physical Examination*, 8e. St. Louis: Mosby.

Ball, J., Dains, J., Flynn, J. et al. (2014b). *Student Laboratory Manual to Accompany Seidel's Guide to Physical Examination*, 8e. St. Louis: Mosby.

Bickley, L. and Szilagyi, P. (2007). *Bates' Guide to Physical Examination and History Taking*, 9e. Philadelphia: Lippincott.

Bickley, L. and Szilagyi, P. (2013). *Bates' Guide to Physical Examination and History Taking*, 11e. New York: Wolters Kluwer/Lippincott Williams & Wilkins.

Collins-Bride, G. and Saxe, J. (2013). *Clinical Guidelines for Advanced Practice Nursing – An Interdisciplinary Approach*, 2e. Burlington, MA: Jones and Bartlett Learning.

Dains, J., Baumann, L., and Scheibel, P. (2012). *Advanced Health Assessment and Clinical Diagnosis in Primary Care*, 4e. St Louis: Elsevier.

Dains, J., Baumann, L., and Scheibel, P. (2015). *Advanced Health Assessment and Clinical Diagnosis in Primary Care*, 5e. St. Louis: Mosby.

Hodkinson, H. (1972). Evaluation of a mental test score for assessment of mental impairment in the elderly. *Age and Ageing* 1: 233–238.

Japp, A. and Robertson, C. (2013). *Macleod's Clinical Diagnosis*. Edinburgh: Churchill Livingstone, Elsevier.

Jarvis, C. (2015). *Physical Examination and Health Assessment*, 7e. Edinburgh: Elsevier.

Kane, R., Ouslander, J., Abrass, A., and Resnick, B. (2013). *Essentials of Clinical Geriatrics*, 7e. New York: McGraw-Hill.

Muché, J.A. (2017). Geriatric Rehabilitation. https://emedicine.medscape.com/article/318521-overview (accessed 28 January 2018).

RNID (2015). Hearing Matters Report. https://www.actiononhearingloss.org.uk/how-we-help/information-and-resources/publications/research-reports/hearing-matters-report (accessed 2 September 2018).

Reuben, D., Herr, K., Pacala, J. et al. (2014). *Geriatrics at Your Fingertips*, 16e. New York: The American Geriatrics Society.

Rhoads, J. and Paterson, S. (2013). *Advanced Health Assessment and Diagnostic Reasoning*, 2e. Burlington: Jones and Bartlett.

Rundio, A. and Lorman, W. (2017). *Lippincott Certification Review: Family Nurse Practitioner & Adult-Gerontology Nurse Practitioner*. London: Wolters Kluwer.

Seidel, H., Ball, J., Dains, J., and Benedict, G. (2010). *Mosby's Physical Examination Handbook*, 7e. St. Louis: Mosby-Year Book.

Seidel, H., Ball, J., Dains, J., and Benedict, G. (2006). *Mosby's Physical Examination Handbook*. St. Louis: Mosby.

Swartz, M. (2014). *Physical Diagnosis: History and Examination*, With Student Consult Online Access, 7e. London: Elsevier.

Swartz, M. (2006). *Physical Diagnosis, History and Examination*, 5e. London: W. B. Saunders.

Talley, N. and O'Connor, S. (2014). *Clinical Examination: A Systematic Guide to Physical Diagnosis*, 7e. London: Churchill Livingstone, Elsevier.

Talley, N. and O'Connor, S. (2006). *Clinical Examination: A Systematic Guide to Physical Diagnosis*, 5e. London: Churchill Livingstone.

Thompson, S. (2002). Older people. In: *Loss and Grief* (ed. N. Thompson), 162–173. Basingstoke: Palgrave.

WHO (1980). *International Classification of Impairments, Disabilities, and Handicaps*. Geneva: World Health Organization.

Chapter 16

Imaging Techniques, Clinical Investigations, and Interpretation

Jennifer Edie

General Procedures

Introduction

This chapter begins with a general description of the main techniques used in imaging and clinical investigations. It addresses the basic principles of diagnostic imaging techniques and is followed by additional specialised investigations in cardiology (supported by Chapter 4), respiratory medicine (supported by Chapter 5), gastroenterology (supported by Chapter 6), and urology and neurology (supported by Chapters 7, 9, and 10).

Diagnostic Imaging

Diagnostic imaging consists of a range of procedures and use of sophisticated equipment to produce high-quality images to view various body organs and systems that aid identification, evaluation, monitoring, and management of disease processes, soft tissue and skeletal abnormalities, and trauma.

The range of techniques includes:

- Ultrasound – uses high-frequency sound. This technique is increasingly used in obstetrics, including foetal monitoring throughout pregnancy, gynaecology, abdominal, paediatrics, cardiac, vascular, and musculoskeletal;
- Plain film radiography – uses X-rays to look through tissue to examine bones, cavities, and foreign objects;
- Fluoroscopy – uses X-rays to image body structures providing a real-time image;
- Angiography – to investigate blood vessels and organ perfusion after injecting a contrast agent which aids visualisation of the cardiovascular system
- Computed tomography (CT) – uses X-rays to provide cross-sectional views (slices) of the body;
- Magnetic resonance imaging (MRI) – builds a two-dimensional (2D) map of different tissue types within the body;

Physical Assessment for Nurses and Healthcare Professionals, Third Edition. Edited by Carol Lynn Cox.
© 2019 John Wiley & Sons Ltd. Published 2019 by John Wiley & Sons Ltd.

- Interventional procedures specialist imaging procedures used to investigate and treat conditions such as vascular disease, cancer, and biopsies of various structures. These procedures can be undertaken using a variety of imaging methods. These procedures can be undertaken using a variety of imaging methods, usually ultrasound, fluoroscopy, angiography, or CT.
- Nuclear medicine (sometimes referred to as radionuclide imaging) – uses radioactive pharmaceuticals which can be administered to examine how the body and organs function.

Ultrasound

High-frequency (2.5–10 MHz) ultrasound waves are produced by the piezoelectric effect within ultrasound transducers. These transducers, which both produce and receive sound waves, are moved over the skin surface or inserted into various body cavities, and images of the underlying organ structures are produced from the reflected sound waves. Structures with very few interfaces, such as fluid-filled structures, allow through transmission of the sound waves and therefore appear black on the screen. Structures with a large number of interfaces, such as soft tissues, cause significant reflection and refraction of the sound waves and therefore appear as varying shades of grey. Dense structures, such as bone, reflect most sound and appear white on the screen. Air causes almost complete attenuation of the sound wave and therefore structures deep to this cannot be visualised because air is not dense like bone, solid tumours, or organs for example.

Ultrasound scanning is a real-time examination and is dependent on the experience of the operator for its accuracy. The diagnosis is made from the real-time examination, although a permanent record of findings can be recorded onto digital storage media. 2D ultrasound image shows anatomical structure and pathology whilst Doppler ultrasound demonstrates blood flow and organ perfusion.

The technique has the advantage of being safe, using nonionising radiation, being repeatable, painless, and requiring little, if any, preparation of the patient. It is also possible to carry out the examination at the patient's bedside and to evaluate a series of organs in a relatively short period of time. For these reasons, it is often used as a first-line imaging method before other procedures are requested.

Ultrasound is used in many different situations, including the following.

Abdomen/Pelvis

- liver – tumours, abscesses, diffuse liver disease, dilated bile ducts, hepatic vasculature
- gall bladder – gallstones, gall bladder wall pathology (Figure 16.1)
- pancreas – tumours, cysts, pancreatitis
- kidneys – size, hydronephrosis, tumours, stones, scarring
- spleen – size, focal abnormalities
- ovaries – size, cysts, tumours
- uterus – pregnancy, tumours, endometrium
- aorta – aneurysm
- bowel – inflammation, tumours, abscesses
- bladder – size, tumours
- prostate – size, tumours

Brain

- possible in the infant before the anterior fontanelle closes; carotid and vertebral artery to investigate blood flow to brain in cases of TIA, atherosclerotic disease

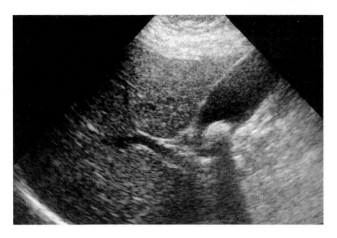

Figure 16.1   Ultrasound scan showing a stone within gall bladder, casting an acoustic shadow.

Heart
- cardiac anatomy, function, heart disease

Blood Vessels
- aneurysms, stenosis, clots in veins

Neck
- thyroid – characterisation of masses

Scrotum
- tumours, inflammation, trauma

Musculoskeletal
- joint effusions, soft-tissue masses, sports injuries

Breast
- tumours, characterisation of masses

Plain Film Radiography

A radiograph is an image of the internal structures of the body and is produced by exposure to radiation (X-rays) with the image being recorded on a film or in digital form and displayed on a computer screen

Conventional X-rays visualise four basic radiographic densities: air, metal, fat, and water. Air densities are black; metal densities (the most common of which are calcium and barium) are white with well-defined edges; fat and water densities are dark and midgrey.

There can be difficulty in visualising a three-dimensional (3D) structure from a 2D film. One helpful rule in deciding where a lesion is situated is to note which, if any, adjacent normal landmarks are obliterated. For example, a water density lesion that obliterates the right border of the heart must lie in the right middle lobe and not the lower lobe. A different view, e.g. lateral chest radiograph, is needed to be certain of the position of densities.

Apart from skeletal imaging of limbs and spine, the most common radiographic examinations are the chest radiograph and abdominal radiograph.

Chest Radiograph

Use a systematic approach to evaluate the image.

- Posteroanterior (PA) chest radiograph is the standard view (anteroposterior (AP) is done only when the patient is in a bed) (Figure 16.2). The correct name for the usual chest study is 'a PA chest radiograph'. This means that the anteriorly situated heart is as close to the film as possible and its image will be minimally enlarged. Generally, this view is taken with the patient standing facing towards the X-ray film
- When reviewing the image (Figure 16.3) follow a logical progression from centre of film to periphery.
  - Interfaces are seen only in silhouette when adjacent tissues have different attenuation properties of X-rays; thus the heart border becomes invisible when there is collapse or consolidation in adjacent lung

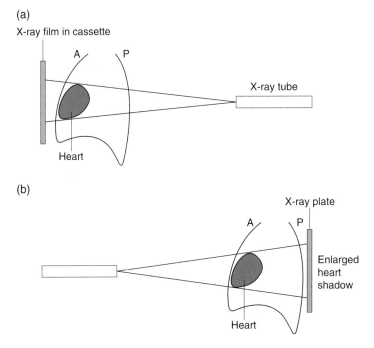

Figure 16.2   (a) A normal posteroanterior (PA) chest radiograph; (b) An anteroposterior (AP) chest radiograph of patient in bed.

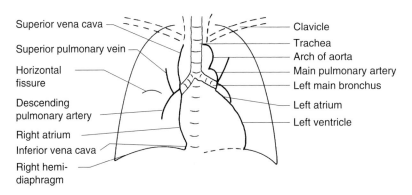

Figure 16.3   Outline of cardiothoracic structures that may be visualised on a chest radiograph. Review particularly lungs, apices, costophrenic angles, hilar, behind heart.

- Technical factors
  - positioning – apices and costophrenic angles should be on the film
  - inspiration – at least six posterior ribs seen above right diaphragm
  - penetration –midcardiac intervertebral disc spaces visible
  - rotation – medial end of clavicles equidistant from spinous processes
  - note any catheters, tubes, pacing wires, pneumothorax
- Heart
  - size
    - normal < 50% cardiothoracic ratio (maximum diameter heart maximum internal diameter of thoracic ribs as percent)
    - males < 15.5 cm, females < 15 cm diameter
  - shape – any chamber enlarged?
    - PA radiograph: LV and RA
    - lateral radiograph: RV and LA
  - calcification – in valves (better seen on lateral chest X-ray) or arteries
- Pericardium
  - globular suggests pericardial effusion (general examination of the patient will show distended neck veins and muffled heart sounds)
  - calcification suggests tuberculosis
- Aorta
  - large in aneurysms, small in atrial septal defect
  - calcification in intima, > 6 mm inside outer wall suggests dissection
- Mediastinum
  - ? widening – look at lateral chest X-ray to locate
- Hila
  - right at horizontal fissure, left 0–2.5 cm higher
    - displacement suggests loss of lung volume, e.g. *collapse, fibrosis*
  - enlargement
    - if lobulated – a mass or lymph nodes
    - ? vascular dilation
  - density – ? mass projected over hilum
- Pulmonary vessels
  - large in intracardiac or peripheral shunts – prominent in outer third (plethora)
  - large in *pulmonary hypertension* with small vessels in outer third (pruning) – *shunts, hypoxia, emboli, chronic lung disease*
  - segmental avascularity – *pulmonary emboli*
  - small in *congenital heart disease, right ventricular/pulmonary artery atresia*
- Lung parenchyma
  - lungs should be equally transradiant (black)
  - alveolar shadows – ill defined or confluent and dense
    - air bronchogram – water, pus, blood, tumour around patent bronchi, often seen end on, as a circle, near hila
  - nodular shadows, e.g. *granuloma, tuberculosis*
  - reticular shadows – *fibrotic lung disease;* note uniformity, symmetry, unilateral or bilateral, upper or lower zones.
  - masses
    - define position (request lateral chest radiograph), edge, shape, size
    - *tumour, abscess, embolus, infection*
- Pleura
  - fluid
    - homogeneous, opaque shadow, usually with lateral meniscus
    - if air–fluid interface, *empyema* or after thoracocentesis

- o pneumothorax
  - — peripheral space devoid of markings with edge of lung visible
  - — look for mediastinal (shift) displacement – *tension pneumothorax*
- o masses
  - — lobulated shadows – loculated fluid or tumour
- Skeleton
  - o sclerosis, focal – ? *metastases*, e.g. *breast, prostate, stomach, kidney, thyroid, lymphoma*
    - — *myelofibrosis, Paget's disease*
  - o lytic – ? *metastases, e.g. lung, colorectal, myeloma*
  - o osteopenia (only visible when advanced) – osteoporosis and osteomalacia cannot be distinguished on radiographs, except Looser's zones (pseudofracture) in osteomalacia
  - o look for fractures
- Other areas
  - o hiatus hernia, behind heart
  - o left lower lobe collapse (pneumothorax), behind heart
  - o lungs behind dome of diaphragm
  - o gas below diaphragm on erect chest radiograph – *perforated viscus, recent surgery*
  - o apices – ? lung visible above clavicle

Abdominal Radiograph

388

This is less satisfactory than chest radiography because there are fewer contrasting densities as most of the tissues being imaged are soft tissues. Air in the gut is helpful, as are the psoas lines. Try to find as many organ outlines as possible.

- supine (AP) radiograph is the standard view.
- erect radiograph:
  - o for air–fluid levels (AFLs)
  - o < five short AFLs normal
  - o many – *obstruction*
  - o also in *paralytic ileus, coeliac disease, jejunal diverticula*
- Visceral organs (Figure 16.4)
  - o liver
    - — usually < 18 cm long – inferior surface outlined by fat
    - — ? gas in biliary tree centrally
  - o spleen – enlargement displaces stomach gas bubble to midline
  - o kidneys – normally 3–3.5 vertebrae long

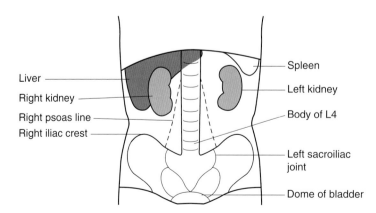

Figure 16.4　Outline of visceral organs that may be visualised on an abdominal radiograph.

- Bowel gas pattern
  - stomach
    - normally small air bubble (gastric bubble)
    - dilated in *pyloric stenosis* and *proximal small-bowel obstruction*
  - small bowel
    - central position
    - small loops, valvulae across lumen, no faeces
    - dilated when > 3.5 cm proximally, > 2.5 cm distally – suggests *obstruction*
  - large bowel
    - vertical in flanks and across top of abdomen
    - wider loops, haustral folds do not cross lumen +/− faeces
    - dilated when > 5.5 cm – suggests obstruction
    - > 9 cm – suggests perforation risk
    - hernial orifices – ? bowel air pattern below femoral neck indicates hernia
- Abnormal gas
  - pneumoperitoneum
  - both sides of bowel defined as thin lines
  - loss of liver density from gas anteriorly
  - bowel wall – thin streaks of gas suggest infarction or gas-producing bacteria
- Abnormal calcification
  - 30% of gallstones are radiopaque – can be anywhere in abdomen
  - pancreas calcification – follows oblique line of pancreas and suggests *chronic pancreatitis*
  - renal stones – usually radiopaque
  - nephrocalcinosis – *medullary sponge kidney* or *metabolic calcinosis*
  - in phleboliths or faecoliths in diverticulae
- Other soft tissues
  - psoas lines
    - outlined by retroperitoneal fat
    - absent in 20% of normal patients
    - unilateral absence suggests *retroperitoneal mass* or *haematoma*
  - ascites
    - uniformly grey appearance
    - bowel gas 'floats' centrally (abdominal examination shows tympani on percussion centrally with lateral dullness)

389

Fluoroscopy

Fluoroscopy is a procedure that uses radiation to produce a real-time image of parts of the body, and shows anatomy and function. In association with fluoroscopy, a contrast agent may be used to outline parts of the body which would otherwise not show up well on the images; the most common being barium studies of the GI tract and vascular studies using iodine-based contrast agents (see angiography below). Fluoroscopy can also be used to guide various interventional procedures, both vascular (e.g. angioplasty and embolisation) and nonvascular (e.g. biopsy, ablation, stone removal).

Angiography

Angiography is a procedure that uses radiation to investigate and produce a series of images of the cardiovascular system after injecting an iodine-based contrast agent, usually via a catheter in the femoral artery (Figure 16.5):

- cardiac angiography, e.g. *anatomical and functional information of cardiac chambers and valves*
- coronary arteriography, e.g. *coronary artery disease*

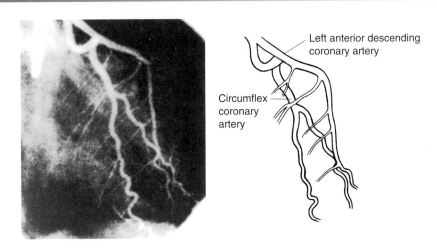

Figure 16.5   Left coronary artery angiogram viewed from right.

- cerebral angiography, e.g. *aneurysm* after *subarachnoid haemorrhage*
- carotid angiography e.g. *stenoses*
- pulmonary angiography, e.g. *pulmonary embolus* or *fistula*
- renal angiography, e.g. *renal artery stenosis, arteriovenous fistula, renal perfusion*
- aortography and iliofemoral angiography, e.g. *aortic aneurysm, iliofemoral artery atheroma*
- leg venogram, e.g. *deep venous thrombosis*

In many cases, Doppler ultrasound is used as the first-line vascular investigation before angiography is considered as it has less risk associated and does not involve the use of contrast agents or insertion of catheters. Also because of advances in technology and image acquisition times, there is increased use of CT or MRI with contrast agents to show cardiovascular structures.

Computed Tomography

CT scanning uses X-rays to take a series of images of the body and produce very detailed cross-sectional images of the inside of the body. There is an X-ray beam that rotates around the patient and an array of sensors on the opposite side that detects the amount of radiation passing through the patient (Figure 16.6). Attenuation of X-rays depends on tissue – water is arbitrary 0, black is −1000 and white is +1000 Hounsfield units. Different 'windows' are chosen to display different characteristics, e.g. soft-tissue window, lung window, bone window. CT can be used:

- for organs and masses in abdomen and thorax
- to diagnose tumours, infarcts, and bleeds in cerebral hemispheres
- for posterior fossa – lesions less easy to visualise because of bony base of skull
- to visualise disc prolapse and neoplasm in spinal cord, but adjacent bones interfere; intrathecal contrast medium is often required for cord tumours

Variants of CT:

- intravenous contrast
  - iodine based
  - opacifies blood vessels
  - shows leaky vessels or increased number of vessels

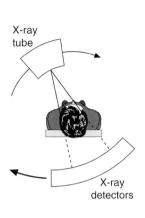

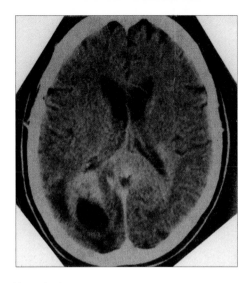

Figure 16.6   Axial CT scan across cerebral hemispheres.

- oral contrast
  - usually barium based
  - opacifies gut contents
- spiral/helical CT
  - X-ray tube constantly rotated with patient moving
  - computer segments into slices
  - advantages – faster, more detail, can use intravenous contrast medium
  - becoming the investigation of choice for pulmonary embolism
  - multislice CT which takes a number of CT 'slices' at the same time to speed up the scanning process
- CT angiography
  - evaluate the vascular system, using intravenous contrast agent and take series of images of relevant body area showing various phases of perfusion
- 3D CT
  - a series of individual CT slices can be combined to produce a 'volume' image that can be viewed as a 3D image

Magnetic Resonance Imaging

MRI uses a strong magnetic field and radiowaves to produce detailed cross-sectional images of the inside of the body. The images the scans produce are usually 2D but, in some cases, several scans can be taken to build up a 3D image that can be displayed on a computer screen. N.B. Because of the strong magnetic field patients with pacemakers should not be subjected to MRI, and patients with metal implants may not be able to undergo MRI; this must be discussed with a radiologist.

The patient is positioned within a superconducting magnet that provides a strong external magnetic field (Figure 16.7). The axes of individual hydrogen ions usually lie at random but can be lined up at a particular angle by a strong magnetic field (position 'a'). When subjected to a 2nd radiofrequency magnetic field the angle is changed (to position 'b'). When the radiowaves cease, position 'a' is restored by the continuing magnetic field and a radiowave is emitted and detected.

Hydrogen is the most plentiful element in the body. MRI can detect differences between the concentration of hydrogen ions in different tissues, notably fat (—CH_2—) and water (HOH).

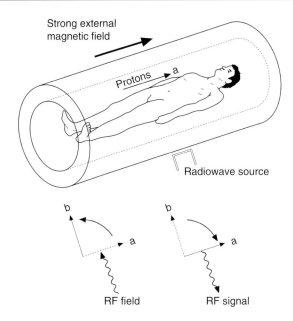

Figure 16.7   Magnetic resonance imaging.

(a)   (b)

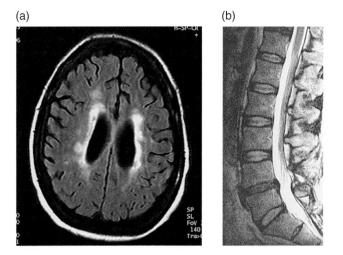

Figure 16.8   (a) MRI (axial section) of the brain. The central white areas are areas of demyelination in multiple sclerosis and subcutaneous fat is white. (b) MRI (sagittal section) of the lumbar spine showing white central spinal fluid surrounding the spinal cord.

MRI scans can show muscles, joints, bone marrow, blood vessels, nerves, and other structures within the body.

Excellent for examination of the head and spinal cord:

- the brain for demonstrating tumours, multiple areas of demyelination of white matter in multiple sclerosis (Figure 16.8), in spinal cord lesions, including disc prolapse
- bone and soft-tissue tumours

Images can be obtained using a variety of imaging sequences that accentuate different characteristics:

- spin echo T_1-weighted
  - depends on fat content of tissues, good for defining anatomy
  - fat – white (bright), myelin sheath of white matter brighter than grey matter,
  - fluid – dark, e.g. CSF
  - cortical bone – black
- spin echo T_2-weighted
  - depends on water content of tissues being imaged, good for evaluating pathology (infection, tumour, inflammation) as these lesions often contain water
  - fat – grey, so white matter darker than grey matter
  - fluid – white (bright), e.g. CSF
- proton density
  - signal intensity depends on number of protons per unit area in the tissue
  - high proton density – bright (CSF)
  - low protons – dark
- FLAIR (fluid-attenuated inversion recovery) sequence
  - similar to T2 but bright signal from CSF is suppressed.
- gradient echo
  - flowing blood – white
  - used for MRI angiography to evaluate the vascular system, with or without contrast agent, and no radiation exposure
- intravenous contrast
  - gadolinium based
  - leaky vessels from inflammation
  - increased number of vessels from neoplasm
- oral contrast
  - to label bowel
- intravenous contrast
  - gadolinium based
  - leaky vessels from inflammation
  - increased number of vessels from neoplasm
- oral contrast
  - to label bowel

Interventional Radiology

- Allows management of disease via minimally invasive therapy.
- Procedures done under image guidance using ultrasound, fluoroscopy, CT, or MRI.
- Vascular procedures include angioplasty (balloon dilation of vessels), stenting (metal stents to splint open vascular lumen), embolisation (to manage bleeding using coils, gel foam, etc.)
- Nonvascular procedures include biopsy (for tumour diagnosis), drain insertion, radiofrequency ablation (targeted destruction of tumour tissue), stenting (insertion of stent to hold open structure such as oesophagus, colon, bronchi), percutaneous transhepatic cholangiography (relief of biliary obstruction by dilation, stenting or drain insertion), urinary (to relieve a pelviureteric junction obstruction, extract calculi).

Nuclear Medicine

Nuclear medicine, sometimes referred to as radionuclide imaging, uses radioactive isotopes (mostly technetium 99 m) coupled to appropriate pharmaceuticals or monoclonal antibodies designed to seek out different organ systems or pathology to obtain images of the body.

A gamma camera is used to detect the radiation emitted and produces images that give functional rather than anatomical information. These isotopes can be introduced via a number of routes depending on the organs to be examined. They are sensitive, but not specific.

Lesions show up on images as either photon-abundant areas (as in bone or brain) or photon-deficient areas (as in liver, lung, hearts, etc.).

The following are the more common investigations routinely available:

- bone scan
  - any cause of increased bone turnover or altered blood flow to bone, e.g. tumour, infection, trauma, infarction.
  - used mostly for detection of metastases.
- ventilation/perfusion scans
  - diagnosis of pulmonary emboli using perfusion scintigraphy, when emboli cause defects which do not correspond to water densities in the same position on simultaneous chest radiographs.
  - usually indicated only when chronic obstructive airways disease is present.
- cardiovascular scan
  - for the measurement of ventricular function, e.g. ejection fractions, and for examining myocardial integrity.
  - ischaemia or scarring causes 'cold' areas on myocardial scintigrams.
  - studies are usually carried out at rest and after exercise (Figure 16.9).
- renal scans
  - static renal imaging provides good definition of the cortical outline and relative distribution of functional tissue.
  - dynamic renal imaging provides information relating to renal vascularity, renal function, and excretion.
- cerebral scan
  - for the detection of abnormalities associated with certain neuropsychiatric disorders, notably the dementias, schizophrenia, and epilepsy.
- thyroid scan
  - for estimation of the size, shape, and position of the gland, detecting the presence of 'hot' thyrotoxic nodules or 'cold' nodules caused by adenoma, carcinoma, cysts, haemorrhage, or any combination thereof. Iodine uptake can also be estimated simultaneously.
- other areas
  - tracers are also available for detecting certain tumours, notably lymphoma, colonic carcinoma, ovarian carcinoma, and malignant melanoma.
  - labelled red cells can detect sites of gastrointestinal bleeding. Oesophageal and gastric emptying studies are also available.

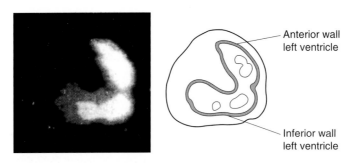

Figure 16.9   Thallium 201 study of the heart.

- Positron emission tomography (PET)
  - uses a radiotracer – 18-F-dioxyglucose (FDG) where FDG uptake correlates with glucose metabolism. Malignant tumours actively metabolise glucose making it possible to image tumours using this technique.
- Single photon emission computed tomography (SPECT)
  - Imaging that gives functional information, e.g. uptake of isotopes by tumours (which helps to identify lesions missed by other imaging techniques), myocardial perfusion, and functional brain imaging.

PET and SPECT are nuclear medicine imaging techniques that provide metabolic and functional information. Often combined with CT to produce more detailed anatomical and metabolic information (PET/CT or SPECT/CT).

Endoscopy

An endoscopy is a procedure where the internal organs are directly visualised, usually with a flexible fibreoptic endoscope. An endoscope is a thin, long, flexible tube that contains a light source and a video camera, so that images of the inside of the body can be relayed to an external monitor (screen).

Gastroscopy

A flexible scope is inserted via the patient's mouth after intravenous diazepam for direct vision of oesophagus, stomach, and duodenum. Refer to endoscopic retrograde cholangiopancreatography (ERCP) in this chapter.

Proctoscopy

With the patient lying in a left lateral position, with knees and hips flexed, a short tube is introduced through the patient's anus with a removable obturator lubricated with a gel. This is used to investigate:

- rectal bleeding – haemorrhoids or anal carcinoma.

Sigmoidoscopy

With the patient in left lateral position, either a rigid tube with a removable obturator or a flexible fibreoptic endoscope is introduced. Bowel is kept patent with air from a hand pump. This is used to investigate:

- bleeding, diarrhoea, or constipation – ulcerative colitis, other inflammatory bowel disease, or carcinoma
- inflamed area or lumps that can be biopsied.

Colonoscopy

After the bowel is emptied with an oral purgative and a washout if necessary, the whole of the colon and possibly the terminal ileum can be examined. This is used to investigate:

- bleeding, diarrhoea, or constipation – *inflammatory bowel disease, polyps,* or *carcinoma.*

Bronchoscopy

After intravenous diazepam, the major bronchi are observed. This is used to investigate:

- haemoptysis or suspected bronchial obstruction – *bronchial carcinoma* and for clearing *obstructed bronchi*, e.g. peanuts, plug of mucus.

Laparoscopy

After general anaesthetic, organs can be observed through a small abdominal incision, aspirated for cells or organisms, or biopsied. Laparoscopic surgery includes sterilisation, ova collection for *in vitro* fertilisation, and laparoscopic cholecystectomy.

Cystoscopy

After local anaesthetic, a cystoscope is inserted into the urethral meatus. This is used to investigate:

- urinary bleeding or poor flow – *bladder tumours*
- under direct vision, catheters can be inserted into ureters for retrograde pyelograms.

Colposcopy

Examination of cervix, usually to take a cervical smear. This is used to investigate:

- premalignant changes or cancer.

Needle Biopsy

Core Biopsy

A small core of tissue (30 × 1 mm) is obtained through needle puncture of organs for histological diagnosis. This is used to investigate:

- liver – *cirrhosis, alcoholic liver disease, chronic active hepatitis*
- kidney – glomerulonephritis, interstitial nephritis
- lung – *fibrosis, tumours, tuberculosis.*

Fine-Needle Aspiration

A technique to obtain cells for diagnosis of tumours or for microbiological diagnosis. The needle position is guided by ultrasound, CT scan or MRI scan. For investigation of many unexplained lumps, e.g. pancreas or breast lumps, to diagnose carcinoma.

Cardiac Investigations

Electrocardiogram

The electrocardiogram (ECG/EKG) tracings arise from the electrical changes, depolarisation, and repolarisation that accompany muscle contraction. With knowledge of the relative position of the leads to the electrodes, the ECG/EKG tracings provide direct information about the cardiac muscle and its activity (see Chapter 4). Six standard leads – I, II, II, aVR, aVL, aVF- are recorded from the limb electrodes (aV = augmented voltage) and examine the heart from the different directions Figure 16.10. The standard leads examine the heart in the vertical plane.

Chest Radiograph

X-ray of the chest, posteroanterior (PA), anteroposterior (AP), and lateral. See earlier in this chapter.

Exercise Electrocardiography (Stress Testing)

- Exercise may reveal cardiac dysfunction not apparent at rest.
- Most commonly used in suspected coronary artery disease.

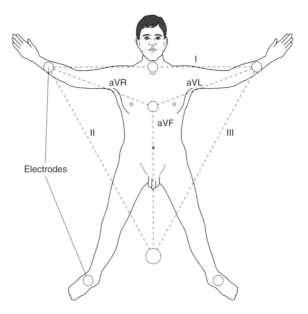

Figure 16.10   The positioning of the limb electrodes and the six standard leads.

Connected to a 12-lead electrocardiograph (ECG) machine, with resuscitation equipment available, the patient exercises at an increasing workload on a treadmill (or bicycle). Bruce protocol: three minute stages of increasing belt speed and treadmill gradient. Take ECG every minute, blood pressure every three minutes. This assesses:

- exercise capacity
- haemodynamic response
- symptoms
- ECG changes.

Exercise for as long as possible stopping when there are:

- marked symptoms
- severe ECG changes
- ventricular arrhythmias
- fall in blood pressure.

Myocardial ischaemia causes ST segment depression. A high false-positive rate occurs in absence of angina (c. 20%). False-positive incidence depends on age and sex, with young females having the highest rate, even in the presence of typical symptoms of angina.

Clinically important abnormalities are:

- horizontal or downward sloping ST depression (Figure 16.11)
- deep ST depression
- ST changes with typical anginal symptoms.

A definitely negative test at a high workload denotes an excellent prognosis.

- Angiography is indicated only if a low workload is achieved before important abnormalities occur.
- Medical treatment of angina may be appropriate if three or four stages are completed.

(a)

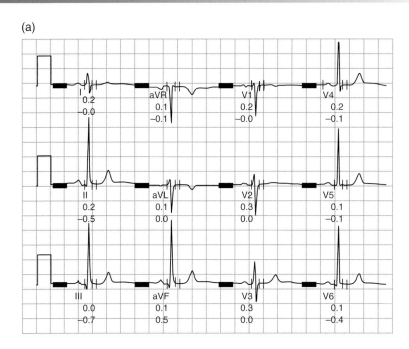

(b)

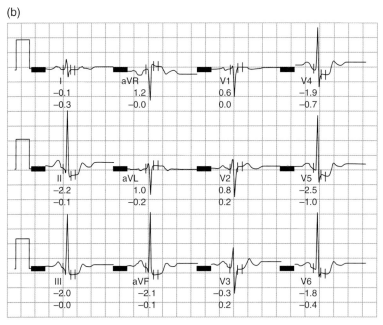

Figure 16.11   Example of a strongly positive exercise test – signal averaged recordings before exercise (a) and at peak effort (b). There is a marked horizontal ST depression in the inferolateral leads II, III, aVF, and V$_{4-6}$.

Echocardiography

This visualises structures and function of the heart. Uses ultrasound (2.5–7.5 MHz) to reflect from interfaces in the heart, e.g. ventricle and atrial walls, heart, valves, major vessels. The higher frequency gives better discrimination but lower tissue penetration. The time delay between transmission and reception indicates depth.

Two-Dimensional Echocardiography

Two-dimensional echocardiography (Figure 16.12) uses a scanning ultrasound beam that is swept backwards and forwards across a 45° or 60° arc to construct an image of the anatomy of the heart.

2D echocardiography is excellent for demonstrating:

- valvular anatomy
- ventricular function, e.g. poor contraction, low ejection fraction, akinetic segment, paradoxical motion in aneurysm
- structural abnormalities:
    - pericardial effusion
    - ventricular hypertrophy
    - congenital heart disease.

Quantifying valvular function is better achieved by Doppler echocardiography.

M-Mode Echocardiography

M-mode echocardiography (Figure 16.13) uses a single pencil beam of ultrasound, and movements of the heart in that beam are visualised on moving sensitised paper or on a monitor. It predates 2D echocardiography but is useful for measuring ventricular diameters in systole/diastole.

Doppler Echocardiography

- Doppler ultrasound provides functional assessment to complement the anatomical assessment of 2D echocardiography.

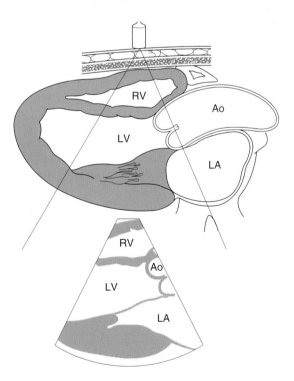

Figure 16.12 Outline of two-dimensional echocardiograph (ultrasound scan). Ao, aorta; LA, left atrium; LV, left ventricle; RV, right ventricle.

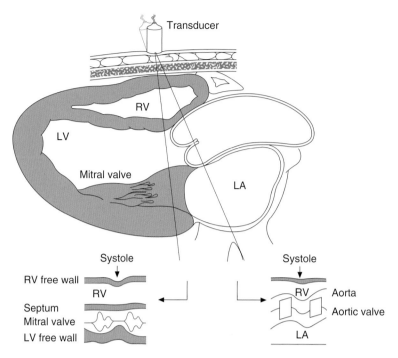

Figure 16.13 Outline of M-mode echocardiographs, with two examples showing mitral and aortic valves opening and closing. LA, left atrium; LV, left ventricle; RV, right ventricle.

- Velocity of blood movement in the heart and circulation assessed by Doppler shift (frequency changes due to movement of red blood cells)
- Produces a spectral (graphic) trace demonstrating velocity changes during the cardiac cycle
- Blood accelerates through an obstruction, e.g. a stenosed valve. The peak velocity is proportional to the haemodynamic gradient.
- Reverse flow pattern in valvular reflux.

Colour-Flow Doppler Echocardiography

- Rapid method of detecting abnormal blood flow due to a leaking valve or an intracardiac shunt, e.g. ventricular septal defect.
- Ultrasound machine calculates the direction and velocity of flow, pixel by pixel, within a segment of the image and codes it in colour – red and blue depending on direction of blood flow
- It superimposes colour flow on the 2D image.

Nuclear Medicine

Radionuclides can be used in the assessment of cardiac disease in three main ways:

Myocardial Perfusion Scintigraphy

- Demonstrates abnormal blood flow in coronary artery disease in conjunction with exercise testing. Thallium 201 is extracted from the blood in proportion to flow.
- Ischaemic myocardium appears as a cold spot on the scan taken immediately after injection of thallium.

- If the area is not infarcted, the cold spot 'fills in' as thallium redistributes in the following four hours.
- Thallium scanning is a more reliable diagnostic investigation than exercise testing and the number and extent of defects correlate with prognosis.

Radionuclide Ventriculography (Multiple Gated Acquisition [MUGA] Scanning)

- Assesses ventricle function.

The patient's blood (usually red blood cells) is labelled with technetium 99 m (half-life six hours). A gamma camera and a computer generate a moving image of the heart by 'gating' the computer to the patient's ECG.

Systolic function of the left ventricle is quantified by the ejection fraction (normally 0.50–0.70):

$$\text{Ejection fraction} = \frac{\text{stroke volume}}{\text{end-diastolic volume}}$$

i.e. the proportion of the total diastolic volume that is ejected in systole.

Images can be collected during exercise as well as at rest, to assess the effect of stress on left ventricular function.

Pyrophosphate Scanning

- Demonstrates recent myocardial infarction, e.g. 1–10 days after event.

Technetium 99 m pyrophosphate is taken up by areas of myocardial infarction producing a hot spot, maximal at three days.

Indicated when:

- the ECG is too abnormal to demonstrate infarction (e.g. left bundle-branch block)
- the patient has presented after the plasma enzyme changes, e.g. at three days

Cardiac Angiography (Cardiac Catheterisation)

An invasive assessment of cardiac function and disease in which fine tubes are passed, with mild sedation under operating theatre conditions:

- retrograde through arteries to left side of heart and coronary arteries
- anterograde through veins to right side of heart and pulmonary arteries
  - to make diagnosis, e.g. is valve critically stenosed?
  - is chest pain due to coronary artery disease?
  - to plan cardiac surgery, particularly coronary artery bypass grafting.

It entails a major radiation dose. Major complications (1 in 2000 cases):

- access artery dissection (2%)
- myocardial infarction (0.1%)
- air or cholesterol emboli can cause stroke or myocardial infarction
- death (0.01%).

Risks must be outweighed by the benefit the patient receives.

The commonest approach is cannulation of the right femoral vessels by the Seldinger technique. A percutaneous fine gauge needle punctures the vessel, through which a soft guide wire is passed. The needle is withdrawn and an introducer sheath and catheter are

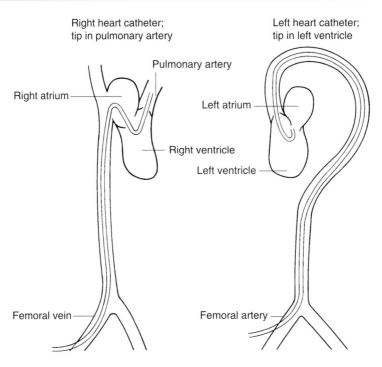

Right heart catheter;
tip in pulmonary artery

Left heart catheter;
tip in left ventricle

Pulmonary artery

Right atrium

Left atrium

Right ventricle

Left ventricle

Femoral vein

Femoral artery

Figure 16.14   Cardiac catheterisation.

inserted over the guide wire that is then withdrawn. Haemostasis is achieved by compression. The technique is not suitable if the patient is on anticoagulant drugs or has severe peripheral vascular disease or an abdominal aortic aneurysm (Figure 16.14).

Alternative approach: brachial vessels at elbow through a skin incision. Closure of arterotomy by sutures allows use in anticoagulated patients.

Pressure Measurements

Cardiac haemodynamics and gradients across individual valves, e.g. by pulling the catheter back across the aortic valve, whilst systolic pressure is recorded (Figure 16.15).

Mitral stenosis is quantified by the diastolic pressure difference between the left ventricle (left heart catheter) and left atrium measured indirectly via the right heart catheter in the 'wedge' position – passed through the pulmonary artery to occlude a pulmonary arteriole so the pressure at the tip reflects the left atrial pressure transmitted through the pulmonary capillaries (Figure 16.16).

The cardiac output is calculated either by the Fick principle (cardiac output is inversely proportional to difference between systemic arterial and mixed venous blood oxygen saturation) or by the thermodilution technique.

Radio-Opaque Contrast

Radio-opaque contrast (iodine based) is:

- injected into chambers to assess their systolic function and to detect valve regurgitation, e.g. left ventricular injection for mitral regurgitation
- injected into coronary ostia to detect coronary artery disease, with X-ray images multiple projections.

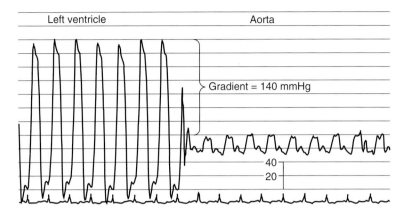

Figure 16.15 Aortic stenosis. The systolic pressure falls as the catheter tip leaves the left ventricle, crossing the stenosed aortic valve. Diastolic pressure is prevented from falling by the aortic valve.

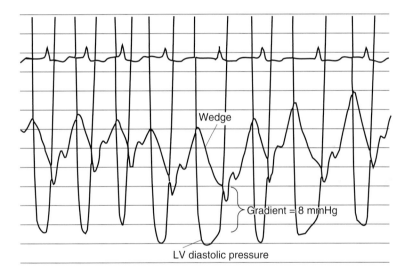

Figure 16.16 Mitral stenosis. Left ventricular (LV) pressure trace expanded to show low diastolic pressures. A pressure difference between the wedge trace and LV diastolic trace reflects obstruction to flow into the left ventricle due to mitral stenosis. The rhythm is atrial fibrillation.

Computed Tomography

See earlier in this chapter.

- CT angiography (CTA) – use of an iodine-based contrast agent to enhance the coronary vessels

Magnetic Resonance Imaging

See earlier in this chapter.

- MR angiography (MRA) – longer scan times than CTA, can be performed with or without contrast agents, but patients with pacemakers cannot be scanned.

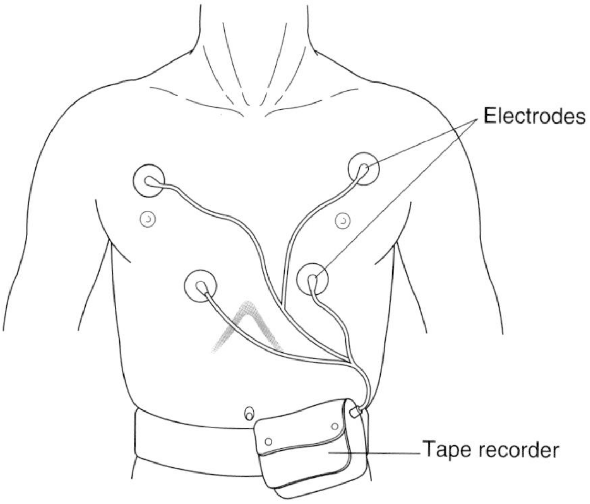

Figure 16.17   The arrangement for the 24-hour ECG tape recorder.

Twenty-Four-Hour ECG Tape Recording

ECG worn for 24 hours (or 48 hours) (Figure 16.17) obtains on tape a continuous ECG recording during normal activities. For diagnosis of:

- palpitations
- dizzy spells
- light-headedness or blackouts of possible cardiac origin

    May show episodes of:

- atrial asystole
- atrial or ventricular tachycardias
- complete heart block
- ST segment changes during angina or silent ischaemia

Twenty-Four-Hour Blood Pressure Recording

Blood pressure is measured intermittently with an upper arm cuff and microphone, with recording on a tape. Allows evaluation of blood pressure during everyday activities without the 'white coat' effect of anxiety at the doctor's surgery increasing measured blood pressure.

Hypertension is defined as daytime average > 140/ > 90 mmHg. Absence of lower blood pressure during the night ('dip') suggests secondary hypertension.

Respiratory Investigations
pH and Arterial Blood Gases

See Chapter 5 for values in type I and type II respiratory failure. Normal ranges (Figure 16.18):

- pH 7.35–7.45
- P_{CO_2} 4.6–6.0 kPa
- P_{O_2} 12–14 kPa
- HCO_3–22–26 mmol l^{-1}
- base excess is the amount of acid required to titrate pH to 7.4

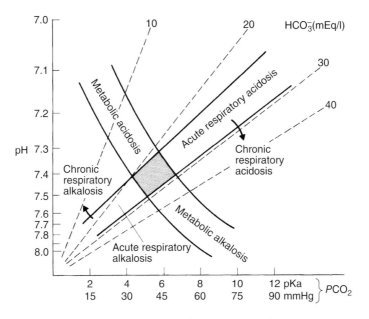

Figure 16.18   Descriptive clinical terms. Shaded area is normal range.

In ventilatory failure:

- Po_2 low
- Pco_2 high

In respiratory failure from lung disease often:

- Po_2 low
- normal Pco_2 due to high carbon dioxide (CO_2) solubility and efficient transfer in lungs

For example, in asthma, raised CO_2 signifies tiredness and decreased ventilation from reduced muscular effort.

Respiratory Acidosis

CO_2 retention from:

- respiratory disease with right-to-left shunt
- ventilatory failure
  - neuromuscular disease
  - physical causes, e.g. flail chest, kyphoscoliosis

Raised CO_2 leads to increased bicarbonate:

$$CO_2 + H_2O = H_2CO_3 = H^+ + HCO_3^-.$$

In chronic respiratory failure, renal compensation by excretion of H^+ and retention of HCO_3^- leads to further increased HCO_3^- (i.e. maintenance of normal pH with compensatory metabolic alkalosis).

Respiratory Alkalosis

CO_2 blown off by hyperventilation due to:

- hysteria
- brainstem stimulation (rare)

In respiratory alkalosis:

- Po_2 normal
- Pco_2 low

If chronic, compensated by metabolic acidosis with renal retention of H⁺ and excretion of HCO_3^-.

Metabolic Acidosis

Excess H⁺ in blood:

- ketosis – 3-OH butyric acid accumulation in diabetes or starvation
- uraemia – lack of renal H⁺ excretion
- renal tubular acidosis – lack of H⁺ or NH_4^+ excretion
- acid ingestion – aspirin
- lactic acid accumulation – shock, hypoxia, exercise, biguanide
- formic acid accumulation – methanol intake
- loss of base – diarrhoea

Usually compensatory respiratory alkalosis, e.g. Kussmaul respiration of diabetic coma (hyperventilation with deep breathing):

- Po_2 normal
- Pco_2 low
- to assist diagnosis, measure anion gap

$$\left[Na^+\right]+\left[K^+\right]-\left[Cl^-\right]-\left[HCO_3^-\right]=7-16\,mmol\,l^{-1}$$

If anion gap > 16 mmol l⁻¹, unestimated anions are present, e.g. 3-OH butyrate, lactate, formate.

Metabolic Alkalosis

Loss of H⁺ due to:

- prolonged vomiting
- potassium depletion – secondary to renal tubular potassium–hydrogen exchange
- ingestion of base – old-fashioned sodium bicarbonate therapy of peptic ulcers

Usually compensatory respiratory acidosis with hypoventilation:

- Po_2 low
- Pco_2 high

Peak Flow (Figure 16.19)

- Blow into machine as hard and fast as you can.
- Records in litres per minute. Useful for diagnosing and observing asthma. Normal range is 300–500 l min⁻¹.
- Improvement with β-agonist, e.g. isoprenaline, indicates reversible airway disease, i.e. asthma.

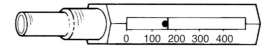

Figure 16.19   Peak flow machine.

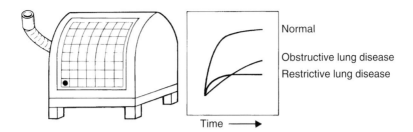

Figure 16.20 A vitalograph.

Spirometry (Figure 16.20)
- Blow into machine, a vitalograph, as hard as you can – measures pattern of airflow during forced expiration.
- To distinguish between restrictive lung disease, e.g. *emphysema, fibrosis* and *obstructive lung disease*, e.g. *asthma, chronic obstructive airways disease.*

Skin Testing for Allergens
Drops of a weak allergen solution are placed on to the skin and a superficial prick of the skin, with a short lancet though the liquid, inoculates the epidermis. Special lancets coated with freeze-dried allergen can be used. A local wheal indicates an allergic response.

Carbon Monoxide Transfer Factor
The rate of uptake of carbon monoxide from inspired gas determines the lung diffusion capacity. It is reduced in alveolar diseases, e.g. *pulmonary fibrosis.*

Chest Radiograph
See earlier in this chapter

Ventilation/Perfusion Scan
Ventilat-ion (V) Scan
Inhalation of an isotope allows image of parenchyma of the lungs to be taken by a gamma camera.

Perfusion (P) Scan
Injection of isotope into the bloodstream demonstrates the blood flow in the lungs.

Mismatch of the scans is used to diagnose pulmonary embolism, i.e. air reaches all parts of the lung, whilst the blood does not (Figure 16.21). Matching defects occur with other lung pathologies, e.g. *emphysema.*

N.B. A perfusion scan showing an area of ischaemia with a normal chest X-ray is generally sufficient to diagnose a pulmonary embolus. A *V/Q* scan is needed if there is other lung pathology suspected or on X-ray (e.g. chronic bronchitis/emphysema), but in practice the results are difficult to interpret.

Computed Tomography
See earlier in this chapter.

- Can be used to detect pleural effusions, tumours. Computed tomography pulmonary angiography (CTPA) – used to detect pulmonary embolism

(a)   (b)

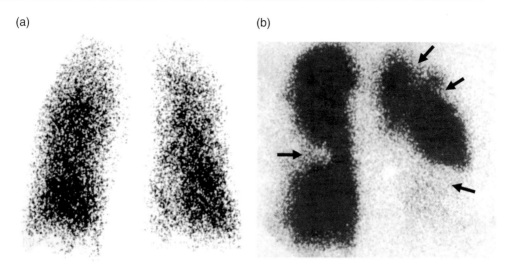

Figure 16.21   *V/Q* scan of pulmonary embolism: (a) ventilation scan – normal; (b) perfusion scan (arrows mark perfusion defects).

Bronchoscopy

Flexible bronchoscopy – under mild sedation, e.g. intravenous diazepam with local anaesthetic spray to pharynx and larynx. Vision by fibreoptics.

- Obstructions can be visualised.
- Biopsies can be taken for neoplasms.
- Aspiration samples, sometimes after lavage with saline, can be taken for organisms and malignant cells.

Gastrointestinal Investigations
Abdominal Radiograph

X-ray of the abdomen which uses a small dose of ionising radiation to create pictures of the contents of the abdominal cavity. The stomach, liver, intestines, and spleen can be evaluated and a diagnosis can be determined from the findings (see earlier in this chapter).

Abdominal Ultrasound

See earlier in this chapter. Ultrasound is used as a first-line investigation for generalised abdominal problems in order to rule out non-GI related problems. It has the advantage over plain abdominal radiography of not using radiation. The results can then help to identify the next imaging procedure if it is required.

Upper Gastrointestinal Endoscopy

A flexible fibreoptic tube is introduced into the oesophagus, stomach, and duodenum after mild sedation, e.g. intravenous diazepam, with local anaesthetic to pharynx.
Direct vision of the gastrointestinal tract to investigate:

- dysphagia – oesophageal tumour or stricture
- haematemasis or melaena – oesophageal varices, gastric and duodenal ulcers, superficial gastric erosions, gastric carcinoma
- epigastric pain – peptic ulcer, oesophagitis, gastritis, duodenitis
- unexplained weight loss – gastric carcinoma

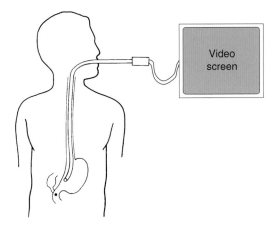

Figure 16.22 Endoscopic retrograde cholangiopancreatography.

Endoscopic Retrograde Cholangiopancreatography (ERCP) (Figure 16.22)

Through a fibreoptic endoscope, with an image on a video, under direct vision, a tube is inserted through the ampulla of Vater at the opening of the common bile duct, and introduction of a radiopaque contrast medium allows X-ray visualisation of:

- **biliary tree**, for stones, tumours, strictures, irregularities
- **pancreatic ducts**, for chronic pancreatitis, dilated ducts, or distortion from a tumour

The endoscope can be used for surgery, including sphincterotomy of ampulla for removal of gallstones in the bile duct or the introduction of a rigid tube, a stent, through a constricting tumour to allow biliary drainage.

Barium Swallow, Meal, Enema

Barium is drunk (swallow for oesophagus, meal for stomach/duodenum) or introduced rectally (enema) or via a catheter into the duodenum (small-bowel enema). Real-time images of barium coating the mucosa are viewed using fluoroscopy and then images are taken. Air may be introduced to distend organs and to give double-contrast images.

It outlines physical abnormalities:

- strictures, e.g. *fibrosis, carcinomata*
- filling defects, e.g. *polyps, carcinomata*
- craters, e.g. *ulcers, diverticula*
- mucosal irregularities
- mucosal folds radiating from *peptic ulcer*
- clefts in *Crohn's disease of ileum and colon*
- featureless mucosa of *early ulcerative colitis*
- islands of mucosa in *severe ulcerative colitis*

An irregularity on a single film needs to be seen on other views before an abnormality is confirmed, as peristalsis or gut contents can mimic defects.

Hydrogen Breath Tests

- Lactulose breath test for bacterial overgrowth. Oral lactulose is given, and excess gut flora in the small bowel or blind loop causes prompt metabolism to provide exhaled hydrogen.
- Lactose breath test for lactase deficiency.
  - Oral lactose with subnormal exhaled hydrogen.

Computed Tomography

See earlier in this chapter. Can be used to detect tumours, IBD, bowel perforation.

- CT colonography–multiple scans of abdomen, used to reconstruct 3D image of bowel.

Renal Investigations

Urine Testing

Testing the urine is part of the routine physical examination. It is most simply done using one of the combination dipsticks.

- Dip the stick in the urine and compare the colours with the key at the times specified. Of particular interest are:
  - pH
  - protein content (N.B. does not detect Bence Jones protein)
  - ketones
  - glucose
  - bilirubin
  - urobilinogen
  - blood/haemoglobin.

Urine Microscopy

Urine should be sent to the laboratory (sterile) for 'M, C, and S':

- M (microscopy) – for the presence of red cells, white cells, casts, and pathogens
- C (culture) – using appropriate media to detect bacteria and other pathogens
- S (sensitivity) – to determine the sensitivity of bacteria to antibiotics

Creatinine Clearance

Precise measurements of the glomerular filtration rate are made isotopically, e.g. chromium EDTA clearance. The creatinine clearance is easier to organise, although less accurate.

- Collect a blood sample for plasma creatinine.
- Collect a 24-hour urine sample for creatinine.

$$\text{Formula}: \frac{U \times V}{P \times T}$$

$$\underbrace{\frac{\text{(mmol)}}{\text{Plasma creatinine}}}_{\substack{\text{Urine creatinine} \\ \text{(mmol)}}} \times \underbrace{\frac{\text{(ml)} \times 10^{3}}{\text{Duration collection}}}_{\substack{\text{Urine volume} \\ \text{(min)}}} = \text{Clearance}\left(\text{ml min}^{-1}\right)$$

Normal value: 80–120 ml min^{-1}.

Abdominal Radiograph

See earlier in this chapter

Abdominal Ultrasound

See earlier in this chapter. In many cases ultrasound is used as a first-line investigation for generalised abdominal/pelvic problems in order to rule out nonurinary tract related problems and has the advantage over plain abdominal radiography of not using radiation. The results can then help to identify the next imaging procedure if it is required.

Intravenous Urogram

An initial plain film to show renal or ureteric stones. Contrast medium is injected intravenously, concentrated in the kidney and excreted.

- nephrogram phase – kidneys are outlined
    - observe position, size, shape, filling defects, e.g. tumour
- excretion phase – renal pelvis
    - renal papillae may be lost from chronic pyelonephritis, papillary necrosis
    - calyces blunted from hydronephrosis
    - pelviureteric obstruction – large pelvis, normal ureters
- ureters – observe position – displaced by other pathology?
    - size – dilated from obstruction or recent infection
    - irregularities – may be contractions and need to be checked in sequential films

Computed Tomography

See earlier in this chapter

- CT angiography – to examine blood flow in renal artery disease and suitability for transplants

Nuclear Medicine

See earlier in this chapter

- DMSA scan

Static imaging where images are obtained two to three hours after intravenous injection of 99mTc DMSA. Provides information regarding the cortical morphology of the kidneys and used for evaluation of cortical scarring and distribution of functional tissue.

- DTPA scan

Dynamic imaging is performed most often with 99mTc DTPA. Provides information relating to renal vascularity, renal function, excretion and any obstructive pathology involving the kidneys.

Neurological Investigations

Electroencephalogram

Approximately 22 electrodes are applied to the scalp in standard positions and cerebral electrical activity is amplified and recorded. There are marked normal variations and differences between awake and sleep.

Main Uses

- epilepsy
    - primary, generalised epilepsy – generalised spike and slow-wave discharges
    - partial epilepsy – focal spikes
- disorders of consciousness or coma
    - encephalopathy
    - encephalitis
    - dementia

The main value of this technique is in showing episodes of abnormal waves compatible with epilepsy. Large normal variation makes interpretation difficult.

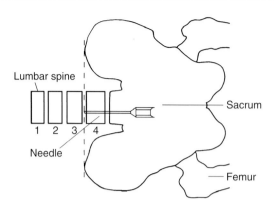

Figure 16.23   The lumbar puncture needle is positioned between L3 and L4 to one side of the supraspinous ligament.

Lumbar Puncture

A needle is introduced between the lumbar vertebrae (Figure 16.23), through the dura into the subarachnoid space, and cerebrospinal fluid is obtained for examination. Normal cerebrospinal fluid is completely clear.

The major diagnostic value of this technique is in:

- subarachnoid haemorrhage – uniformly red, whereas blood from a 'traumatic' tap is in the 1st specimen.
- xanthochromia – yellow stain from haemoglobin breakdown.
- meningitis – pyogenic, turbid fluid, white cells, organisms on culture, low glucose, and raised protein.
- raised pressure may indicate a tumour.

Ultrasound

Use of Doppler ultrasound to visualise carotid blood flow to investigate atherosclerotic disease

Angiography

See earlier in this chapter

Computed Tomography

See earlier in this chapter

- To look for intracranial haemorrhage (acute phase), cerebral infarct, tumours

Magnetic Resonance Imaging

See earlier in this chapter

- To look for intracranial haemorrhage (subacute and chronic), tumours (more sensitive and specific than CT).
- Excellent visualisation of spinal cord, nerve roots, intervertebral discs, and surrounding soft tissues. Spinal tumours, multiple sclerosis, disc herniation, and cord compression.

Nuclear Medicine

See earlier in this chapter

- SPECT – for functional brain imaging

Myelogram

- Contrast medium is injected into cerebrospinal fluid in subarachnoid space to demonstrate thoracic or cervical disc prolapses or cord tumours. Largely replaced by MRI.

Lumbar Radiculogram

- Contrast medium is injected to demonstrate lumbar disc prolapses. Largely replaced by MRI.

Further Reading

Adam, A., Dixon, A., Gillard, J. et al. (2015). *Grainger & Allison's Diagnostic Radiology: A Textbook of Medical Imaging*, 6e. Elsevier.

Ashford, R. and Evans, N. (2001). *Surgical Critical Care*. London: Greenwich Medical Media.

Chowdhury, R., Wilson, I., Rofe, C., and Lloyd-Jones, G. (2010). *Radiology at a Glance*. Wiley-Blackwell.

Hatton, C. and Blackwood, R. (2003). *Lecture Notes on Clinical Skills*, 4e. Oxford: Blackwell Science.

Jones, S. and Taylor, E. (2006). *Imaging for Nurses*. Oxford: Blackwell.

Lisle, D. (2012). *Imaging for Students*, 4e. Arnold Publishers.

Swartz, M. (2014). *Physical Diagnosis, History and Examination*, 7e. London: W. B. Saunders.

Talley, N. and O'Connor, S. (2009). *Clinical Examination: A Systematic Guide to Physical Diagnosis*, 6e. London: Churchill Livingstone.

Watson, N. (2014). *Chapman & Nakielny's Guide to Radiological Procedures*, 6e. Elsevier.

Chapter 17

Basic Examination, Notes, and Diagnostic Principles

Carol Lynn Cox and Brandy Lunsford

Basic Examination

Introduction

In practice, you cannot attempt to elicit every single physical sign for each system. Your examination will be guided by the patient's chief complaint and presenting history. Basic signs should be sought on every examination, and if there is any hint of abnormality, additional physical signs can be elicited to confirm your suspicion (Bickley and Szilagyi 2007, 2013; Collins-Bride and Saxe 2013; Dains et al. 2012, 2015; Japp and Robertson 2013; Jarvis 2015; Seidel et al. 2006, 2010; Swartz 2006, 2014).

Listed below are the basic examinations of the systems which will enable you to complete a routine examination adequately but not excessively.

- General examination
  - general appearance
  - is the patient well or ill?
  - look at temperature chart or take patient's temperature
  - any obvious abnormality?
  - mental health state, mood, behaviour
- General and cardiovascular system
  - observation – dyspnoea, distress
  - O_2 saturation
  - blood pressure
  - hands
    - temperature
    - nails, e.g. clubbing, leukonychia, koilonychias, palmar erythema

Physical Assessment for Nurses and Healthcare Professionals, Third Edition. Edited by Carol Lynn Cox.
© 2019 John Wiley & Sons Ltd. Published 2019 by John Wiley & Sons Ltd.

- pulse – rate, rhythm, character
- axillae – lymph nodes
- neck – lymph nodes
- face and eyes – anaemia, jaundice
- tongue and mucus membranes – central cyanosis
- jugular venous pulse (JVP)/distension (JVD) – height and v wave
- apex beat/point of maximal impulse (PMI) – position and character
- parasternal – heave or thrills
- stethoscope
    - heart sounds (S_1 and S_2), added sounds (clicks or snaps), splits (? physiological split), murmurs
    - listen in all five areas with stethoscope using the bell and diaphragm
    - lay patient on left side, with the bell of stethoscope listen for mitral stenosis (MS)
    - sit patient up, have them lean forwards and breathe out, with bell of stethoscope listen for aortic incompetence (AI)

- **Respiratory system**
    - observation (scars, lesions, ecchymoses)
    - trachea – position
    - front of chest
        - movement (respiratory excursion; flail)
        - palpate (lumps, crepitus, fremitus)
        - percuss – compare sides
        - auscultate – compare sides
    - back of chest
        - movement (respiratory excursion)
        - palpate (lumps, crepitus, fremitus)
        - percuss – particularly level of bases (diaphragmatic excursion); compare sides
        - auscultate – compare sides
    - examine sputum
- **Examine spine** (? lordosis, kyphosis, scoliosis, gibbus)
- **Abdomen**
    - lay patient flat (knees bent to relax abdomen)
    - look at abdomen – ask if pain or tenderness
    - auscultate in all four quadrants (include aortic, iliac and femoral arteries/? bruits)
    - palpate abdomen gently
        - generally all over? masses
        - liver – then percuss
        - spleen – then percuss
        - kidneys
        - (shifting dullness – ascites if indicated)
    - feel femoral pulses and inguinal lymph nodes
    - hernia
    - males – genitals
    - per rectum (PR; only if given permission) – usually at end of examination
    - per vaginam (PV; only if given permission) – usually at end of examination
- **Legs**
    - observation
    - arterial pulses (joints if indicated)
    - neurology

– reflexes	– knees	tone	only if indicated
	– ankles	power	
	– plantar responses	coordination	
– sensation	– pinprick	position	
	– vibration	cotton-wool	
		temperature	

- Arms
  - posture: outstretched hands, eyes closed, rapid finger movements
  - finger–nose coordination

– reflexes	– triceps	tone	only if indicated
	– biceps	power	
	– supinator		
		vibration	
– sensation	– pinprick	position	
		cotton-wool	
		temperature	

- Cranial nerves
  - I (if indicated)
  - II: eyes
    - reading print/acuity
    - fields
    - pupils – torch and accommodation
    - ophthalmoscope – sclera, cornea, anterior chamber, and posterior fundi
  - III, IV, VI: eye movements (EOM)
    - 'Do you see double?'
    - note nystagmus
  - V, VII
    - open mouth
    - grit teeth – feel masseters
    - sensation – cotton-wool
    - (corneal reflex – if indicated)
    - (taste – if indicated)
  - VIII: hearing
    - watch at each ear
    - (Rinne, Weber tests if indicated)
  - IX, X: fauces movement
  - XI: shrug shoulders
  - XII: put out tongue
- Walk – look at gait
- Hernia and varicose veins

Example of Notes

You may find the SOAPIER (Subjective, Objective, Assessment, Plan, Implementation, Evaluation, Review) format or POMR (Problem Oriented Medical Record) useful in documenting your findings (Clark 1999; Jarvis 2015; Swartz 2006, 2014).

Patient's name:	Age:	Occupation:

Date of admission:
Complains of (chief complaint):
- list, in patient's words

History of present illness:
- detailed description of each symptom (even if appears irrelevant) (Note language barriers that may have an impact on documentation.)
- last well
- chronological order, with both actual date of onset, and time previous to admission
- (may include history from informant – in which case, state this is so)
- then detail other questions which seem relevant to possible differential diagnoses
- then **functional enquiry**, 'check' system for other symptoms
- (minimal statement in notes – weight, appetite, digestion, bowels, micturition, menstruation, if appropriate)

Past history:
- chronological order

Family history:
- include genogram

Personal and social history:
- must include details of home circumstances, dependents, patient's occupation
- effect of illness on life and its relevance to foreseeable discharge of patient
- smoking, alcohol, drug misuse, medications

Medications:
- list all medications the patient is presently taking

Allergies:
Physical examination:
- general appearance
- then record findings according to systems

Minimal statement:
Healthy, well-nourished woman (or man)
Afebrile, not anaemic, icteric, or cyanosed
No enlargement of lymph nodes
No clubbing
Breasts/chest and thyroid normal

Cerebrovascular system (CVS):	Blood pressure, pulse rate, and rhythm
	JVP not raised
	Apex position
	Heart sounds 1 and 2, no murmurs
Respiratory system:	Cyanosis (present/absent)
	O_2 saturation
	Chest and movements normal
	Fremitus normal
	Percussion note normal
	Breath sounds bilateral/vesicular
	No other (adventitious) sounds

Abdominal system:	Tongue and mucus membranes normal
	Abdomen normal, no tenderness
	Liver, spleen, kidneys, bladder impalpable
	No masses felt
	Hernial orifices normal
	Rectal examination normal
	Vaginal examination not performed
	Testes normal
Central nervous system (CNS):	Alert and intelligent
	Pupils equal, regular, react equally to light and accommodation (PERRLA)
	Fundi normal
	Normal eye movements
	Other cranial nerves normal
	Limbs normal
	Knee jerks + +
	Ankle jerks + +
	Plantar reflexes ↓ ↓
	Touch and vibration normal
	Spine and joints normal
	Gait normal
	Pulses (including dorsalis pedis, posterior tibial, and popliteal) palpable

Summary

Write a few sentences only:

- salient positive features of history and examination
- relevant negative information
- home circumstances
- patient's mental state
  - understanding of illness
  - specific concerns

Problem List and Diagnoses

After your history and examination, make a list of:

- the diagnoses you have been able to make
- problems or abnormal findings which need explaining.

For example:

- symptoms or signs
- anxiety
- poor social background
- laboratory results
- drug sensitivities

It is best to separate the current problems of actual or potential clinical significance requiring treatment or follow-up from the inactive problems. An example is:

Active problems	Date
1. Unexplained episodes of fainting	one week
2. Angina	since 2012
3. Hypertension – blood pressure 190/100 mmHg	2012
4. Chronic renal failure – plasma creatinine 200 µmol l^{-1}	August 2014
5. Widower, unemployed, lives on own	
6. Anxious about possibility of being injured in a fall	
7. Smokes 40 cigarettes per day	

Inactive problems	Date
1. Thyrotoxicosis treated by partial thyroidectomy	2000
2. ACE inhibitor-induced cough	2011

When you initially begin examining patients you will have difficulty knowing which problems to put down separately and which can be covered under one diagnosis and a single entry. It is therefore advisable to rewrite the problem list if a problem resolves or can be explained by a diagnosis. When you are more experienced, it will be appropriate to fill out the problems on a complete problem list at the front of the notes. Use medical diagnoses in the medical notes.

Active problems	Date	Inactive problems	Date
Include symptoms, signs, unexplained abnormal investigations, social and psychiatric problems		Include major past illness, operation, or hypersensitivities; do not include problems requiring active care	

From the problem list, you should be able to make:

- differential diagnoses, including that which you think is most likely. Remember:
  - common diseases occur commonly
  - an unusual manifestation of a common disease is more likely than an uncommon disease
  - do not necessarily be put off by some aspect which does not fit
- possible diagnostic investigations you feel are appropriate
- management and therapy you think are appropriate
- prognostic implications

Diagnoses

The diagnostic terms which are used often relate to different levels of understanding:

Disordered function	Immobile painful joint	Breathlessness	Angina
	↑	↑	↑
Structural lesion	Osteoarthritis	Anaemia	Narrow coronary artery
	↑	↑	↑
Pathology	Iron-deposition fibrosis (haemochromatosis)	Iron deficiency	Aortitis
	↑	↑	↑
Aetiology	Inherited disorder of iron metabolism – homozygous for C282Y with A-H	Bleeding duodenal ulcer	*Treponema pallidum* (syphilis)

Different problems require diagnoses at different levels, which may change as further information becomes available. Thus, a patient initially may be diagnosed as *pyrexia of unknown origin*. After a plain X-ray of the abdomen, the patient may be found to have a *renal mass* which on a computed tomography (CT) scan becomes *perinephric abscess*, which from blood cultures is found to be *Staphylococcus aureus* infection. For a complete diagnosis all aspects should be known, but often this is not possible (Bickley and Szilagyi 2013; Collins-Bride and Saxe 2013; Dains et al. 2012, 2015; Japp and Robertson 2013; Jarvis 2015; Seidel et al. 2006, 2010; Swartz 2006, 2014).

Note that many terms are used as a diagnosis but, in fact, cover considerable ignorance, e.g. *diabetes mellitus* (originally 'sweet-tasting urine', but now also diagnosed by high plasma glucose) is no more than a descriptive term of disordered function. *Sarcoid* relates to a pattern of symptoms and a pathology of noncaseating granulomata, of which the aetiology is unknown.

Progress Notes

The electronic patient record has become the norm in most healthcare environments. In the general practice surgery, clinic, or primary care facility, full progress notes should give a complete picture of:

- how the diagnosis was established
- how the patient was treated
- the evolution of the illness
- any complications that occurred

These notes are as important as the account of the original examination. In acute cases, record daily changes in signs and symptoms. In chronic cases, the relevant systems should be reexamined at least once a week and the findings recorded.

It is useful to separate different aspects of the illness:

- symptoms
- signs
- laboratory investigations
- general assessment, e.g. apparent response to therapy
- further plans, which would include educating the patient and his family about the illness

Objective findings such as alterations in weight, improvement in colour, pulse, character of respirations, or fluid intake and output are more valuable than purely subjective statements such as 'General improvement from previous examination'.

When appropriate, daily blood pressure readings or analyses of the urine should be recorded.

An account of all procedures such as aspirations of chest should be included.

Specifically record:

- the findings and comments of the physician, surgeon, or advanced registered nurse practitioner (ARNP) managing the case
- results of a case conference
- an opinion from another department

Serial Investigations

The results of these should be collected together in a table on a special sheet. When any large series of investigations is made, e.g. serial blood counts, erythrocyte sedimentation rates, or multiple biochemical analyses, the results can also be expressed by a graph.

Operation Notes

If you are working in a team where patients are undergoing surgical treatment, you may be required to write an operation note following surgery. An operation note must be written immediately after the operation. Do not trust your memory for any length of time as several similar problems may be operated on at one session. Even if you are distracted by an emergency, the notes must be written up the same day as the operation. These notes should contain definite statements on the following facts:

- name of surgeon performing the operation and the surgical assistant
- name of anaesthetist and anaesthetic used
- type and dimension of incision used
- pathological condition found and mention of anatomical variations
- operative procedures carried out
- method of repair of wound and suture materials used
- whether drainage used, material used, and whether sutured to wound
- type of dressing used.

Postoperative Notes

Within the 1st two days after an operation note:

- the general condition of the patient
- any complication or troublesome symptom, e.g. pain, haemorrhage, vomiting, distension, etc.
- any treatment.

Discharge Note from Hospital

A full statement of the patient's condition on discharge should be written:

- final diagnosis
- active problems
- medication and other therapies
- plan
- what the patient has been told: education (patient teaching) given on medications, diagnosis and other pertinent information (e.g. blood pressure monitoring)

- specific follow-up points, e.g. persistent depressive disorder
- where the patient has gone, and what help is available
- when the patient is next being seen
- an estimate of the prognosis.

References

Bickley, L. and Szilagyi, P. (2007). *Bates' Guide to Physical Examination and History Taking*, 9e. Philadelphia: Lippincott.

Bickley, L. and Szilagyi, P. (2013). *Bates' Guide to Physical Examination and History Taking*, 11e. New York: Wolters Kluwer/Lippincott Williams & Wilkins.

Clark, C. (1999). Taking a history. In: *Nurse Practitioners, Clinical Skills and Professional Issues* (ed. M. Walsh, A. Crumbie and S. Reveley). Oxford: Butterworth Heinemann.

Collins-Bride, G. and Saxe, J. (2013). *Clinical Guidelines for Advanced Practice Nursing – An Interdisciplinary Approach*, 2e. Burlington, MA: Jones and Bartlett Learning.

Dains, J., Baumann, L., and Scheibel, P. (2012). *Advanced Health Assessment and Clinical Diagnosis in Primary Care*, 4e. St. Louis: Elsevier.

Dains, J., Baumann, L., and Scheibel, P. (2015). *Advanced Health Assessment and Clinical Diagnosis in Primary Care*, 5e. St. Louis: Mosby.

Japp, A. and Robertson, C. (2013). *Macleod's Clinical Diagnosis*. Edinburgh: Churchill Livingstone, Elsevier.

Jarvis, C. (2015). *Physical Examination and Health Assessment*, 7e. Edinburgh: Elsevier.

Seidel, H., Ball, J., Dains, J., and Benedict, G. (2006). *Mosby's Physical Examination Handbook*. St. Louis: Mosby.

Seidel, H., Ball, J., Dains, J., and Benedict, G. (2010). *Mosby's Physical Examination Handbook*, 7e. St. Louis: Mosby-Year Book.

Swartz, M. (2006). *Physical Diagnosis, History and Examination*, 5e. London: W. B. Saunders.

Swartz, M. (2014). *Physical Diagnosis: History and Examination*, With Student Consult Online Access, 7e. London: Elsevier.

Chapter 18

Presenting Cases and Communication

Carol Lynn Cox and Brandy Lunsford

Presentations to Healthcare Professionals and Patients

Introduction

Practitioners working within a healthcare system must be able to communicate effectively to other healthcare practitioners for the sake of their patients (Collins-Bride and Saxe 2013; Cox 2010, Cox and Hill 2010; Lack 2012; Rhoads and Paterson 2013). Being an advocate for your patients is one of the most important roles you portray within your practice discipline (Ball et al. 2014a, b; Bickley and Szilagyi 2013; Cox and Hill 2010; Dains et al. 2012, 2015; Japp and Robertson 2013; Jarvis 2015; Seidel et al. 2010; Swartz 2014; Talley and O'Connor 2014). The more practice you get in speaking, the better you will become and the more confident you will appear in front of other healthcare professionals and patients. Confidence displayed by you and an ability to speak lucidly are important aspects of therapy. Their value to the patient is enormous.

Practise talking to yourself in a mirror, avoiding any breaks or interpolating the word 'er', 'uh', or 'um'. Open a textbook, find a subject, and give a little talk on it to yourself. Even if you do not know anything about the subject, you will be able to make up a few coherent sentences once you have practised.

A presentation is not the time to demonstrate you have been thorough and have asked all questions. It a time to show you can intelligently assemble the essential facts.

In all presentations, give the salient positive findings and the relevant negative findings. For example:

- In a patient with progressive dyspnoea, state if patient has ever smoked.
- In a patient with icterus, state whether the patient has been abroad, has had any recent injections or drugs, or contact with other jaundiced patients.

Three types of presentations are likely to be encountered: presentation of a case to a meeting, presentation of a new case on a ward/unit round, and a brief follow-up presentation.

Physical Assessment for Nurses and Healthcare Professionals, Third Edition. Edited by Carol Lynn Cox.
© 2019 John Wiley & Sons Ltd. Published 2019 by John Wiley & Sons Ltd.

Presentation of a Case to a Meeting

Presentation of a case to a group of healthcare practitioners in a meeting must be properly prepared, including visual aids as necessary. The principal details, shown on a PowerPoint® presentation for example, are helpful as a reminder to you, and the audience may more easily remember the details of a case if they 'see' as well as 'hear' them. An advantage of PowerPoint is the ability to print out the full presentation as a series of slides with spaces for the audience to write notes. Remember to keep narrative on the slides succinct. You can elaborate with your own narrative as you speak.

- Practise your presentation from beginning to end several times. Leave nothing to chance.
- Do not speak to the screen; speak to the audience.
- Do not stand in front of the data projector so that the screen is blocked by your shadow.
- Do not crack jokes, unless you are confident they are appropriate.
- Do not make sweeping statements.
- Do not make any statements that you cannot defend with references (medical research).
- Remember what you are advised to do in a court of law – dress up, stand up, speak up, shut up.
- Read up about the disease or problem beforehand so that you can answer any questions raised by the audience.
- Read recent leading articles, review or research publications on the subject and refer to these during your presentation.

In many clinical settings it is expected that you present an apposite, original article. Be prepared to evaluate and criticise the manuscript. If your seniors or colleagues cannot provide you with references, look up the subject in search engines such as CHBD, CINAHL, Medline Plus, EMBASE, Global Health, GoPubMed, HubMed, PubMed, PubPsych, British Nursing Index, Retina Medical Search, ASSIA, Cochrane Library, *Index Medicus*, or recently published textbooks (published references should be within the past five years). Always ask the librarian for advice. Laboriously repeating standard information from a textbook is often a turn-off. A recent series or research paper is more educational for you and more interesting for the audience.

A PowerPoint slide or overhead should summarise any presentation:

Mr. A. B. Age: *x* years Brief description, e.g. occupation

Complains of

(state in patient's words – for *x* period)

History of present complaint

- essential details
- other relevant information, e.g. risk factors
- relevant negative information relating to possible diagnoses
- extent to which symptoms or disease limit normal activity
- other symptoms – mention briefly

Past history

- briefly mention inactive problems
- historical information about active problems, or inactive problems relevant to present illness
- record allergies, including type of reaction to drugs

Family history

- brief information about parents, otherwise detail only if relevant
  (Present a genogram for the audience to review.)

Social history
- brief unless relevant
- give family social background
- occupation and previous occupations
- any other special problems
- tobacco or ethanol abuse, past or present

Treatment
- note all drugs with doses

Chief complaint
- note in the patient's words what the patient indicates the problem is

  On examination

General description
- introductory descriptive sentence, e.g. well, obese man (indicate body mass index)
- review of systems as indicated from the patient's perspective (e.g. no complaint of skin problems or hair loss)
- clinical signs relevant to disease
- relevant negative findings
  Remember these findings should be descriptive data rather than your interpretation.

  Problem list
  Differential diagnoses
  (Put in order of likelihood.)

427

Investigations
- relevant positive findings
- relevant negative findings
- tables or graphs for repetitive data
- scan an electrocardiogram or temperature chart for the PowerPoint presentation or photocopy an electrocardiogram or temperature chart for distribution to the audience

  Progress report
  Plan
  Subjects which often are discussed after your presentation are:

- other differential diagnoses
- other features of presumed diagnosis that might have been present or require investigation
- pathophysiological mechanisms
- mechanisms of action of drugs and possible side effects.

Presentation of a New Case on a Ward/Unit Round

- Good written notes are of great assistance. Do not read your notes word for word – use your notes as a reference.
- Highlight, underline, or asterisk key features you wish to refer to or write up a separate notecard for reference.
- Talk formally and avoid speaking too quickly or too slowly. Speak to the whole assembled group rather than a tête-à-tête with the doctor/consultant.
- Stand upright and look presentable – it helps to make you appear confident.
- If you are interrupted by a discussion, note where you are and be ready to resume, repeating the last sentence before proceeding.

History

The format will be similar to that on PowerPoint or an overhead, with emphasis on positive findings and relevant negative information. A full description of the initial main symptom is usually required.

Examination

Once your history is complete the doctor/consultant may ask for the relevant clinical signs only. Still add relevant negative signs you think are important.

Summary

Be prepared to give a problem list and differential diagnoses.

If you are presenting the patient at the bedside, ensure the patient is comfortable. If the patient wishes to make an additional point or clarification, it is best to welcome this. If it is relevant it can be helpful. If irrelevant, politely say to the patient you will come back to them in a moment, after you have presented the findings. Do not appear to disagree with the patient in the patient's presence.

Brief Follow-Up Presentation

Give a brief, orienting introduction to provide a framework on which other information can be placed. For example:

A xx-year-old man who was admitted xx days ago.
Long-standing problems include xxxxx (list briefly).
Presented with xx symptoms for x period.
On examination had xx signs.
Initial diagnosis of xx was confirmed/supported by/not supported by xx investigations.
He was treated by xx.
Since then xx progress:
- symptoms
- examination
  Start with general description and temperature chart and, if relevant, investigations.
If there are multiple active problems, describe each separately, e.g.
- 1st in regard to the xxxx
- 2nd in regard to the xxxx
The outstanding problems are xxxx.
The plan is xxxx.

Aides-Mémoire

These are basic lists that provide brief reminders when presenting patients and diseases. Organising your thoughts along structured lines is helpful.

History

- principal symptom(s)
- history of present illness
- note chronology
- present situation

- functional enquiry
- past history
- family history
- personal and social history

Pain or Other Symptoms

- site
- radiation
- character
- severity
- onset/duration
- frequency/periodicity or constant
- precipitating factors
- relieving factors
- associated symptoms
- getting worse or better

Lumps

Inspection

- site
- size
- shape
- surface
- surroundings

Palpation

- soft/solid consistency
- surroundings – fixed/mobile
- tender
- pulsatility
- transmission of illumination

Local Lymph Nodes

Delineate nodes in the occipital region, cervical region, neck, axillary, or groin, for example.

About the Disease

- incidence
- geographical area
- gender/age
- aetiology
- pathology
  - macroscopic
  - microscopic
- pathophysiology
- symptoms
- signs
- therapy
- prognosis

Causes of Disease
- genetic
- infective
  - virus
  - bacterial
  - fungal
  - parasitic
- neoplastic
  - cancer
    - primary
    - secondary
  - lymphoma
- vascular
  - atheroma
  - hypertension
  - other, e.g. arteritis
- infiltrative
  - fibrosis
  - amyloid
  - granuloma
- autoimmune
- endocrine
- degenerative
- environmental
  - trauma
  - iatrogenic – drug side effects
  - poisoning
- malnutrition
  - general
  - specific, e.g. vitamin deficiency
  - perinatal with effects on subsequent development

Diagnostic Labels
- aetiology, e.g. tuberculosis, genetic

  ↓

- pathology, e.g. sarcoid, amyloid

  ↓

- disordered function, e.g. hypertension, diabetes

  ↓

- symptoms or signs, e.g. jaundice, erythema nodosum

People – Including Patients

A significant number of disasters, a great deal of irritation, and a lot of unpleasantness could be avoided in the general practice surgery, outpatient clinics, primary care facilities, and hospitals by proper communication. You must remember that you are part of a multidisciplinary team, all of whom significantly help the patient. You must be able to communicate properly with the medical staff, nursing staff, physiotherapists, occupational therapists, administrators, ancillary staff, and, above all, the patients.

Remember these points.

- Time – when you talk to anyone, try not to appear in a rush or they will lose concentration and not listen. A little time taken to talk to somebody properly will help enormously. One minute spent sitting down can seem like five minutes to the patient; five minutes standing up can seem like one minute.
- Silence – in normal social interaction we tend to avoid silences. In a conversation, as soon as one person stops talking (or even before) the other person jumps in to say their bit. When interviewing patients, it is often useful, if you wish to encourage the patient to talk further, to remain silent a moment longer than would be natural. An encouraging nod of the head or an echoing of the patient's last word or two (reflection) may also encourage the patient to talk further.
- Listen – active listening is not easy but essential for good communication. Many people stop talking but not all appear to be listening. Sitting down with the patient is advantageous, both in helping you to concentrate and in transmitting to the patient that you are willing to listen.
- Smile and use facilitative body language – grumpiness or irritation is the best way to stop a patient talking. A smile and display of interest will often encourage a patient to tell you problems they would not normally do. This behaviour helps everybody to relax.
- Reassurance – if you appear confident and relaxed this helps others to feel the same. Being calm without excessive body movements can help. Note how a good advanced nurse practitioner has a reassuring word for patients and allows others in the team to feel they are (or are capable of) working effectively.
- Advocacy – you are the patient's advocate. Advocacy is essential in order to preserve the practitioner–patient relationship.

431

Diabetes Case

You are being presented with the following case. How would you interview this man? What would you discern to be his presenting problem? How would you go about examining this man? What are your primary concerns? What should be documented? How would you present this case?

Mr. A. is a retired 69-year-old man with a five-year history of type 2 diabetes. He presents with recent weight gain and elevated glucose between 200 and 275. He has increased his physical activity over the last eight months but hasn't lost any weight. He has gained 22 pounds over the last eight months. Mr. A is currently prescribed glyburide 5 mg daily, but stopped taking it because of dizziness, sweating, and mild agitation, especially in the late afternoon. He does not check his blood glucose. His diet history reveals excessive carbohydrate intake. Mr. A hasn't seen a dietician.

References

Ball, J., Dains, J., Flynn, J. et al. (2014a). *Seidel's Guide to Physical Examination*, 8e. St. Louis: Mosby.

Ball, J., Dains, J., Flynn, J. et al. (2014b). *Student Laboratory Manual to Accompany Seidel's Guide to Physical Examination*, 8e. St. Louis: Mosby.

Bickley, L. and Szilagyi, P. (2013). *Bates' Guide to Physical Examination and History Taking*, 11e. New York: Wolters Kluwer/Lippincott Williams & Wilkins.

Collins-Bride, G. and Saxe, J. (2013). *Clinical Guidelines for Advanced Practice Nursing – An Interdisciplinary Approach*, 2e. Burlington, MA: Jones and Bartlett Learning.

Cox, C. (2010). *Physical Assessment for Nurses*, 2e. Oxford: Wiley Blackwell.

Cox, C. and Hill, M. (2010). *Professional Issues in Primary Care Nursing*. Oxford: Wiley Blackwell.

Dains, J., Baumann, L., and Scheibel, P. (2012). *Advanced Health Assessment and Clinical Diagnosis in Primary Care*, 4e. St. Louis: Elsevier.

Dains, J., Baumann, L., and Scheibel, P. (2015). *Advanced Health Assessment and Clinical Diagnosis in Primary Care*, 5e. St. Louis: Mosby.

Japp, A. and Robertson, C. (2013). *Macleod's Clinical Diagnosis*. Edinburgh: Churchill Livingstone, Elsevier.

Jarvis, C. (2015). *Physical Examination and Health Assessment*, 7e. Edinburgh: Elsevier.

Lack, V. (2012). Consultation skills. In: *Advanced Practice in Healthcare* (ed. C. Cox, M. Hill and V. Lack), 39–56. London: Routledge.

Rhoads, J. and Paterson, S. (2013). *Advanced Health Assessment and Diagnostic Reasoning*, 2e. Burlington: Jones and Bartlett.

Seidel, H., Ball, J., Dains, J., and Benedict, G. (2010). *Mosby's Physical Examination Handbook*, 7e. St. Louis: Mosby-Year Book.

Swartz, M. (2014). *Physical Diagnosis: History and Examination, with Student Consult Online Access*, 7e. London: Elsevier.

Talley, N. and O'Connor, S. (2014). *Clinical Examination: A Systematic Guide to Physical Diagnosis*, 7e. London: Churchill Livingstone, Elsevier.

Appendices

Appendix A: Jaeger Reading Chart

Jaeger types assess visual acuity for close tasks. They provide the easiest quick method of assessment. The patient should wear the spectacles normally required for reading. Ask the patient to read the smallest type she can; if read with few mistakes, ask her to read the next size down. Record the size of type that can be read with each eye separately.

Hope, they say, deserts us at no period of our existence. From First to last, and in the face of smarting disillusions we continue to expect good fortune, better health, and better conduct; and that so confidently, that we judge it needless to deserve them. I think it improbable that I shall ever write like Shakespeare, conduct an army like Hannibal, or distinguish

Here we recognise the thoughts of our boyhood; and our boyhood ceased – well, when? – not, I think, at twenty: nor, perhaps, altogether at twenty-five: nor yet at thirty: and possibly to be quite frank, we are still in the thick of that arcadian period. For as the race of man, after centuries of civilisation, still keeps

I have always suspected public taste to be a mongrel product, out of affectation by dogmatism; and felt sure, if you could only find an honest man of no special literary bent, he would tell you he thought much of Shakespeare bombastic and most absurd, and all of him written in very

If you look back on your own education, I am sure it will not be the full, vivid, instructive hours of truancy that you regret: and you would rather cancel some lacklustre period between sleep and waking in the class. For my own part, I have attended

There is a sort of dead-alive, hackneyed people about, who are scarcely conscious of living except in the exercise of some conventional occupation.

Books are good enough in their own way, but they are a mighty bloodless substitute for life. It seems a pity to sit, like the Lady of Shalott, peering into a mirror,

The other day, a ragged, barefoot boy ran down the street after a marble, with so jolly an air that he set every one he passed

A happy man or woman is a better thing to find than a

"How now, young fellow, what dost thou

"Truly, sir, I

Reference

Hatton, C. and Blackwood, R. (2003) *Lecture Notes on Clinical Skills*, Fourth Edition. Oxford: Blackwell Sciences LTD

Appendix B: Visual Acuity 3 Meter/21 Foot Chart

The 3m Snellen chart should be held 3 m (21 feet) from the patient, with good lighting, with each of the patient's eyes covered in turn. Use the patient's usual spectacles/glasses for this distance. If the patient cannot read 6/6 (United Kingdom) or 20/20 (North America) (e.g. 6/12 = UK or 20/12 = NA is best vision in one eye), repeat without spectacles/glasses and with a 'pinhole' that largely nullifies refractive errors. Note for each eye the best acuity obtained and the method used, e.g. L 6/9 R 6/6 with spectacles or L 20/7 R 20/7 with glasses.

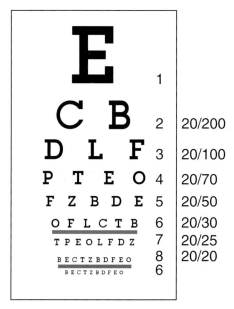

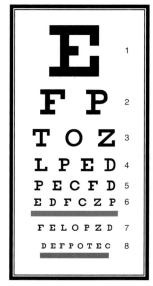

Reference

Hatton, C. and Blackwood, R. (2003) *Lecture Notes on Clinical Skills*, Fourth Edition. Oxford: Blackwell Sciences LTD

Appendix C: Hodkinson Ten-Point Mental Test Score

A simple test of impaired cognitive function (see Chapter 15).

1. Age	Must be correct
2. Time	Without looking at clock or watch, and correct to nearest hour
3. 42 West Street	Give this (or similar) address twice, ask patient to repeat immediately (to check it has registered), and test recall at end of procedure
4. Recognise two people	Point at nurse and other, ask: 'Who is that person? What does she/he do?'
5. Year	Exact, except in January when previous year is accepted
6. Name of place	May ask type of place or area of town
7. Date of birth	Exact
8. Start of World War I	Exact year
9. Name of present monarch	
10. Count from 20 to 1	Backwards, may prompt with 20/19/18, no other prompts; patient may hesitate and self-correct but no other errors (tests concentration)
Check recall of address (question 3 above)	
Total score out of 10	

Communication problems (e.g. *deafness*, *dysphasia*) or abnormal mood (e.g. *depression*) may affect the mental test score, and should be noted. (Source: After Qureshi and Hodkinson (1974).)

Reference

Qureshi, K. and Hodkinson, H. (1974). Evaluation of a ten-question mental test in the institutional elderly. *Age and Ageing* 3: 152.

Appendix D: Barthel Index of Activities of Daily Living

An assessment of disabilities affecting key functions that influence a person's mobility, self-care, and independence (see Chapter 15).

Bowels
0 = incontinent (or needs to be given enema)
1 = occasional accident (once per week or less)
2 = continent (for preceding week)

Bladder
0 = incontinent or catheterised and unable to manage alone
1 = occasional accident (once per day or less)
2 = continent (for preceding week)

Feeding
0 = unable
1 = needs help cutting, spreading butter, etc.
2 = independent

Grooming
0 = needs help with personal care
1 = independent face/hair/teeth/shaving (implements provided)

Dressing
0 = dependent
1 = needs help but can do about half unaided
2 = independent (including buttons, zips, laces, etc.)

Transfer bed to chair and back
0 = unable, no sitting balance
1 = major help (one strong/skilled or two people), can sit up
2 = minor help from one person (physical or verbal)
3 = independent

Toilet use
0 = dependent
1 = needs some help, but can do something alone
2 = independent (on and off, dressing, wiping)

Mobility around house or ward, indoors
0 = immobile
1 = wheelchair independent, including corners
2 = walks with help of one person (physical, verbal, supervision)
3 = independent (but may use any aid, e.g. stick)

Stairs
0 = unable
1 = needs help (physical, verbal, carrying aid)
2 = independent

Bathing
0 = dependent
1 = independent (in and out of bath or shower)

Total score out of 20

Guidelines for the Barthel Index of Activities of Daily Living (ADL)

1. The index should be used as a record of what a patient does, not what a patient *can* do.
2. The main aim is to establish the degree of independence from any help, physical or verbal, however minor and for whatever reason.
3. The need for supervision renders the patient not independent.
4. A patient's performance should be established using the best available evidence. The patient, friends/relatives and nurses are the usual sources, but direct observation and common sense are also important. Direct testing is not necessary.
5. Usually the patient's performance over the preceding 24–48 hours is important, but occasionally longer periods will be relevant.

6. Middle categories imply that the patient supplies over 50% of the effort.
7. The use of aids to be independent is allowed.

(*Source*: After Collin et al. (1988).)

Reference

After Collin, C., Wade, D.T., Davies, S., and Horne, V. (1988). The Barthel ADL index: a reliability study. *International Disability Studies* 10: 61–63.

Appendix E: Mini-Mental State Examination (MMSE)

The purpose of the Mini-Mental State Examination (MMSE) is to determine the mental status of a patient. It should be incorporated into mental health and neurological assessments as well as being an essential component of examinations in which dementia is suspected in the older adult. The MMSE may be viewed as the psychological equivalent of a physical examination. Through utilisation of the MMSE it is possible to evaluate both quantitatively and qualitatively a range of mental functions and behaviours at specific points in time (House 2016). The MMSE is beneficial in obtaining important information related to cognitive functioning that is used in formulating a diagnosis and discerning a disorder's progression and response to treatment. In addition to the scores obtained from the various tests shown here, observations of the patient during the interview should become part of the MMSE, which begins when the healthcare professional initially meets the patient. Information gathered includes the patient's behaviours, thinking, and mood. The healthcare professional's informal and formal observations should be integrated from the assessment tools shown in this appendix. The sum total of these tools provide substantial information about the patient's attention span, memory, and organisation of thought.

The MMSEs shown here include information about appearance, motor activity, speech, affect, thought content, thought process, perception, intellect, and insight.

Major Elements of the Mental Status Examination

Appearance: Age, sex, race, body build, posture, eye contact, dress, grooming, manner, attentiveness to examiner, distinguishing features, prominent physical abnormalities, emotional facial expression, alertness.

Motor: Retardation, agitation, abnormal movements, gait, catatonia.

Speech: Rate, rhythm, volume, amount, articulation, spontaneity.

Affect: Stability, range, appropriateness, intensity, affect, mood.

Thought content: Suicidal ideation, death wishes, homicidal ideation, depressive cognitions, obsessions, ruminations, phobias, ideas of reference, paranoid ideation, magical ideation, delusions, overvalued ideas.

Thought process: Associations, coherence, logic, stream, clang associations, perseveration, neologism, blocking, attention.

Perception: Hallucinations, illusions, depersonalization, derealisation, déjà vu, jamais vu.

Intellect: Global impression: average, above average, below average.

Insight: Awareness of illness.

Source: Adapted from Zimmerman (1994: 121–122) and House (2016).

Mini-Mental State Examination

Maximum score	Patient's score	Orientation
5		What is the (year) (season) (date) (day) (month)?
5		Where are we: (state) (country) (town) (hospital) (floor)?
		Registration
3		Name three objects: take one second to say each. Then ask patient to repeat them. Give one point for each correct answer.
		Attention and calculation
5		Serials 7 s from 100. One point for each correct answer. Stop after five answers. Alternatively, spell "world" backwards.
3		**Recall**
		Ask for the three objects named above. One point for each correct answer.
		Language
2		Ask patient to name a pencil and watch. (two points)
2		Repeat the following: "No ifs, ands, or buts." (two points)
3		Follow a three-stage command: "Take a paper in your right hand, fold it in half, and put it on the table." (three points)
1		Read and obey the following: Close your eyes (one point)
1		Write a sentence (one point)
1		Copy a drawing of intersecting pentagons (one point)
Maximum Total = 30 (Guide: Mild > 21; Moderate = 10–20; Severe < or = 9)	Actual Score =	

Source: Adapted from Folstein et al. (1975).

References

Folstein, M.F., Folstein, S.E., and PR, M.H. (1975). Mini-Mental State: A practical method for grading the cognitive states of patients for the clinician. *J Psychiatr Res* 12: 189–198.

House, R. (2016). The Mental Status Examination. http://www.brown.edu/Courses/BI_278/Other/Clerkship/Didactics/Readings/THE%20MENTAL%20STATUS%20EXAMINATION.pdf (accessed 17 August 2016).

Zimmerman, M. (1994). *Interviewing Guide for Evaluating DSM-IV Psychiatric Disorders and the Mental Status Examination,* 121–122. Philadelphia: Psychiatric Press Products.

Appendix F: Glasgow Coma Scale

The Glasgow Coma Scale (GCS) is a neurological scale that is considered, internationally, to be the key instrument used to determine and record the conscious state of a patient.

Glasgow Coma Scale

Category	Score
Eyes open (E) Spontaneously 4 To speech 3 To pain 2 None 1	
Best motor response (M) Obeys command 5 Localises pain 4 Flexion to pain 3 Extension to pain 2 None 1	
Best verbal response (V) Oriented 5 Confused 4 Inappropriate words 3 Incomprehensible sounds 2 None 1	
Summed coma scale $= E + M + V$	

Reference

Smith, S., Duell, D. and Martin, B. (2008) *Clinical Nursing Skills, Basic to Advanced Skills*. London: Pearson Education LTD, p. 293.

Appendix G: Warning Signs of Alzheimer's Disease

The example shown here is a good instrument for determining the executive function of a patient with potential Alzheimer's disease.

Ten Warning Signs of Alzheimer's Disease

Normal aging events	Possible Alzheimer's disease
Periodically/temporarily forgetting a person's name	Unable to remember the person discussed or seen later
Forgetting food cooking on the stove until after the meal has finished	Forgetting a meal has been prepared
Substitution of fit words because the individual is unable to remember the right word	Speaking in incomprehensible sentences
Forgetting where the person is going	Getting lost on the person's own street – unable to find their way home
Speaking on the telephone and forgetting to watch a child they are responsible for watching	Forgetting a child is present
Experiencing trouble balancing a checkbook	No longer knows what numbers mean
Misplacing an item until retracing their steps	Putting an item in the wrong place (e.g. a wallet in the refrigerator)
Feeling the day has been depressing	Experiencing rapid mood shifts (e.g. getting angry about something inappropriately and then laughing inappropriately)

Normal aging events	Possible Alzheimer's disease
Changes in personality over time	Significant change in personality (e.g. a kind and considerate person becomes cruel and verbally abusive or inappropriate)
Getting tired of household chores but does go back and complete them later on	Does not know that household chores need to be done or caring about them

Source: Adapted from Needham (2014).

Reference

Needham, J. (2014). *Alzheimer's Disease*. Sacramento, CA: NetCE.

Appendix H: Trigger Symptoms Indicative of Dementia

Dementia is a common feature in the ageing process. When assessing a patient for dementia consider whether the patient has difficulty in any of the following areas whilst also considering how long the symptoms have been present, whether they are abrupt or gradual in onset, and whether there has been continuous or stepwise deterioration.

Trigger Symptoms of Dementia

Area of concern	Trigger symptoms
Learning/Retaining New Information	More repetitive; trouble remembering recent conversations, events, or appointments; and more frequently misplaces items
Handling Complex Activities	Difficulty following a complex train of thought, undertaking tasks that require numerous steps (e.g. balancing a checkbook)
Ability to Reason	Unable to develop a reasonable plan to resolve problems at work or at home (e.g. what to do if the kitchen sink overflows or demonstrates an uncharacteristic disregard for social norms)
Special Abilities and Orientation	Difficulty driving, putting objects in the wrong location (e.g. putting milk from the refrigerator in the bedroom closet) or finding their way to and from familiar places. In addition, fails to arrive at the right time for appointments; has difficulty discussing current events and is untidy in dress or inappropriately dressed.
Language	Difficulty in finding the correct words to express what they want to say and with following conversations (when hearing is not a problem)
Behaviour	Is passive and less responsive; is more irritable than in the past and is more suspicious (e.g. refuses having a cleaner come to clean because they might take something) and also misinterprets visual or auditory stimuli.

Source: Adapted from Folstein et al. (1975) and Ferris et al. (1997).

References

Ferris, S., Mackell, J., Mohs, R. et al. (1997). A multicenter evaluation of new treatment efficacy instruments for Alzheimer's disease clinical trials: overview and general results. *Alzheimer Disease Association Disorder* 11 (supplement 1): S1–S12.

Folstein, M., Folstein, S., and McHugh, R. (1975). "Mini-Mental State": a practical method for grading the cognitive state of patients for the clinician. *Journal of Psychiatric Review* 12: 189–198.

Index

Page numbers in *italic* indicate figures and those in **bold** indicate tables.